App Use and Patient Empowerment in Diabetes Self-Management

Nicola Brew-Sam

App Use and Patient Empowerment in Diabetes Self-Management

Advancing Theory-Guided mHealth Research

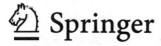 Springer

Nicola Brew-Sam
Regensburg, Germany

Dissertation Philosophische Fakultät der Universität Erfurt, 2019

ISBN 978-3-658-29356-7   ISBN 978-3-658-29357-4   (eBook)
https://doi.org/10.1007/978-3-658-29357-4

This Springer imprint is published by the registered company Springer Fachmedien Wiesbaden GmbH part of Springer Nature.
The registered company address is: Abraham-Lincoln-Str. 46, 65189 Wiesbaden, Germany

Acknowledgements

I would like to express my special appreciation and thanks to my supervisors Professor Constanze Rossmann (University of Erfurt, Germany) and Associate Professor Arul Indrasen Chib (NTU Singapore). You have been tremendous mentors for me. I would like to thank you for encouraging my research and for providing incredible feedback on my thesis, as well as on the related journal papers. Your advice on both research as well as on my career have been invaluable.

I would like to thank all TOUCH support group members and Diabetes Singapore (former DSS) support group members for the outstanding support when I recruited study participants and collected data for my Ph.D. thesis in Singapore.

Moreover, a special thanks to all study participants who took the time for participating in my studies, despite their limited available time and sometimes hard life circumstances dealing with their diabetes. I have never met people who are kinder and stronger than you are, and I wish you all the best for the future!

Finally, special thanks to my family and friends. Words cannot express how grateful I am to my husband, my parents, my mother-in law, and my friends who supported me on my way and who sometimes had to make sacrifices on my behalf.

Nicola Brew-Sam

Research funding for the studies was provided by Nanyang Technological University (Singapore) research grant M4081081.

An ethical review and approval was provided by the Nanyang Technological University Review Board (IRB-2016-01-012).

Copyright

Table of Contents

1. Introduction 1
2. Background on Diabetes Self-Management 7
3. Defining and Categorizing Diabetes Apps for Self-Management 17
4. Diabetes App Use – Previous mHealth Research 29
5. Anteceding Factors of Diabetes App Use 39
6. Summarizing mHealth Research Gaps I: Alternative Theory is Needed............. 51
7. Empowerment as an Antecedent of Diabetes App Use 53
8. Summarizing mHealth Research Gaps II: Empowerment and Diabetes
    App Use 85
9. Summarizing Model on Empowerment and Diabetes App Use 89
10. Research Questions and Hypotheses 93
11. Overview of the Research Design 97
12. Study 1 – Diabetes App Features Corresponding to Indicators of
    Empowerment: An App Feature and Quality Analysis 101
13. Study 2 – Interviews on App Use for Diabetes Self-Management
    and the Relevance of Empowerment 131
14. Study 3 – An Online Survey on Empowerment as an Antecedent of
    Diabetes App Use 197
15. Discussion and Deriving Research Gaps 243
16. Learning from Research Results – Implications for Research and Diabetes
    Care Practice 265
17. Summarizing Research Limitations 273
18. Conclusion 275

Table of Contents

1. **Introduction** 1

    1.1.   The Urgency of Self-Management in Diabetes Care 1

    1.2.   Research Interest: Empowerment as an Anteceding Factor of Diabetes
            App Use for Self-Management 2

    1.3.   Chapter Overview 5

2. **Background on Diabetes Self-Management** 7

    2.1.   What is Diabetes? – Types of Diabetes Mellitus 7

    2.2.   Diabetes Self-Management – Definition and Development 9

    2.3.   Factors Influencing Diabetes Self-Management 12

3. **Defining and Categorizing Diabetes Apps for Self-Management** 17

    3.1.   Diabetes Apps for Self-Management as Second Generation
            mHealth Tools 17

    3.2.   Purpose, Types and Features of Diabetes Apps for Self-Management 20

    3.3.   Shortcomings of Diabetes Apps and Diabetes App Quality 23

4. **Diabetes App Use – Previous mHealth Research** 29

    4.1.   Defining Diabetes App "Use" 29

    4.2.   Categorizing Studies on Diabetes App Use:
            The Inputs-Mechanisms-Outputs Pathway 30

            4.2.1. Input: Feasibility and Accessibility Studies 32

            4.2.2. Output: Diabetes App Usage Effect Studies 35

            4.2.3. Mechanisms: Lacking Research on Antecedents of Health
                    App Use 38

5. **Anteceding Factors of Diabetes App Use** 39

    5.1.   Defining "Antecedents" of mHealth Use 39

    5.2.   The Relevance of Studies Looking into Antecedents of mHealth Use 40

    5.3.   Previous Studies Looking into Antecedents of mHealth Use 41

5.4.   Antecedents of the Unified Theory of Acceptance and Use of
         Technology 42

5.5.   Shortcomings of the Unified Theory of Acceptance and Use 45

6.   Summarizing mHealth Research Gaps I: Alternative Theory is Needed 51

7.   Empowerment as an Antecedent of Diabetes App Use...................................53

7.1.   The Empowerment Approach in Psychology and Management
         Research..53

        7.1.1.   Psychological Empowerment 56

        7.1.2.   Behavioral Empowerment 59

        7.1.3.   Empowerment as a Motivational Approach 66

        7.1.4.   Empowerment and Self-Determination 68

7.2.   Empowerment and its Relevance for Diabetes Self-Management 70

7.3.   Empowerment and Diabetes App Use...73

        7.3.1.   Research on Empowerment and Diabetes App Use:
                   Outcome Perspectives..73

        7.3.2.   Understanding the Overall Process of Empowerment and
                   Diabetes App Use 78

        7.3.3.   Empowerment as an Antecedent of Diabetes App Use 80

8.   Summarizing mHealth Research Gaps II: Empowerment and Diabetes
App Use 85

8.1.   Empowerment as a Multi-Dimensional Antecedent of Diabetes
         App Use 85

8.2.   Two Research Perspectives on Empowerment as an Antecedent of
         Diabetes App Use 86

9.   Summarizing Model on Empowerment and Diabetes App Use.....................89

10.   Research Questions and Hypotheses 93

11. Overview of the Research Design **97**

    11.1. mHealth Research on Diabetes App Use in Singapore............................97

    11.2. Research Procedure...98

12. Study 1 – Diabetes App Features Corresponding to Indicators of

    Empowerment: An App Feature and Quality Analysis.................................**101**

    12.1. Method..102

        12.1.1. Operationalization...102

        12.1.2. App Collection Procedure...104

        12.1.3. Pretesting and Coding Procedure...107

        12.1.4. Data Analysis...110

    12.2. Results..110

        12.2.1. Features and Types of Diabetes Apps 110

        12.2.2. App Features Corresponding to Psychological

                Empowerment Indicators...111

        12.2.3. App Features Corresponding to Behavioral

                Empowerment Indicators...115

        12.2.4. Diabetes App Quality Assessment...117

        12.2.5. MySugr App Series Chosen for Study 2...................................120

    12.3. Discussion...122

    12.4. Study Limitations...126

    12.5. Conclusion..128

13. Study 2 – Interviews on App Use for Diabetes Self-Management

    and the Relevance of Empowerment...**131**

    13.1. Method..131

        13.1.1. Operationalization...133

        13.1.2. Sampling and Data Collection Procedure..................................136

        13.1.3. Data Analysis – Thematic Analysis..137

        13.1.4. Data Analysis – Diabetes App User Typology..........................140

    13.2. Results..141

        13.2.1. Sample Description..141

13.2.2. Diabetes App Use in the Sample 146

13.2.3. Potential Antecedents of Diabetes App Use
Represented in the Interviews................................150

13.2.4. Diabetes App (Non-) User Group Differences – Typology.......164

13.3. Discussion..190

13.4. Study Limitations...193

13.5. Conclusion 195

**14. Study 3 – An Online Survey on Empowerment as an Antecedent of
Diabetes App Use..197**

14.1. Method...197

14.1.1. Operationalization..199

14.1.2. Pretest and Sampling 201

14.1.3. Data Analysis...203

14.2. Results..206

14.2.1. Sample Description..206

14.2.2. Diabetes App Use 209

14.2.3. Types of Diabetes App (Non-) Users – Results from
Hierarchical Cluster Analysis...............................211

14.2.4. Differences between Diabetes App Users and Non-Users –
Hypotheses...223

14.2.5. Most Relevant Factors' Strength of Influence on
Diabetes App Use 226

14.3. Discussion..233

14.4. Study Limitations...239

14.5. Conclusion 241

15. Discussion and Deriving Research Gaps............................243

15.1. Summary on Study Results from Studies 1 to 3 243

15.2. What does Empowerment Explain?.............................249

15.2.1. Empowerment and Diabetes App Use.......................249

15.2.2. Empowerment and Other Influencing Factors...............251

15.3. The Value of Empowerment for mHealth Research.............................258

15.4. The Operationalization of Empowerment..260

16. **Learning from Research Results – Implications for Research and Diabetes Care Practice...265**

16.1. Implications for Other Health Domains...265

16.2. Advancing Methodology 266

16.3. Implications for Diabetes Care – The Practical Value of Diabetes Apps..267

16.4. Designing Diabetes Apps for Specific Target Groups..........................270

17. **Summarizing Research Limitations 273**

18. **Conclusion..275**

List of Figures

Figure 1.   The Unified Theory of Acceptance and Use of Technology by
             Venkatesh et al. (2003). 44

Figure 2.   The process of empowerment and mHealth (app) use for diabetes
             self-management. 91

Figure 3.   Types of diabetes apps in the sample (Study 1) 112

Figure 4.   MySugr app series (2016/2017). 121

Figure 5.   Hypotheses on empowerment as an antecedent of diabetes app
             use in addition to other anteceding factors (Study 3). 198

Figure 6.   Dendrogram using Ward Linkage – hierarchical cluster analysis
             for app users (Study 3). 213

Figure 7.   Elbow criterion – hierarchical cluster analysis for app users
             (Study 3). 213

Figure 8.   Dendrogram using Ward Linkage – hierarchical cluster analysis
             for app non-users (Study 3). 217

Figure 9.   Elbow criterion – hierarchical cluster analysis for app non-users
             (Study 3). 217

Figure 10.   Hypotheses results regarding the process between empowerment
             and diabetes app use (Study 3). 227

Figure 11.   Suggested mediators and moderators of the relationship between
             empowerment as an antecedent factor and diabetes app use. 253

List of Tables

Table 1.   Factors Influencing Diabetes Self-Management 14

Table 2.   Factors Influencing Technology Use from the Unified Theory of
            Acceptance and Use of Technology 45

Table 3.   Empowerment Dimensions...65

Table 4.   Research Questions and Hypotheses 96

Table 5.   App Quality Assessment (Study 1) 105

Table 6.   Diabetes App Inclusion Criteria (Study 1) 108

Table 7.   Diabetes App Collection Procedure Results (Study 1).........................108

Table 8.   Diabetes App Features and Characteristics (Study 1) 113

Table 9.   App Features Corresponding to Empowerment Dimensions
            (Study 1) 116

Table 10.   Diabetes App Quality Scores from Adapted MARS (Study 1)...........118

Table 11.   Apps Rated Best in Quality – Overall Adapted MARS Score
            (Study 1) 119

Table 12.   App Downloads and User Ratings (Study 1)..119

Table 13.   Interview Participants (Study 2) 144

Table 14.   Sample Description (Study 2)..145

Table 15.   Diabetes App (Non-) Use Categories in the Sample (Study 2) 149

Table 16.   Factor Collection Summary (Study 2)..152

Table 17.   Diabetes App (Non-) User Typology (Study 2) 164

Table 18.   Types of App (Non-) Users Compared for Factors Potentially
            Influencing App Use (Study 2)..172

Table 19.   Summary on Hypotheses Deriving from Study 2 Results....................189

Table 20.   Sample Description (Study 3)..208

Table 21.   Diabetes Apps in the Sample (Study 3)..210

Table 22.   Pearson Correlation for Clustering Variables (Study 3)......................212

Table 23.   Two-Cluster Result for Diabetes App Users – Mean Group
            Differences (Study 3)..214

Table 24.   Two Cluster Result for Diabetes App Non-Users – Mean Group
             Differences (Study 3)..219
Table 25.   Summarized Results from Hierarchical Cluster Analysis
             (Study 3) 221
Table 26.   Mean Diabetes App User and Non-User Group Differences
             (Study 3) 225
Table 27.   Summary of Hypotheses Testing Results (Study 3).............................228

List of Abbreviations

App	smart device application
BG	blood glucose
CA	content analysis
DAFNE	dose adjusting for normal eating (program)
DNE	diabetes nurse educator
eHealth	electronic health
GP	general practitioner
HCP	healthcare professional
HIS	health information seeking
mHealth	mobile health, the use of mobile communications for health information and services (Nacinovich, 2011)
MPA	Mobile Phone Appropriation (model)
SDT	Self-Determination Theory
SMS	short message service
T1DM	type 1 diabetes mellitus
T2DM	type 2 diabetes mellitus
UTAUT	Unified Theory of the Acceptance and Use of Technology

Abstract

Objectives. With increasing prevalence rates of diabetes, new strategies have to be found to address the challenges faced by the diabetes care sector and by society regarding larger patient numbers, delays in diagnoses, and increasing complications in diabetes patients. Research has shown that mere symptom treatment at a late disease stage is not cost-effective and does not reduce mortality. Thus, with a change in perspective required, diabetes care approaches have started to place greater emphasis on self-management by patients instead of medical treatment only. Self-management includes a range of behaviors, like blood sugar testing, physical exercise, or medication adherence, and recently has started to include technology-supported behaviors in addition to traditional self-management. With mobile (smart) tools ("mHealth") for the support of self-management developing rapidly, a large number of diabetes applications for self-management are now available on the app market. However, their effectiveness has not yet been fully proven, with previous effect reviews showing no or only marginal use effects on health behaviors and health outcomes. There is still a lack of research into the underlying processes and mechanisms behind app use that could help explain this lack in usage outcomes. Knowledge of underlying mechanisms of app use is essential to the design of high-quality apps and interventions based on these processes, and to prove their (use) effects. To increase knowledge about mechanisms of diabetes app adoption and use, their antecedents need to be understood.

Empowerment – as a multi-dimensional approach including both psychological and behavioral dimensions and as a fundamental motivational antecedent of chronic disease self-management – is examined as a potential antecedent of diabetes app use complementing other anteceding factors from technology adoption theory as well as from self-management theory. In this way, this research aims at taking one step back from mHealth use effect studies in order to understand underlying mechanisms of mHealth use in greater depth. A model of potential processes relating empowerment to diabetes app use is suggested, to situate the perspective on empowerment as an antecedent into the overall self-management context.

Methods and Results. The research design included three studies conducted in Singapore, with high diabetes prevalence rates and high technological affinity in the Singaporean population. It is argued that both an examination of diabetes app characteristics (app features, app quality) and an examination of a (non-) app user perspective were required. This is because app characteristics like app quality were expected to influence app use, in addition to app (non-) user attitudes and empowerment-related user preconditions. Along this line of argumentation, Study 1 looked into characteristics of diabetes apps, while Studies 2 and 3 were dedicated to the examination of a diabetes app (non-) user perspective.

Study 1 examined how features of 121 diabetes apps for self-management corresponded with theoretical indicators of empowerment, to be able to discuss the app potential for empowered self-management (app perspective). Additionally, app quality was analyzed using an existing shortened quality assessment scale (Mobile App Rating Scale), with app quality having been proven to influence aspects of app use. Study 1 results showed that the majority of the analyzed diabetes apps offered a very narrow range of limited features only partly corresponding with indicators of psychological and behavioral empowerment. Moreover, most diabetes apps were found to show low app quality, as evaluated with a shortened version of the Mobile App Rating Scale. Overall the potential of the apps for empowered self-management could only be summarized as limited, with the state of the apps failing to live up to the promises of health apps. From the few apps with high quality and a larger range of features supporting empowerment dimensions available in the sample, one app series was chosen for further research in studies 2 and 3 (MySugr Series).

For explanatory and illustrative purposes, the selected app series was included in *Study 2* which used 21 semi-structured face-to-face interviews with both type 1 and type 2 diabetes patients to identify diabetes app (non-) use in this sample, and to draw first conclusions about the relevance of empowerment for diabetes app use. From the data, a diabetes app user and non-user typology was developed to examine differences in app use regarding empowerment, in addition to other technology adoption factors and self-management factors. In this way, first conclusions about empowerment as a potential antecedent factor of diabetes app use could be drawn. Study 2 results highlighted differences between diabetes app user and non-user types, including differences in empowerment dimensions. App (non-) user types found included non-users of diabetes apps that were generally interested in the app use but faced high usage barriers, non-users without interest in diabetes apps, short-term adopters of diabetes apps, diabetes app switchers, and long-term users. The group of interested non-users showed a high risk for diabetes complications and lower psychological and behavioral empowerment in comparison with all diabetes app user groups. Generally, there was a tendency towards higher psychological and behavioral empowerment in users than in non-users of diabetes apps. In addition to empowerment, other factors like the type/medical specialty of the supervising healthcare professional or age were revealed as additional explanatory factors for (non-) user differences. For example, older non-users without interest in diabetes apps showed equally high psychological empowerment despite lower behavioral empowerment by general practitioners when compared to user groups, but high self-management experience and independent self-care at the same time. A first preliminary proof was delivered that empowerment was relevant for diabetes app use in addition to other factors. Hypotheses regarding the relationship between empowerment dimensions, other antecedents, and the use of diabetes apps were developed from Study 2 to be tested in Study 3.

Study 3 included an online survey with a sample of 65 type 1 and type 2 diabetes patients, and used cluster analytical methods to test the preliminary Study 2 diabetes app (non-) user typology, as well as binary logistic regression to compare the strength of influence of various anteceding factors on the likelihood of diabetes app use. Study 3 results demonstrated that the Study 2 user and non-user typology could be confirmed to a high degree, with minor differences compared with Study 2 results. Moreover, binary logistic regression showed that only the factors *perceived health status*, *type/medical specialty of supervising healthcare professional*, and *social influence by private social networks* as an indicator of behavioral empowerment, significantly predicted diabetes app use. While a better perceived health status and supervision by diabetes specialists significantly increased the chance of diabetes app use, social support from private social networks significantly decreased the likelihood of app use.

Conclusion. The three studies delivered initial proof that certain empowerment dimensions were antecedents of diabetes app use in addition to other influencing factors (e.g., the perceived health status, the type/medical specialty of supervising healthcare professional). Overall, the three studies confirmed a general relevance of empowerment for diabetes app use. Especially behavioral empowerment by private social patient networks could be shown to play a crucial role for technology-supported self-management, despite its minor role in previous empowerment approaches in diabetes or mHealth research. However, further research suitable for an examination of causal relationships is needed. Suggestions for future research are outlined, implications for the measurement of empowerment are presented, and practical suggestions based on the results are introduced.

1 Introduction

1.1 The Urgency of Self-Management in Diabetes Care

> Diabetes mellitus is one of the most common non-communicable long-term conditions in the world and is linked to high mortality, morbidity, loss of quality of life and high social and economic cost. Diabetes presents a serious health challenge, as it is a significant cause of ill health and premature death. (Wilkinson, Whitehead, & Ritchie, 2014, p. 111)

The World Health Organization published statistics in 2014 showing that 347 million individuals suffer from diabetes worldwide, with rising tendencies (World Health Organization, 2015). Even though diabetes is usually referred to as a "rich-men's-disease" or a "disease of affluence" (F. B. Hu, 2011), the WHO states that more than 80% of people with diabetes live in low- and middle-income countries (World Health Organization, 2015). Thus, diabetes has become a global problem. Mathers and Loncar (2006) predict that diabetes will move from rank eleven of the fifteen leading causes of death in 2002 to rank seven in 2030. In addition, the WHO projects "that diabetes deaths will double between 2005 and 2030" (World Health Organization, 2015).

These numbers show that society will face serious issues regarding diabetes and other lifestyle-related diseases in the future, with numbers of patients and risk groups increasing drastically in both developed and developing countries (International Diabetes Federation, 2010, 2014b). With healthcare costs skyrocketing for long-term diabetes care, new strategies have to be found to stop the financial burden (e.g., Diabetes Prevention Program Research Group, 2012; World Health Organization, 2016a). To address this financial pressure, mere medical diabetes symptom treatment is not sufficient anymore (especially starting at a late disease stage) because this approach has not been proven to lower healthcare costs long-term (e.g., Diabetes Prevention Program Research Group, 2012; World Health Organization, 2016a). Approaches focusing on medication have to be complemented by other approaches focusing on diabetes prevention (risk groups for developing diabetes) and diabetes lifestyle interventions (risk groups and diabetes patients). Cost-effective lifestyle interventions can improve diabetes outcomes in all types of diabetes patients (World Health Organization,

N. Brew-Sam, *App Use and Patient Empowerment in Diabetes Self-Management*, https://doi.org/10.1007/978-3-658-29357-4_1

2016a). According to the World Health Organization (2016a), these interventions mainly emphasize diabetes self-management, including blood glucose (BG) control (diet, physical activity, medication), blood pressure control, as well as adherence to regular screenings (eyes, kidneys, feet). It is crucial for a diabetes patient to self-manage the chronic condition him-/herself, because the disease has to be taken care of daily for a long period of time to avoid negative long-term health consequences (see American Diabetes Association, 2014). In diabetes, healthcare professionals cannot constantly accompany patients, but usually provide feedback during regular HbA1c checkups every 3-4 months (Goh et al., 2014).

Past (diabetes) research looking into doctor-patient relationships has shown a shift from a paternalistic approach of regarding healthcare providers as solely responsible for disease outcomes towards a collaborative approach between the patient and the healthcare professional with much stronger self-responsibility given to the patient, thus promoting self-management (Snoek, 2007). If self-management is poor due to existing self-care barriers, long-term complications in patients have proven to be more serious (Glasgow, Toobert, & Gillette, 2001; Wilkinson et al., 2014). Therefore, life-style-related self-management approaches are at the center of chronic disease care.

1.2   Research Interest: Empowerment as an Anteceding Factor of Diabetes App Use for Self-Management

With a stronger focus on self-management, strategies and tools supporting the self-management processes gained relevance in diabetes care (Solomon, 2008). Technology for self-management developed rapidly, and mobile self-management solutions appeared with the emergence of mobile phones and mobile smart devices (Lucas, 2015). With health apps entering the mobile smart device market, apps for diabetes self-management sprang up in large numbers. Diabetes smart device apps delivered promising options for technology-supported self-management, e.g., for diabetes monitoring using diabetes diary/logbook apps (e.g., the MySugr Logbook, https://mysugr.com). Diabetes logbook apps can be used to track and monitor blood glucose values and other health data by the patient as part of overall self-management.

The availability of objective ways to monitor the disease helps to carry out self-management successfully (Tattersall, 2002).

Despite an available research tradition looking into the use of diabetes-specific apps for self-management as well as usage effects (see Chapter 4), the effectiveness of diabetes app use for self-management is not clear yet. Previous mobile interventions for diabetes management, as well as app use effect studies, were frequently conducted without a theoretical foundation on app adoption and use processes (see Chapter 4.2.2 and following chapters). Theory-based knowledge on adoption and usage processes is fundamental to enable the design of high-quality apps based on these processes that are able to show strong effects. Thus, before looking into app usage effects, it is necessary to take one step back to understand diabetes app adoption and use processes in greater depth.

To increase knowledge about underlying mechanisms of diabetes app adoption and use, antecedents of app use need to be understood. Previous research on mHealth use has mainly followed an adoption paradigm, and frequently looked into antecedent factors based on or similar to factors from the well-known Unified Theory of Acceptance and Use of Technology (UTAUT, Venkatesh, Morris, Davis, & Davis, 2003), which is a summary of eight previous models. The UTAUT mentions four factors – performance expectancy, effort expectancy, social influence, and facilitating conditions – as influencing user acceptance and usage behavior, and four factors – gender, age, experience, and voluntariness of use – as key moderating variables. However, when applied to a chronic disease self-management context, there are several shortcomings of the antecedent factors included in the UTAUT. A comprehensive consideration of intrinsic and extrinsic motivational factors, especially relevant in terms of intrinsic individual (psychological) patient factors influencing self-management, as well as extrinsic healthcare provider/professional (HCP) factors (social influence), is missing.

Empowerment as a fundamental motivational approach for chronic disease self-management is suggested as a potential antecedent that can address shortcomings of technology adoption models regarding intrinsic and extrinsic motivational aspects, as well as general mHealth research gaps regarding (alternative) theories for explaining mHealth use in the context of disease self-management. Empowerment is defined as a multi-dimensional motivational approach, differing from related motivational concepts by including both intrinsic psychological (feeling of empowerment) and extrinsic behavioral dimensions (social support by HCPs and by private social networks) (M. Lee & Koh, 2001). In contrast to the few previous mHealth studies looking into empowerment as an outcome of mHealth use, the research aims to examine whether empowerment with its psychological and behavioral dimensions is a relevant antecedent of diabetes app use, complementing other anteceding factors from technology adoption and self-management theory. A model was developed of potential processes relating to empowerment and diabetes app use, to situate empowerment as an antecedent in the overall self-management context.

The theory and the studies showed that both an examination of diabetes app characteristics and an examination of an app user perspective were required when trying to understand empowerment as an antecedent of diabetes app use. Regarding the first, updated knowledge about diabetes app features, app types and app quality were needed as a foundation for understanding user perspectives on diabetes app use. Thus, Study 1 focused on app characteristics and app features and looked into 121 diabetes apps as tools providing the technological foundation for app use, and how they differed in quality and in potential for empowered self-management. The study investigated how diabetes app features corresponded to theoretical indicators of empowerment. From there, following an exploratory and interpretive approach, the potential of diabetes apps for empowerment and for self-management was discussed. Studies 2 and 3 focused on the user perspective of diabetes apps, and examined empowerment of patients in relation to reported diabetes app use. Study 2 used one selected app from Study 1 to discuss previous diabetes app use with 21 diabetes patients in semi-structured face-to-face interviews. To examine the influence of reported psychological and behavioral empowerment on diabetes app use as a first step, a diabetes app user and non-user typology was used in Study 2 to examine differences in app use regarding empowerment and in addition to other factors from technology adoption and self-management theory. Hypotheses regarding the relationship between empowerment dimensions, other antecedents, and the use of diabetes apps were developed from Study 2 to be tested in Study 3. Study 3 used cluster analytical methods to test the preliminary Study 2 diabetes app (non-) user typology in a sample of 65 diabetes patients (online survey), as well as used binary logistic regression to compare the strength of influence of various anteceding factors on the likelihood of diabetes app use.

1.3   Chapter Overview

Chapter 2 delivers background information on diabetes and on self-management as part of diabetes care. It emphasizes the relevance of motivation as a precondition for successful diabetes self-management behaviors, before the focus is put on mobile apps for diabetes self-management in Chapter 3. In Chapter 4, a closer look is directed towards previous research on the use of apps for diabetes self-management and usage effects, as well as research gaps relating to an understanding of diabetes app usage processes. The relevance of investigating antecedents of diabetes app use to understand usage processes in greater detail is outlined in Chapter 5. Following an adoption paradigm in mHealth research, anteceding factors from the Unified Theory of Acceptance and Use of Technology (UTAUT) as a summary of eight previous models are introduced in Chapter 5. Shortcomings (regarding motivational antecedents) of the UTAUT are described when applying the theory to a diabetes self-management context, and overall theoretical research gaps are summarized in Chapter 6. To close the research gaps regarding the outlined theoretical shortcomings, empowerment is introduced as an antecedent of diabetes app use in Chapter 7, with empowerment being a fundamental motivational precondition for self-management behaviors. Chapter 7 delivers a conceptual empowerment definition and distinction from related concepts, and argues why empowerment is a motivational approach that is both relevant for diabetes self-management behaviors and diabetes app use. It then introduces previous research on empowerment in the context of mHealth use. It explains why the view has to be expanded from a usage outcome perspective towards a broader perspective on empowerment and diabetes app use, including an understanding of empowerment as an antecedent of diabetes app use. Chapter 8 summarizes research gaps regarding empowerment and diabetes app use, and outlines that empowerment should be investigated as a multi-dimensional antecedent of diabetes app use. Moreover, it is argued that several research perspectives are needed in that context, including both an app perspective and an app user perspective. Following the research gaps, Chapter 9 summarizes the research interest and the described processes from previous chapters in a graphic model. Resulting research questions and hypotheses on empowerment as an antecedent of diabetes app use are introduced in Chapter 10. Chapter 11 delivers an overview on the empirical research design to test the hypotheses and to answer the research questions. The methods, research procedures, findings, and study limitations of the three studies conducted to answer the research questions are comprehensively presented in Chapters 12 to 14. An overall discussion of the findings is presented in Chapter 15. This chapter also points towards defining research gaps from the findings. Finally, suggestions for practical and scientific implications are presented in Chapter 16. Chapter 17 summarizes the main research limitations, before Chapter 18 delivers an overall conclusion.

2 Background on Diabetes Self-Management

2.1 What is Diabetes? – Types of Diabetes Mellitus

According to the American Diabetes Association, the term "diabetes" comprises a group of metabolic diseases. Their common characteristic is high blood glucose that results from defects in insulin secretion and action (American Diabetes Association, 2010). In this condition, the body shows inability to use blood sugar for energy, resulting in hyperglycemia (high blood glucose) (National Diabetes Information Clearinghouse, 2011). Hyperglycemia is associated with physical long-term damage, especially the dysfunction and failure of organs like the eyes, the kidneys, the nerves, the heart, and the blood vessels (American Diabetes Association, 2010). Diabetes is subsumed under the broader category of chronic diseases due to the fact that the disease develops over a long period of time and affects the patient's life long-term.

Usually most cases of diabetes are assigned to one of two broad categories, type 1 (T1DM) or type 2 (T2DM) diabetes mellitus (American Diabetes Association, 2010). T1DM, often called "insulin-dependent diabetes", is an autoimmune disease and is characterized by an absolute deficiency of insulin secretion. The autoimmune disease leads to the destruction of cells of the pancreas, where the hormone insulin usually is produced (American Diabetes Association, 2010). The progress of the cell destruction can vary in patients, but in a large number of cases the disease already shows in childhood. Common complications include skin, eye, and foot complications, high blood pressure (hypertension), kidney disease (nephropathy), nerve damage (neuropathy), stomach complications, heart disease, stroke, and others (American Diabetes Association, 2015). Furthermore, both hyperglycemia and hypoglycemia, which are extremely high or extremely low blood glucose levels, can occur. Risk factors for developing T1DM are family history of diabetes type 1, environmental factors, and viral infections to some extent (International Diabetes Federation, 2014a). Because of the final complete lack of insulin, T1DM patients sooner or later have to supply their bodies with insulin through injections and therefore are called insulin-dependent. In total, patients suffering from T1DM account for only five to ten percent of all diabetes patients.

N. Brew-Sam, *App Use and Patient Empowerment in Diabetes Self-Management*, https://doi.org/10.1007/978-3-658-29357-4_2

The more prevalent T2DM (90-95%), which sometimes is referred to as "non-insulin-dependent diabetes", is caused by a "combination of resistance to insulin action and an inadequate compensatory insulin secretory response" (American Diabetes Association, 2010, p. 62). Thus the pancreas produces a sufficient amount of the hormone insulin, but the effect of insulin is reduced due to the respective degree of insulin resistance. Even though the pancreas produces more insulin after a while, the resistance prevents insulin effectiveness. This has negative effects for several other organs in the long run, but might not be detected for a period of time, because insulin resistance usually causes no clinical symptoms over many years (American Diabetes Association, 2010). T2DM usually develops gradually with symptoms slowly showing in later disease stages. The causes of insulin resistance are mainly lifestyle related. The risk for T2DM increases with body weight, age and a lack of physical activity and can be decreased by an adaption of a healthy lifestyle and additional medication. According to the International Diabetes Federation (2014a) several risk factors have been associated with T2DM, among other things family history of diabetes, overweight, an unhealthy diet, physical inactivity, increasing age, high blood pressure, ethnicity, the history of gestational diabetes (diabetes during pregnancy), and poor nutrition during pregnancy. Similar to T1DM there is a genetic disposition for the development of T2DM, but in contrast to T1DM environmental influences are much more crucial for the disease development (American Diabetes Association, 2010).

> While there are a number of factors that influence the development of type 2 diabetes, it is evident that the most influential are lifestyle behaviours commonly associated with urbanisation. These include consumption of processed foods, for example foods with a high fat content, sugar- sweetened beverages and highly refined carbohydrates. At the same time, modern lifestyles are characterised by physical inactivity and long sedentary periods. Together these behaviours are associated with an increased risk of being overweight or obese and the development of type 2 diabetes. (International Diabetes Federation, 2015a, p. 104)

Other forms of diabetes include gestational diabetes (occurring during pregnancy), and other less common forms listed on Diabetes Digital Media (2017). Moreover, pre-diabetes "is characterized by the presence of blood glucose levels that are higher than normal but not yet high enough to be classified as diabetes" (Diabetes Digital Media, 2017). Diabetes self-management in all types of diabetes is crucial, especially in the strongly lifestyle-related T2DM. The focus in this thesis is mainly on T1DM and T2DM being the most common types of diabetes.

Diabetes treatment includes a variety of strategies to keep a diabetes patient's BG levels stable, or to improve them where possible (Diabetes Digital Media, 2018). Treatment is usually adapted by the healthcare team for an individual and should include medical, psychosocial and lifestyle strategies (Diabetes Digital Media, 2018). Insulin-dependent diabetes (mainly type 1) is treated using a combination of strict diet, planned exercise, regular insulin injections, and BG testing. Non-insulin-dependent diabetes (mainly type 2) is treated in a similar way with diet, exercise, BG testing, and in some cases oral medication and/or insulin (Diabetes Digital Media, 2018). Apart from medical approaches (oral medication and insulin), the relevance of lifestyle approaches in diabetes treatment – including effective self-management of the disease by the patient – is steadily increasing.

> Improved glycemic control is partly related to advances in medical treatment, but optimal outcomes are also directly tied to an individual's ability to engage in consistent self-management behaviors. This requires the involvement of the individual and their family over the course of the disease, engaging in a multitude of disease management behaviors, and the ability to address concurrent or associated psychosocial challenges. (Hunter, 2016, p. 517)

The following chapter goes into further detail about self-management as part of diabetes treatment, its development from paternalistic to participatory care approaches, and its relevance for diabetes outcomes.

2.2 Diabetes Self-Management – Definition and Development

Self-management approaches gained relevance with the introduction of home blood glucose monitoring possibilities in the 1970s, leading to a shift from a mere healthcare professional's (HCP) responsibility to a stronger self-responsibility on the part of the patient (Snoek, 2007). In the earlier diabetes care approach, healthcare professionals were exclusively considered responsible for diagnosis and treatment of diabetes, with a prescriptive approach following the "do as I say" or the "doctor knows best" principle (Funnell & Anderson, 2004). In this approach, the HCPs aimed at patient compliance, even if it came at the cost of patient's quality of life. It was assumed that the benefits of compliance outweigh the impacts of guidelines and recommendations on the patient's quality of life (Funnell & Anderson, 2004). This approach is often referred to as "medical paternalism" (Chin, 2002). However, following this approach to diabetes care non-compliance rates were shown to be high, and rethinking became necessary (Funnell & Anderson, 2004). It had to be recognized that even though the HCPs know best about diabetes facts and treatment options, it is the patients themselves who have knowledge about their individual context of life (Funnell & Anderson, 2004). Only the diabetes patients themselves know which diabetes management strategy will match their individual lifestyle. According to R. M. Anderson and Funnell (2010) "collaboration is necessary to develop plans that fit both the patients' diabetes and their lives" (p. 279). Diabetes self-management became the core of the management of this chronic disease, with diabetes patients being the decision-makers in control of their daily diabetes self-management (Funnell & Anderson, 2004). The traditional paternalistic approach was replaced by a collaborative approach in diabetes management (Funnell & Anderson, 2004). Feeling responsible *for* the patients changed towards feeling responsible *to* them (Funnell & Anderson, 2004).

The amendment to the ethical code of the American Medical Association displays the shifts towards self-management that took place, and thus is a good example that illustrates the changes. The "obligations of patients to their physicians" in the original AMA Code of Medical Ethics talks about an implicit and prompt obedience of the patient to the prescriptions of the physician, and warns about the patient's "crude opinions" (American Medical Association, 1847). In contrast, the current AMA Code of Medical Ethics (based on a report 1992/93) explains in the "opinions on the patient-physician relationship" (American Medical Association, 2015, section 10.00) that health and well-being depend on a collaborative effort between the patient and the physician (opinion 10.01). It stresses the mutual cooperation between the patient and the health professional, and attributes the right of the patient to receive information, as well as the right to make treatment decisions (among other rights). Furthermore, the current code "recognizes the human capacity to self-govern" (opinion 10.02) and therefore explicitly points towards self-management.

Clark and colleagues started to develop a framework for conceptualizing disease management in 1988, and developed it further in the following years (Clark & Houle, 2009). In their work, patient self-management is defined as "the conscious use of strategies to manipulate situations to reduce the impact of disease on daily life" (p. 27). Thus, diabetes self-management includes all behaviors that are related to the active management of the chronic disease by the patient him- or herself. Preventing the development or the worsening of diabetes usually is achieved by the reduction of body weight through increased physical activity and diet, as well as certain forms of medication (American Diabetes Association, 2010). Gomersall, Madill, and Summers (2011) conducted a meta-synthesis of 38 papers on diabetes self-management. They found that "self-managing diabetes includes, for example, adopting lower-fat diets and regular exercise. To control diabetes, the individual patient must oversee his or her daily behavior, and long-held habits often have to be changed. Self-management therefore implies an intrapersonal understanding of diabetes control" (p. 854). The Self-Care Behaviors Framework by the American Association of Diabetes Educators (AADE) specifies seven essential self-care behaviors for disease management: healthy eating, being active, blood glucose monitoring, taking medication, problem solving, reducing risks, and healthy coping (American Association of Diabetes Educators, 2017). Other behaviors include foot and eye care and regular check-up adherence (Goh et al., 2014).

Problem solving, reducing risks, and healthy coping relate to the psychological aspects of diabetes care. Problem solving for example includes dealing with unexpected events by analyzing the situation, while reducing risks includes taking control, and healthy coping relates to dealing with stress (American Association of Diabetes Educators, 2017). In their meta-synthesis, Gomersall et al. (2011) report that "diabetes management requires a number of behavioral and dietary adaptations that are often difficult for people to incorporate into preexisting life contexts" (p. 865). As part of self-management, psychological aspects of diabetes care increasingly gained attention in addition to behavioral aspects (Hunter, 2016; Mathiesen et al., 2017; Peyrot et al., 2005). The DAWN study was able to show that psychological problems are common in diabetes patients worldwide (Peyrot et al., 2005), and that problems like depression need to be addressed to improve diabetes self-management outcomes. Psychological care is frequently not included in average care plans, but attention is increasingly paid to the relevance of psychosocial aspects of diabetes self-management. According to Hunter (2016, p. 517) more psychologists with training for diabetes are needed to be able to include psychological support in diabetes care.

Diabetes self-management includes two major relevant aspects: first, it includes the patient's self-management behaviors as well as underlying psychological aspects, and secondly, it includes aspects of social support from other individuals (e.g., HCPs). This can also be shown more clearly by looking into factors influencing diabetes self-management outcomes, as argued in the following chapter.

2.3 Factors Influencing Diabetes Self-Management

For collaborative diabetes care approaches to work, studies investigated factors that might support or hinder successful diabetes self-management. Wilkinson et al. (2014) conducted a systematic literature review of qualitative research findings on factors that influence the ability for diabetes self-management in T1DM and T2DM patients. Several factors in both patients and the diabetes care system were found to be relevant for enabling the diabetes patient to execute, change or maintain self-management behaviors (factors see Table 1). Ahola and Groop (2013) call these two categories "individual related" and "environment related" factors, while K. M. Rodriguez (2013) simply speak of "intrinsic" and "extrinsic" factors. The authors of all three papers (Ahola & Groop, 2013; K. M. Rodriguez, 2013; Wilkinson et al., 2014) also speak of "barriers" towards self-management, hindering the execution of self-management behaviors when not fulfilled. Barriers are "factors that impede diabetes self-management and quality of life" (Glasgow et al., 2001, p. 39). All three papers show similar results, and were seen as exemplary research on factors influencing diabetes self-management because they deliver comprehensive overviews on influencing factors while most other papers mainly look into single factors or a smaller number of factors (e.g., Ahmed et al., 2010; Lorant & Dauvrin, 2012; Mathiesen et al., 2017; Murphy, Casey, Dinneen, Lawton, & Brown, 2011; Naeem, 2016; Peyrot et al., 2005; Trentini, Malgaroli, Camerini, Di Serio, & Schulz, 2015).

Following the three papers (Table 1), on the one hand personal/individual factors influencing diabetes self-management include personal and health beliefs and attitudes, as well as coping and learning skills (e.g., problem solving abilities, literacy, knowledge, and learning abilities). Additionally, psychological factors like depression, anxiety, other emotions, empowerment, self-efficacy, or motivation are relevant for self-management, as well as individual physical factors (e.g., health status, other diseases) and practical factors (e.g., socioeconomic factors).

On the other hand, provider and care system factors include access factors, like access to good HCPs and healthcare facilities. Care factors further include characteristics of care, like the quality of care, the individualization of care, or the influence of competing care interests and duties on self-management. Communication and clinical relationships are of relevance as well, with differing decision-making and communication approaches being possible between HCPs and patients. Moreover, diabetes-specific education influences self-management, with diabetes knowledge and self-management skills being taught to patients. Social support is also relevant, including support from HCPs, families and relatives to manage diabetes successfully. Table 1 summarizes all factors supporting or hindering diabetes self-management as mentioned in the three papers (Ahola & Groop, 2013; K. M. Rodriguez, 2013; Wilkinson et al., 2014).

Table 1. Factors Influencing Diabetes Self-Management

	Wilkinson et al. (2014)		Ahola and Groop (2013)	Rodriguez (2013)
	Factors	Explanation/examples	Factors	Factors
Personal/ individual related/ intrinsic factors	Individual adaptability	Ability to problem solve, adapt, find balance and manage diabetes at home, work and in social situations	Coping and problem solving skills	
	Learning experience	Experiential learning – Individuals base decisions on results from previous learning	Knowledge, Health literacy	Diabetes knowledge and technical skill, functional health literacy
	Personal beliefs	Cultural and spiritual beliefs about food, exercise, body image, family, life, illness, death	Health Beliefs	Health Beliefs, attitudes
	Physical factors	Symptoms impacting ability to undertake self-care activities; lack of energy	Forgetting, excess use of alcohol, other interfering diseases	
	Practical factors	Monetary limitations, equipment malfunction, or having others to care for	Socio-economic factors (here environmental)	Financial considerations (here extrinsic)
	Psychological factors	Mental and emotional processes, e.g., frustration about inability to achieve goals	Empowerment, motivation, self-efficacy, locus of control, depression, anxiety	Self-efficacy
Provider/ care system/ environment related/ extrinsic factors	Access factors	Consistency of healthcare provider, e.g., access to same HCP at each visit; lack of HCP time	Distance to the site of healthcare, factors related to the availability of good quality healthcare, nutritious foods, exercise opportunities, etc.	Access to effective diabetes healthcare delivery
	Care factors	Individualized care, lack of care quality	Other competing interests and duties	
	Communication	Difficulty in communicating with HCP, respectful communication, shared decision-making		Clinical relationships
	Education	Consistent education and information from different HCP, conflicting advice, sustained knowledge building on previous knowledge		
	Support	Meaningful support from HCP, lack of support from significant others (e.g., family), others become self-management partners	Social support	Family and community support systems

Note. Factors extracted and summarized from the three selected studies and reviews

Regarding (1) personal factors, Ahola and Groop (2013) point out that special atten-tion has to be paid to motivation as a major factor in self-management (also see Mur-phy et al., 2011). According to Oftedal, Bru, and Karlsen (2011) "previous research has suggested that motivational problems are probably one of the main reasons for poor diabetes management" (p. 735). Motivation is defined as "a driving force or forces responsible for the initiation, persistence, direction, and vigour of goal-directed behaviour" (Colman, 2015, p. 479). Both Oftedal et al. (2011) and Ahola and Groop (2013) distinguish two types of motivation in the context of diabetes self-management, namely intrinsic and extrinsic motivation. "Intrinsic motivation… refers to doing something because it is inherently interesting or enjoyable, and extrinsic mo-tivation… refers to doing something because it leads to a separable outcome" (Ryan & Deci, 2000, p. 55). Extrinsic motivation for example includes providing incentives or rewards to trigger motivation (Benabou & Tirole, 2003), or motivation provided by the healthcare team in diabetes self-management (Ahola & Groop, 2013). Ahola and Groop (2013) state that generally, intrinsic motivation is more important in active dia-betes self-management than extrinsic motivation. Research has shown that intrinsic motivation can provide effective long-term motivation, whereas extrinsic motivation alone only shows success for short-term motivation, or even fully fails to motivate (Benabou & Tirole, 2003). Mere extrinsic motivation may even lead to negative rein-forcement in the long run, while intrinsic motivation is promising long-term (Benabou & Tirole, 2003). Studies have shown that "individuals who are primarily motivated by external factors (i.e., external rewards) have less chance of attaining a healthy diet and maintaining physical activity than those whose motivation is mainly intrinsic" (Of-tedal et al., 2011, p. 735/736). Especially for health behavior changes it is necessary that patients are mainly internally motivated instead of being externally motivated only (R. M. Anderson & Funnell, 2010; Williams, Grow, Freedman, Ryan, & Deci, 1996). However, Oftedal et al. (2011) investigated how intrinsic motivation relates to diet and exercise in type 2 diabetes patients, and their results imply that important ex-trinsic factors additionally play "a significant role in determining dietary behaviour" (p. 735). Thus, both intrinsic and extrinsic motivation have to be focused on in diabe-tes self-management, with an emphasis on intrinsic motivation.

As potential sources of extrinsic motivation and as (2) external factors in diabetes care and support, HCPs play a significant role in diabetes management despite the change from paternalistic towards collaborative approaches. Diabetes self-management still takes place within a HCP-patient relationship, and thus the role of HCPs did not become superfluous but merely changed. Self-management without HCP support has shown to be negatively related to diabetes outcomes. Wysocki et al. (1996) investigated excessive autonomy in self-care in 100 young diabetes patients using a cross-sectional study design. They measured differences in three levels of self-care autonomy (constrained, appropriate, or excessive self-care autonomy) regarding treatment adherence, diabetes knowledge, glycemic control, and hospitalization rates. Their results showed that the group of excessive self-care reported less treatment adherence, less knowledge, and less glycemic control. "Excessive self-care autonomy increased with age and was less common among intact two-parent families" (p. 119).

HCPs both educate the patient as a first step, and provide self-management support as a second step (Funnell & Anderson, 2004). Knowledge about diabetes self-management provides a foundation for executing self-management appropriately (Ahola & Groop, 2013). Diabetes knowledge relates to aspects of health literacy (Schulz & Nakamoto, 2013). However, knowledge itself is not sufficient to achieve improved self-management outcomes if supportive and collaborative interaction between HCPs and the patient is missing (Norris, Engelgau, & Narayan, 2001). In the process of diabetes self-management, the HCP has an important role as the patient's advisor and partner, who motivates the patient to adhere to prescriptions and recommendations (Shetty, Chamukuttan, Nanditha, Raj, & Ramachandran, 2011). HCPs' recommendations are required to fit the patient's goals, priorities, and lifestyle (Funnell & Anderson, 2004). For example, factors like age or profession might influence the patient's ability to follow health professionals' recommendations to exercise regularly.

After having laid out the background on diabetes and diabetes self-management, the following Chapter 3 looks into diabetes apps as technological tools for self-management, previous research on diabetes apps, and classifies these tools within overall mHealth research.

3 Defining and Categorizing Diabetes Apps for Self-Management

With technological development in recent years, diabetes care started to develop technological devices for diabetes self-management that went beyond blood glucose (BG) meters for BG testing. Technology entered the diabetes market with a focus on supplementing HCP diabetes care and supporting self-management by providing educational and motivational support (Hunt, 2015). "As patients become more technologically savvy, devices become more available, and new technologies emerge, the variety of technological self-management strategies increases" (p. 226). According to Hunt, technology for self-management can support all self-management activities including BG and complication monitoring, medication, healthy eating, exercise, and problem-solving. Available technology includes a combination of connected medical devices designed for diabetes patients to use at home (e.g., connected glucose meters), diabetes apps that assist in self-management (e.g., diabetes diaries), service-oriented diabetes apps which make recommendations based on collected data, and telemedical services for diabetes patients (Statista, 2018). By 2020, the number of users of electronic health solutions for diabetes is expected to rise to 13.7 million (Statista, 2018).

Mobile smart devices and mobile internet-based technology for diabetes self-management have increasingly gained relevance with respective technological development. The number of available diabetes apps for self-management is heavily increasing in app stores every year (Research2guidance, 2014b, 2016). With the availability of diabetes apps for self-management, research on the potential of these mobile tools for self-management was initiated. The following chapters will introduce characteristics of diabetes apps for self-management, as well as connected research.

3.1 Diabetes Apps for Self-Management as Second Generation mHealth Tools

Apps for diabetes self-management are second generation mHealth tools. In health communication, the term *mHealth* (short for "mobile Health") refers to mobile communication tools, and "the use of mobile communications for health information and services" (Nacinovich, 2011, p. 1). Rossmann and Karnowski (2014) similarly describe mHealth as the use of mobile information and communication technologies for

N. Brew-Sam, *App Use and Patient Empowerment in Diabetes
Self-Management*, https://doi.org/10.1007/978_3_658_29357_4_3

healthcare and health promotion. The World Health Organization delivers further details about mHealth in their explanation of the field of mobile health:

> The Global Observatory for eHealth (GOe) defined mHealth or mobile health as medical and public health practice supported by mobile devices, such as mobile phones, patient monitoring devices, personal digital assistants (PDAs), and other wireless devices. mHealth involves the use and capitalization on a mobile phone's core utility of voice and short messaging service (SMS) as well as more complex functionalities and applications including general packet radio service (GPRS), third and fourth generation mobile telecommunications (3G and 4G systems), global positioning system (GPS), and Bluetooth technology. (World Health Organization, 2011, p. 6)

The World Health Organization describes mHealth as a component (and further development) of eHealth (electronic health) (World Health Organization, 2011). However, with the development of cloud-based online systems the differences between eHealth and mHealth get more and more blurred. Online channels are steadily merging and online content is increasingly available anywhere from any mobile or stationary device, accessible through online clouds and independent of devices.

mHealth tools can be distinguished depending on the operating systems available (Danaher, Brendryen, Seeley, Tyler, & Woolley, 2015). The second generation of mHealth relates to mobile smart devices and uses texting and IVR, but in a more varied and powerful way than first generation tools (Danaher et al., 2015; Knittle et al., 2016). The first mHealth generation refers to tools on simple mobile feature phones including text messaging and interactive voice response (IVR). Studies on first generation tools for disease self-management have for example been published by Fischer et al. (2012), Fortmann et al. (2017), Mayberry, Mulvaney, Johnson, and Osborn (2017), Nelson et al. (2016), and others. In the second generation, "rather than a loosely connected collection of tools that reach out to participants, smartphone apps can be designed to offer participants a cohesive multifaceted program to use" (Danaher et al., 2015, p. 93). Apart from apps, the authors mention functions like email, text notifications, audio or video notifications, recording pictures, audio, and video, discussion forums (social media and instant messaging), and sensor functionalities. This second generation includes apps for disease self-management as for example studied by Chavez et al. (2017), El-Gayar, Timsina, Nawar, and Eid (2013), Fu, McMahon, Gross, Adam, and Wyman (2017), B. E. Holtz et al. (2017), Huckvale, Adomaviciute, Prieto, Leow, and Car (2015), Istepanian, Casiglia, and Gregory (2017), and Wu et al. (2017).

While first generation mHealth tools mainly have intervention character (e.g., text message interventions), this is not necessarily the case for second generation tools. Interventions are programs usually organized by professional providers (e.g., public health professionals, academics, healthcare professionals) and run over a limited period of time, with a specified sample of participants or target group and a defined aim (e.g., assess, improve, maintain, promote or modify health) (compare World Health Organization, 2016b). A typical first generation mHealth intervention is an mHealth text message intervention with SMS being sent to a defined target group over a specified period of time (Hall, Cole-Lewis, & Bernhardt, 2015). As such, text messages are mostly push channels that require little receiver initiative. For background on push-pull approaches in healthcare see Kingsley (1987).

In contrast, second generation mHealth apps are of different character, and are not necessarily included in interventions but also can be accessed by the user him- or herself. Apps are directly offered to the app user in app stores, and thus are marketed "directly to the consumer" (Kingsley, 1987, abstract). As such they can be categorized as "pull" channels (compare Kingsley, 1987), and require own user initiative because the user has to actively download and manage the apps. Apps can be connected to various other devices, like fitness and sleep trackers (wristband), or glucose meters (e.g., iB-GStar Diabetes Manager App, http://mystar.sanofi.de).

Due to differences between first generation text message interventions (as interventions limited to a certain amount of time in which the participants receive regular messages) and second generation apps for self-management that are not necessarily part of an intervention (here, the app use is not limited to a certain time span and requires more user initiative), mHealth results based on text message interventions are only partially applicable to apps (e.g., usage effect study results).

3.2   Purpose, Types and Features of Diabetes Apps for Self-Management

Diabetes apps for self-management are smart device applications that are specifically designed for the support of individuals in their daily disease self-management. They target diabetes patients already suffering from the disease, to enhance their disease treatment, care and disease management (Istepanian et al., 2017).[1] Thus, they fall within the mHealth category diagnostic treatment and support as differentiated from the categories drug adherence and remote monitoring, remote information dissemination, data collection and disease outbreak surveillance by Nacinovich (2011). However, diabetes self-management apps can also include aspects of remote monitoring (e.g., blood glucose monitoring), drug adherence (e.g., adherence to insulin injections), and information dissemination (e.g., information delivered by support groups). Prevention is only included in the sense of preventing a worsening of the health condition (and not prevention of the disease itself). In contrast, preventive mHealth tools (e.g., text-message or online based mHealth campaigns) target diabetes risk groups to change their health behaviors to prevent them from developing diabetes (Beratarrechea et al., 2016; Jindal et al., 2016; Muralidharan, Ranjani, Anjana, Allender, & Mohan, 2017).

Previous research examined the availability of features included in diabetes apps for self-management. App features are app properties that relate to specific activities, e.g., logins, or interactive features like games. The most prevalent features offered on the app market for diabetes in the United Kingdom in 2014 were insulin and medication recording, data export and communication, diet recording, and weight management (Statista, 2014). In a study by Conway, Campbell, Forbes, Cunningham, and Wake (2016) diabetes app features included data storage/graphics, exercise tracking, health/diet, reminders/alarms, and education. Demidowich, Lu, Tamler, and Bloomgarden (2012) examined 42 Android diabetes apps. They found that 86% of the apps included BG recording, while medication tracking was part of 45% of the apps, and insulin dose calculators of 26% of the apps. Approximately half of the analyzed apps were not free-to-download, with an average price of 2.86 USD. Drincic, Prahalad,

---

[1] There are diabetes management apps targeting health professionals (Arnhold, Quade, & Kirch, 2014). However, these apps are not mainly for self-management by patients and are therefore not focused on here.

Greenwood, and Klonoff (2016) introduced a review of commercially available diabetes applications for self-management that were approved by an official source or had proven to be effective in previous research. They found that these diabetes apps included either insulin dose calculators for insulin management, automated feedback on blood glucose analysis, and/or data sharing (e.g., with HCPs or private social networks). Similarly, later on Veazie et al. (2018) published that common diabetes app features included reminders, BG and hemoglobin (HbA1c) tracking, medication use, physical activity, and weight management.

Overall, the majority of studies show very similar feature results. Diabetes apps include a variety of features similar to the functions mentioned by Danaher et al. (2015), like chat functions, notifications, picture recording, sensor connectivity, diary functions, etc.

In a few studies, some diabetes apps showed the option to be connected to external devices like sensors or blood glucose meters (Heintzman, 2016), or used cloud-based systems for health data storage and data exchange (Beckman et al., 2016). Heintzman (2016) "describes 'connected' technologies – such as smartphone apps, and wearable devices and sensors – which comprise part of a new digital ecosystem of data-driven tools that can link patients and their care teams for precision management of diabetes" (p. 35). These technologies combine sources of physiologic, behavioral, and contextual data that can be integrated and analyzed in cloud-based online systems (Heintzman, 2016). He further describes a vision of ideal app-supported self-management that includes a variety of opportunities:

> One can readily envision precision diabetes management driven by robust data collection, synthesis, and analysis (retrospective and real-time), with context-aware individualized guidance presented to the patient and caregivers in a coordinated fashion. A person with diabetes may receive personalized meal and insulin recommendations as in the aforementioned scenario. Furthermore, her spouse may be automatically notified several hours later that her postprandial glycemia was in-range, and may send her a congratulatory text message. In addition, her endocrinologist may receive regular reports including her detailed diet and exercise information alongside all of her diabetes device data, accom-

>panied by a narrative of patterns identified in the data by specialized analytics
>as well as algorithm-based suggestions for changes to her treatment regimen to
>optimize her glucose control – without waiting months for an in-person visit at
>the clinic. All the while, the person with diabetes may elect to have her data
>anonymized and made available to researchers developing the next generation
>of personalized closed-loop AP technologies and other precision medicine in-
>novations leveraging unprecedented, massively parallel n-of-1 data sets.
>(Heintzman, 2016, p. 38)

As shown in both the published features and the definition of self-management in
Chapter 2.2, diabetes app features can support all behaviors included in self-
management activities, like blood sugar monitoring, diet, or exercise with respective
mobile app interfaces, as well as psychological self-management aspects like motivating the patient, and social influence aspects by connecting the user to HCPs and other
user groups.

Regarding the mentioned app features in published studies in the context of self-
management and social influence, the literature mentions both features for self-
management behaviors (diary functions, insulin and medication recording, graphic
analysis, dietary features, automated notifications, etc.) and features for social influence by others (chat functions, data sharing with HCPs, etc.) (e.g., Drincic et al.,
2016). While self-management features are used by the patient user him-/herself, social influence features connect the user to HCPs or other individuals to receive feedback for their own patient disease management[2]. An increasing discussion of social
influence has been noted in mHealth reviews (Chib & Lin, 2018).

It is necessary to distinguish diabetes apps that mainly focus on independent self-
management of the patient from apps that focus on self-management supported by
others (HCP feedback, app inclusion in diabetes programs, etc.) in order to understand
if diabetes apps are effective tools if social influence features are missing, or if social
influence is a necessary requirement for diabetes apps to be effective. None of the

---

[2] Automated feedback falls into the first category with no other individuals needed to provide feedback, but
feedback provided by the system instead, based on data input of the user (thus no social influence).

published studies distinguished between self-management features and social influence features in diabetes apps, and further research is needed into this direction (therefore, Study 1 addresses this aspect, see Chapter 12).

This also at least partly relates to the question of intrinsic and extrinsic motivation for the use of diabetes apps for self-management as elaborated in Chapter 2.3. Social influence features especially support aspects of extrinsic motivation, and an absence of features that relate an app to the HCP-patient relationship might require higher intrinsic motivation in the diabetes patient to use diabetes apps effectively for self-management.

Moreover, apart from looking into app features, diabetes app reviews hardly summarize types of diabetes apps for self-management (e.g., Kao, Chuang, & Chen, 2017, discuss types of health-related apps). Types of apps are broader app categories with apps differing in their purpose and contents (e.g., a fitness app, or a blood glucose diary app). Thus, it is unclear which types of diabetes apps are available for which self-management aspects (self-management in Chapter 2.2, types of diabetes apps are addressed in Study 1). One reason for a lack of a diabetes app typology might be the diversity of apps for diabetes self-management in the high number of diabetes apps available in app stores (Arnhold et al., 2014; Research2guidance, 2014b). Research2guidance provide diabetes app market reports (Research2guidance, 2014b, 2016). In 2014, they reported that there were already more than 1.100 iOS and Android apps on the Apple App Store and Google Play that were specifically designed for diabetes patients (and healthcare professionals) to treat diabetes. The large and ever-growing number of apps for people with diabetes makes an overview over these apps difficult, as well as determining the best app choices (American Association of Diabetes Educators, 2016).

3.3   Shortcomings of Diabetes Apps and Diabetes App Quality

Arnhold et al. (2014) found that the majority of diabetes apps offered similar functionalities and combined only one to two functions in one app. According to them "an application that simultaneously informs and contributes to successful treatment by combining documentation, reminder, and advisory functions was not available" (Arn-hold et al., 2014, p. 9). Similarly, Brzan, Rotman, Pajnkihar, and Klanjsek (2016) found in a review of 65 diabetes management apps that the apps included only few features and concluded that apps with a higher range of features were needed to attract long-term users.

Calculated (composite) usability scores for the apps in Demidowich et al. (2012) were found to show an average score of 11.3 out of 30. Thus, the mean composite usability was relatively low in the apps. Fu et al. (2017) point towards major usability problems in diabetes apps, and low satisfaction ratings. The authors suggest improving user satisfaction, by using behavior change principles as a foundation, and matching apps with user characteristics.

Apart from usability, J. A. Rodriguez and Singh (2018) examined the availability of diabetes apps for vulnerable target groups, investigating diabetes apps for Latinos with low literacy. Their results indicate that only 30% of 92 diabetes apps had app store descriptions in Spanish. Readability levels were above the recommended reading level for health education material. Overall, examined diabetes apps did not cater to the needs of low literacy diabetes patients (J. A. Rodriguez & Singh, 2018). Thus, apart from limited features, there is insufficient targeting of specific diabetes groups.

El-Gayar et al. (2013) report that further "limitations of the applications include lack of personalized feedback; usability issues, particularly the ease of data entry; and integration with patients['] and electronic health records" (p. 247). Årsand et al. (2012) analyzed ten diabetes apps to learn about effective app design. They concluded that app features enabling automatic data transfer, visual and motivational interfaces, low effort opportunities, dynamic usage possibilities including direct contact with the HCP, long-term perspectives, and context sensitive apps were needed.

Diabetes App Quality

Related to these studies, a question increasingly gaining relevance is the question about the quality of diabetes apps, or of health apps in general. Moustakis, Litos, Dalivigas, and Tsironis (2004) describe website quality as customer satisfaction and the level of accomplishment of user expectations (perceptions). Further they state that website quality relates to the criteria *content, navigation, design* and *structure, appearance* and *multimedia,* and *uniqueness.*

Knowledge about health app quality is relevant to evaluate diabetes apps for self-management, as well as to have an explanation for usage numbers. Low usage numbers can point towards insufficient app quality. No study could be found that specifically investigated a relation between app quality and app usage outcomes. However, there are studies examining the role of app or web quality for aspects of usage. Inukollu, Keshamon, Kang, and Inukollu (2014) report that more than a fifth of app users were found to use an app only once after download. They state that "this number denotes that there is an immediate need to amend the quality and the functions provided by the app. If the app is being used only once, then the app betokens that it is not engendering or integrating any value to the user" (p. 20). In a different context, Dutta, Pfister, and Kosmoski (2010) examined the relevance of quality perceptions on attitudes and intentions to use online health-related content, finding that quality plays a crucial role in determining both. Khalid, Shihab, Nagappan, and Hassan (2015) looked into quality perceptions of users by analyzing user complaints about mobile apps, taken from online user reviews on 20 iOS apps. They report that most complaints related to functional errors, crashing apps, and lack of features. Furthermore, they found that in particular privacy issues as well as hidden costs affected user ratings in a negative way.

Studies specifically on the quality of diabetes apps for self-management are still rare, but are increasingly gaining relevance. Health app quality has been investigated in a large number of studies (Bohme, von Osthoff, Frey, & Hubner, 2018; Guo et al., 2017; Kamel Boulos, Brewer, Karimkhani, Buller, & Dellavalle, 2014; Loy, Ali, & Yap, 2016; McMillan, Hickey, Patel, & Mitchell, 2016; Schoeppe et al., 2017), with few specifically focusing on diabetes app quality (Basilico, Marceglia, Bonacina, & Pinciroli, 2016; Chavez et al., 2017; Hoppe, Cade, & Carter, 2017; Ye, Khan, Boren, Simoes, & Kim, 2018). In most papers, a diabetes app quality assessment is part of more general diabetes app reviews (with some exceptions).

Chavez et al. (2017) assessed whether diabetes apps are of sufficient quality to complement diabetes care. They used the Mobile App Rating Scale (MARS) developed by

Hides et al. (2014) to evaluate the quality of 89 popular free-to-download apps for T2DM management. Hides et al. (2014) and Stoyanov et al. (2015) assessed app quality using criteria on entertainment and interactivity delivered by an app (engagement), app functionality, app aesthetics, app information quality, and subjective quality as estimated by the user. A score on the number of diabetes management tasks included in each app was added by Chavez et al. (2017). They found that the 89 diabetes apps rated relatively high for functionality, aesthetics, and engagement, and suboptimal for information, subjective quality, and the overall quality. Moreover, only four apps integrated all six diabetes management tasks (physical activity, nutrition, blood glucose testing, medication or insulin dosage, health feedback, and education), and less than half integrated at least four tasks (Chavez et al., 2017). Similarly, Basilico et al. (2016) reviewed apps for diabetes self-care regarding quality and concluded that advanced features were implemented in only a small percentage of apps. Brzan et al. (2016) tested and evaluated 65 diabetes management apps and concluded that 56 apps did not meet minimal requirements or did not work properly. Only nine apps were evaluated as useful for self-management based on selected criteria.

Looking for an explanation for weak app quality, the consideration of behavior change theory or theory on diabetes management in diabetes app design and the app development might serve as a starting point. A diabetes app review (Italian market) by Rossi and Bigi (2017) summarized that the apps "do not seem to be based on solid theoretical models of behavior change or decision-making, and do not seem to be intended as devices to be integrated in the ecology of the doctor-patient relationship" (p. 1). Furthermore, the authors report that the studied apps displayed weak educational components. Ye, Khan, et al. (2018) assessed diabetes app quality in 173 apps by comparing app features with the AADE7 diabetes management guidelines published by the American Association of Diabetes Educators (2017). They found that the majority of apps supported healthy eating, monitoring, taking medication, and being active, while very few apps supported problem solving, healthy coping, and reducing risks as part of overall self-management. Thus, AADE guidelines were insufficiently considered in diabetes apps and their design. Similarly, Hoppe et al. (2017) found that examined diabetes apps included few functions or behavior change techniques, and that apps with optimum behavior change techniques were of higher quality.

Overall, the studies found lack of quality in many diabetes apps, both regarding their development along behavior change and self-management theory and the features provided. Additionally, challenges like the quantity of available diabetes apps make it tough to identify apps of high quality (American Association of Diabetes Educators, 2016). In conclusion, good health app quality assessment is of high relevance for both users and distributors of health apps (like HCPs recommending apps).

The Quality of Diabetes App Quality Assessment Tools

Looking into the quality of app quality assessment, Grundy, Wang, and Bero (2016) reviewed health app quality assessments and concluded that the majority of studies falsely claimed "to have performed an exhaustive, replicable, and systematic search and data extraction" due to "the nature of commercial app stores' search engines and personalized app content" (p. 1051). They found that most app assessments used "surrogate and one-dimensional outcome measures of app quality" (p. 1051). They point out that research on health app quality still has to be advanced due to the increasing relevance of health apps as a source for health guidance. Instead of quality assessments, outcome evaluations and evidence-based studies are partly more common (also compare Chapter 4.2.2). For example, with a user perception at the center of eHealth or mHealth quality, some studies looked into app quality by investigating user complaints (e.g., Khalid et al., 2015). However, outcome-oriented studies do not replace quality assessment research, but should rather complement it.

Despite health app quality having been operationalized in several publications previously (Bhattarai et al., 2018; Bohme et al., 2018; DiFilippo et al., 2017; Fiore, 2017; Grundy et al., 2016; Guo et al., 2017; Hides et al., 2014; Loy et al., 2016; Paglialonga et al., 2018; Singh et al., 2016; Stoyanov et al., 2015; Wyatt et al., 2015), systematically developed health app quality assessment tools that are generally applicable to all types of health apps are still rare, with many assessment tools specifically addressing certain types of health apps (e.g., K. Anderson, Burford, & Emmerton, 2016; DiFilippo et al., 2017; Guo et al., 2017).

To summarize, an app quality assessment is important, especially for users to distinguish high quality from low quality diabetes apps, as well as for HCPs and other providers to be able to deliver app recommendations based on app quality (Wyatt et al., 2015). For further overviews, Paglialonga et al. (2018) and Grundy et al. (2016) published overviews on methods for identifying apps, as well as for assessing app features and app quality. Moreover, the International Diabetes Federation published a comprehensive statement about diabetes apps for self-management in 2017 (Jacques Rose, Petrut, L'Heveder, & de Sabata, 2017).

After having given an insight into diabetes apps and their quality from previous research, the following chapter considers the usage aspect of diabetes apps for self-management, and previous studies examining app use and app use effects. From there, research gaps will be outlined.

4 Diabetes App Use – Previous mHealth Research

4.1 Defining Diabetes App "Use"

Studies on mHealth use usually provide an empirical operationalization of mHealth "use" (e.g., frequency or intensity of mHealth use in self-administered surveys), but do not provide a theoretical understanding of "use" (e.g., in Humble et al., 2016). There is hardly any definition of "use", assuming that "use" is inherently understandable. According to Wirth, von Pape, and Karnowski (2008), "numerous [mobile communication] studies have taken up the tradition of quantitative adoption research in explaining the adoption of new mobile technologies" (p. 594), and based on the Diffusion of Innovation Paradigm (Rogers, 2003). Diffusion research discusses "innovation attributes, adopter characteristics and their influence on the adoption decision" (Wirth et al., 2008, p. 594). Theories following a technology adoption paradigm mainly look at both the adoption (or acceptance) and the resulting use of technology (e.g., Technology Acceptance Model, Unified Theory of Acceptance and Use of Technology).

Within an adoption paradigm which is also followed here, "adoption" is understood as a binary concept of acceptance (adoption) or rejection (non-adoption) of (mobile) technology, resulting in the use or non-use of technological tools (Wirth et al., 2008). mHealth adoption refers to the starting of an mHealth use, and a resulting acceptance of it, which is the introduction of a user to new technology and his or her beginning to use the technology as part of patient care (Schoville, 2015). Thus, the acceptance of an mHealth tool and the beginning to use it are understood as adoption. Rejection is understood as the counterpart of adoption, and thus the non-adoption of the mHealth tool. In contrast to adoption, and as a result "(maintained) use" can be understood as the result of successful mHealth adoption, as active involvement with an mHealth tool over a certain period of time, replacing the original trial of an mHealth tool with the actual use. Maintained mHealth use is also called "stickiness" in some studies (Furner, Racherla, & Babb, 2016).

Electronic supplementary material The online version of this chapter (https://doi.org/10.1007/978-3-658-29357-4_4) contains supplementary material, which is available to authorized users.

However, maintained use can still be short-term or long-term, depending on the definition of "long-term". For example, a diabetes app can be successfully adopted and used for three weeks or for three years.

To summarize, technology "use" from the adoption perspective includes both the acceptance or adoption of technology and the actual maintained use of it. Thus in the following, diabetes app "use" is understood as the adoption of diabetes apps, as well as the actual maintained use of the apps.

In addition to this general definition of mHealth "use", the mHealth (app) use must be explained in more detail against the background of general diabetes self-management. In Chapter 2.2, it was explained that diabetes self-management includes behaviors that a patient executes as a part of his/her own active management of a disease, in addition to psychological aspects and social influence/support by other individuals. Traditional self-management behaviors include for example blood sugar testing, carb counting, etc. (see Chapter 2.2). These traditional self-management practices can be complemented with technology-supported behaviors such as the use of diabetes self-management apps. Therefore, diabetes app use has to be understood as a "self-management behavior" in the same way as other (traditional and non-technology-supported) behaviors are understood as part of diabetes self-management.

To summarize, diabetes app use is a technology-supported self-management behavior (because "use" is a behavior), that can complement other traditional self-management behaviors executed in the overall diabetes self-management.

In the following, research on diabetes app use is examined further.

4.2   Categorizing Studies on Diabetes App Use: The Inputs-Mechanisms-Outputs
      Pathway

Previous studies on diabetes app use mainly focused on preconditions for the app adoption and use, the use itself, or usage outcomes. Chib, van Velthoven, and Car (2015) propose an *inputs-mechanisms-outputs* heuristic as a tool to categorize mHealth studies. In relation to previous mHealth research on (diabetes) app use and usage effects, this inputs-mechanisms-outputs pathway is useful to categorize previous studies and literature reviews to get an overview of existing research, and to outline research gaps (also see Brew-Sam & Chib, 2020). In the following, the meaning of "input", "mechanisms", and "output" is briefly explained. All three areas are then substantiated in more detail by means of mHealth studies. The studies were selected as examples using a non-systematic search in order to illustrate the state of research in the three areas related to diabetes self-management. The inputs-mechanisms-outputs pathway was specifically applied to mHealth research on diabetes apps for self-management, and to mHealth (app) research in general where no diabetes-specific research was available.

Following Chib et al. (2015), the category "input" summarizes studies on requirements for mHealth implementation, including technology access and use, as well as feasibility studies (in terms of satisfaction, response rates, data accuracy and error rates, or setup costs). These studies (which are available in large numbers on almost all mHealth topics) are usually the first step in understanding a new technology and its use. In most cases, these studies are limited to descriptive analyses.

"Mechanism" studies go one step further and investigate "the reasons for technology adoption, using theoretical models for explanation or validation of the findings" (Chib et al., 2015, p. 7). Here, theory is used to explain aspects of mHealth adoption and use: "Mechanism factors such as psychosocial influences and individual preferences offer explanatory value to understand technology adoption" (Chib et al., 2015, p. 5). Processes and mechanisms are focused on, and dependencies of adoption/use on other factors are investigated.

Finally, "output" summarizes research on mHealth effectiveness (effect studies), like improved patient health outputs and other patient outcomes (e.g., behavior change) deriving from mHealth use, as well as mHealth efficiency such as healthcare process improvements (Chib et al., 2015).

Chib et al. (2015) summarize that the previous published research especially produced mHealth studies focusing on the category "input", while studies on "output" are available but fewer in numbers. In contrast, "mechanisms" of adoption and appropriation of mHealth technology are still underinvestigated and less well understood, despite their importance as evidence for implementation and effectiveness.

4.2.1   Input: Feasibility and Accessibility Studies

With new technology entering the market, the first studies and study reviews tend to look at the respective new mHealth technology in terms of (1) the access to this technology and accessibility, (2) the feasibility and usability of the technology, and the usage potential, as well as (3) the actual usage in descriptive analyses. These descriptive analyses usually precede an examination of "outputs". Overlaps between an investigation of aspects of technology access, feasibility, usability, and actual usage occur, with research studying one of these aspects frequently looking into another as well (e.g. examining access and usability in parallel).

(1) Studies on diabetes app access and accessibility:

Previous studies on diabetes apps looked into *accessibility* and diabetes app *access* by specific target groups (Arnhold et al., 2014; Isaković, Sedlar, Volk, & Bešter, 2016; St George, Delamater, Pulgaron, Daigre, & Sanchez, 2016), as well as accessibility problems caused by the high number of diabetes apps available, including recommendations for selection (Basilico et al., 2016).

St. George et al. (2016) looked into access to and interest in diabetes apps by 50 Hispanic T1DM adolescents. Despite general access to smartphones and most participants expressing high or moderate interest in diabetes apps, only 37% reported using diabetes apps. Digital divide discussions are still part of the literature on access to diabetes apps, for example with older people and people without internet access being excluded from its use, or experiencing high barriers to digital app use (access and usage barriers in older people or vulnerable populations, e.g., Hoque & Sorwar, 2017; Humble et al., 2016; Isaković et al., 2016; Scheibe, Reichelt, Bellmann, & Kirch, 2015; Ye, Boren, Khan, Simoes, & Kim, 2018).

Access to diabetes apps also includes the question of access to apps in commercial app stores as well as the challenge for diabetes patients to select appropriate products, given the plethora of apps available in online stores with no indicators of their quality (other than download figures) (Basilico et al., 2016). Previous studies showed that users searching for apps tend to pick the apps shown in the top positions in the app stores instead of comprehensively comparing them (Dogruel, Joeckel, & Bowman,

2015). Dogruel et al. (2015) conducted an exploratory study on decision-making heuristics for smartphone app selection, and found the following results:

> The current study identified five decision-making heuristics used to download a variety of smartphone apps. Of these, four were variants of a "Take the First" (TtF) heuristic that allowed smartphone users to quickly navigate the app market, by passing a good deal of other informational cues in order to download apps that were simply highly rated or ranked. (Dogruel et al., 2015, p. 125)

Their study showed that users hardly went further than the fifth displayed app in the Google Play Store (top five) for a variety of selected apps (Dogruel et al., 2015). Their study suggests that apps in lower store ranks are not downloaded by users, cannot be found easily, or show low usage and rating numbers. Identifying the problem of app selection, Basilico et al. (2016) suggest a tool that helps diabetes patients to better select an appropriate app for diabetes self-management.

(2) Diabetes app feasibility and usability studies:

Apart from access to diabetes apps, studies examined the feasibility and usability of apps for diabetes self-management (Burner et al., 2018; Fu et al., 2017; Georgsson & Staggers, 2016; Ho, 2015; Isaković et al., 2016; Mayberry, Berg, Harper, & Osborn, 2016; Zapata, Fernandez-Aleman, Idri, & Toval, 2015) or gave overviews of the potential of diabetes app use for self-management (El-Gayar et al., 2013; Eng & Lee, 2013; Heintzman, 2016; Kao et al., 2017).

The usability of diabetes apps is partly measured using usability scores or similar instruments to describe the usability of an app, or to compare the usability of several apps, as for example found in Veazie et al. (2018), or Demidovich et al. (2012). A usability assessment is mostly part of a larger diabetes app quality assessment, as already outlined in Chapter 3. Results on app usability vary largely, depending on the instruments and diabetes apps included in the respective study. Some results on usability have already been presented in Chapter 3.3.

Feasibility studies looking into diabetes apps can be also found in terms of feasibility trials (sometimes randomized controlled feasibility trials). Burner et al. (2018) for example conducted a randomized controlled feasibility trial with diabetes patients in emergency departments to analyze the feasibility of a diabetes mHealth intervention including social support by family and friends. They found that their mHealth program was feasible and acceptable for diabetes care, and promising in terms of improving social support and diabetes outcomes.

Despite some shortcomings regarding diabetes app quality (including usability), in principle, the potential of diabetes apps for self-management is considered high in the literature, due to the possibilities and advantages the diabetes apps can deliver for self-management. Benefits include for example direct and instant contact to HCPs and peer patients through diabetes apps, interactive feedback options, improved self-monitoring possibilities (with independence of location and time), automated data processing (including graphs and notifications etc.), cloud-based interactive systems, and other possibilities related to mobile online diabetes technology. In their review on both diabetes apps for self-management and research articles, El-Gayar et al. (2013) reported the potential of diabetes apps for having positive impacts on diabetes self-management: "Analysis indicates that application usage is associated with improved attitudes favorable to diabetes self-management" (El-Gayar et al., 2013, abstract).

(3) Studies on diabetes app use:

Other studies descriptively investigated diabetes app use, including usage statistics, as well as barriers to adoption and use, perceptions, experiences, etc. (Georgsson & Staggers, 2017; V. Ramirez et al., 2016; Schreier et al., 2012). Despite the potential attributed to diabetes apps in the literature, the use of apps for diabetes self-management is still relatively low, as only 1.2% of owners of smartphones suffering from diabetes used a diabetes app in 2013, with an expected increase to 7.8% worldwide by 2018 (Research2guidance, 2014a). "The ... usage of diabetes apps within the target group is low" (Research2guidance, 2014a).

In addition to usage numbers, user experiences and perceptions are part of app usage studies. Georgsson and Staggers (2017) for example conducted a study on experiences and perceptions of an mHealth diabetes self-management system (Care4Life), with a patient sample that had participated in a previous 6-month randomized controlled trial, and found that diabetes patients reported perceived benefits in using the mHealth system. However, perceptions were highly individual despite a reported homogeneity of the sample.

Nørgaard et al. (2017) analyzed the awareness and use of the diabetes app "Pregnant with Diabetes", using a survey with 139 women with diabetes in Denmark on their perceptions and experiences. Additionally, the researchers collected national and international download numbers for the app, and found that the app had been downloaded over 4000 times in Denmark and oder 27000 times in 183 countries. Based on these data, they concluded that information accessible through diabetes apps has the potential to reach target groups, that diabetes apps are used and are able to reach patients, and that the apps may contribute to improved health outcomes.

In another study, V. Ramirez et al. (2016) assessed the interest in and use of mHealth technology among a culturally diverse patient sample with chronic diseases. They could show that patients used mobile technology, independently of socioeconomic status. Moreover, overall interest in mHealth technology for the management of chronic conditions was high.

To conclude, despite partly low usage numbers and findings on poor app quality, generally the potential of diabetes apps is estimated as high in literature, with usability and feasibility mostly being reported as acceptable or good. However, there are some limitations regarding target groups with limited access to diabetes apps (e.g., older people[3]), limited usability, and/or perceived limited potential of diabetes apps.

Additional research is still needed that looks into user-centered and sociotechnical design principles to improve usability, perceived usefulness, and, ultimately, adoption of the mobile health technology (El-Gayar et al., 2013). The own study aim described in Chapters 9 to 11 pays attention to these aspects.

4.2.2   Output: Diabetes App Usage Effect Studies

Apart from feasibility and accessibility studies, a good number of mHealth effects studies can be found on both text message interventions and health app use (Zhao,

---

[3] It was refrained from using the term *elderly* throughout the thesis to avoid stereotyping. The term elderly is inappropriate and "ageist" as shown by Avers, Brown, Chui, Wong, and Lusardi (2011).

Freeman, & Li, 2016), with some available studies looking into the effects of diabetes app use for self-management.

Table 16 in the Appendix delivers an overview of a search for a variety of diabetes app usage effect studies, including their design and their main results. The majority of the studies reported either no significant improvements in health behaviors or health outcomes after the diabetes app use, or significant improvements with very small effect sizes. Previous mHealth reviews concluded similar results (despite the mentioned difference between health app use that is not necessarily part of an intervention and first generation mHealth interventions, e.g., text message-based). Buhi et al. (2013) report that only six out of 17 studies published statistically significant improvements in blood glucose concentrations in mHealth solutions for diabetes management. Free et al. (2013) summarize in a meta-analysis that "to date, mobile technology-based interventions... that have statistically significant effects are small and of borderline clinical importance" (p. 25).

Some studies found that the use of diabetes apps delivered visible effects for improved health outcomes only when there was additional HCP support. Veazie et al. (2018) reported limited evidence for the use of diabetes apps resulting in short-term health improvements when there was additional HCP support. In a randomized controlled trial, Torbjornsen et al. (2014) did not find significant HbA1c differences between diabetes patients with and without additional health counseling by a nurse after using a diabetes app (few touch application) for four months. However, health service navigation significantly differed in groups with app usage from the ones without app use after four months, with diabetes patients using apps significantly showing better scores. The app users with additional HCP support (health counseling by the nurse) showed significantly higher scores than both the control group (without app use) and the group with app use only (also after adjusting for confounders). This confirms the relevance of social influence in the usage of diabetes apps for self-management. Moreover, this also justifies the importance of both self-management and social influence features in diabetes apps (Chapter 3.2), and the need for an examination of both. Overall, in contrast to some technology-deterministic and optimistic study results on health app use (for diabetes, e.g., Wu et al., 2017), the current trend in reviews on both mHealth intervention effects and intervention-independent health app usage effects includes a more critical view of mHealth effectiveness (Buhi et al., 2013; Chib et al., 2015; Free et al., 2013; Fu et al., 2017; K. R. Jones, Lekhak, & Kaewluang, 2014).

When trying to explain the limited effects of mHealth use, previous studies hint at the general lack of theory in the context of mHealth (app) research (Middelweerd, Mollee, van der Wal, Brug, & te Velde, 2014). Apart from technology adoption theories, there are only few theories applied to mHealth, mainly comprising traditional behavior change theories (K. R. Jones et al., 2014). Free et al. (2013), for example, found that out of 26 mHealth studies, seven used theories as explanatory frameworks. These include different behavior change theories, including Social Cognitive and Learning Theory, Elaboration Likelihood Theory, Protection Motivation Theory, and the Transtheoretical Model (Free et al., 2013, p. 23). The majority of diabetes app effect studies listed in Table 16 in the Appendix reported no theoretical foundation used in the app development or the study design.

Generally, the field of mHealth has been criticized for the lack of a robust theoretical foundation (Free et al., 2013; K. R. Jones et al., 2014; Riley et al., 2011). According to Riley et al. (2011) theory can give mHealth a stronger basis and improve its effectiveness. This is because the use of a theoretical foundation can result in mHealth "that address[es] more comprehensively the potential mechanisms of behavior change" (Riley et al., 2011, p. 66). A theoretical foundation is needed to inform mHealth (app) study design, and practical mHealth implementation to increase effectiveness (Riley et al., 2011). This also could be shown in relation to app quality in Chapter 3.3. "Future research should study how behavior change techniques can be translated into apps. Additionally, future research should examine the effectiveness of apps and which behavior change techniques or combinations of techniques are more effective" (Middelweerd et al., 2014, discussion).

Specifically for diabetes apps for self-management, with studies showing the relevance of social influence to diabetes self-management (Chapter 2.3) and for diabetes app use (Chapter 3.2 on diabetes apps), theory is needed that accounts for the duality of patient-led self-management (also including psychological aspects) and social influence by others.

4.2.3   Mechanisms: Lacking Research on Antecedents of Health App Use

As already mentioned in the overview on the inputs-mechanisms-outputs pathway at the beginning of Chapter 4, underlying factors and *mechanisms* accounting for mHealth technology adoption, use, and usage outputs have been investigated less than mHealth *input* and *output* (Chib et al., 2015; Danaher et al., 2015). Especially in the context of chronic disease self-management, research on underlying mechanisms of mHealth (app) use is still hard to find (Azhar & Dhillon, 2016; Zhu, Liu, Che, & Chen, 2017). Yet research focusing on underlying mechanisms and processes is crucial to be able to explain usage outputs (Black Box approach, Danaher et al., 2015).

> Without an understanding of what structured process (if any) guided the… approach… it is difficult if not impossible to compare more successful programs with less successful programs, understand why various programs had different impacts on different outcomes, or replicate the more successful programs. Such a lack results in a "Black Box" problem, in which the necessary and sufficient mechanisms of change are unknown and therefore difficult to optimize. (R. M. Anderson et al., 2009, p. 2)

As part of understanding underlying mechanisms of diabetes app use, it is relevant to look at research on anteceding factors that influence app adoption and usage processes. Understanding antecedents of diabetes app use contributes to mHealth research collecting knowledge about mechanisms behind health app use. Theory is needed that is able to provide a foundation for studying anteceding factors of diabetes app use in relation to diabetes self-management influenced by HCPs and other individuals.

The following chapters go into further detail regarding these aspects. Chapter 5.1 first defines the term "antecedent" in the context of mHealth adoption and usage, and explains why it is relevant to investigate antecedents of diabetes app use (Chapter 5.2). Chapter 5.3 introduces previous research on antecedents of diabetes app use, as well as related research, before empowerment is introduced as a theoretical approach addressing the gaps in previous mHealth research that relate to an understanding of antecedents of mHealth use for self-management.

5 Anteceding Factors of Diabetes App Use

5.1 Defining "Antecedents" of mHealth Use

With increased knowledge of antecedents of mHealth use (including diabetes apps), processes behind mHealth adoption and use can be understood in greater detail. In this context, the term "antecedent" describes factors influencing mHealth adoption and use. While Lin (2011), Rai, Chen, Pye, and Baird (2013), and Deng (2013) use the term "determinants" in the context of mHealth adoption, others speak of "antecedents" of technology adoption and use (Agarwal & Prasad, 1998; M.-C. Hu, 2012; Odoom, Anning-Dorson, & Acheampong, 2017; Venkatesh & Davis, 1996; Venkatesh et al., 2003), to refer to similar types of influencing variables. Other studies simply speak of influencing factors (Azhar & Dhillon, 2016), or use "determinant" and "antecedent" synonymously (Venkatesh & Davis, 1996). Previous mHealth and technology adoption and usage research is vague about the difference between the two terms. Clarification is needed of which factors are antecedents of technology adoption and use, and which are determinants, and which differences result from this duality. No paper could be found that explicitly explains the difference between the two terms. However, "determinant" and "antecedent" are not synonymous in their meaning. First, while the term "antecedent" includes a time dimension, the term "determinant" doesn't. L. F. Jones (2008) summarizes that "an antecedent variable is an independent variable that precedes other [independent] variables in time. An antecedent variable could affect the independent variable and alter its relationship to the dependent variable" (block 9, objective 4). Second, a variety of effects between independent and dependent variables can result from looking at an antecedent[4]. Literature on technology adoption theory following a technology adoption paradigm uses the term "antecedent" in relation to factors influencing technology use (e.g., Venkatesh et al., 2003).

---

[4] For example, if Z is the dependent variable, and Y is the independent variable, one might want to know what explains Y (L. F. Jones, 2008). The antecedent X might explain Y. Several possibilities result when the effect of X is examined. First, the relationship between Y and Z could remain the same. Second, the relationship between Y and Z could change. Third, "it is also possible that the antecedent variable affects both the independent variable and the dependent variable, with the original relationship disappearing" (L. F. Jones, 2008, bl. 9, obj. 4).

In contrast, a "determinant" is a causal or deciding factor, that (conclusively) causes an outcome. For example, personal, social, economic, and environmental factors influencing a health status are known as determinants of health (Lorant & Dauvrin, 2012; Office of Disease Prevention and Health Promotion, 2014). In this context determinants are not spoken of as antecedents. Yet, in an mHealth context the term "determinant" is not used here, because the term "determinant" first lacks the notion of time, and second it could be understood as a necessary cause of mHealth (app) adoption. In this understanding, successful mHealth adoption could not be achieved if determinants were not fulfilled. An antecedent of mHealth use is a factor preceding mHealth adoption and use, but less compelling than a determinant, with several outcomes in relationships possible[4]. Some preceding factors might not necessarily lead to adoption and use, and thus are not understood to be determining but rather anteceding factors. With processes (of mHealth use) being focused on here, a notion of time is relevant to the concepts as well, with something happening before and something happening after mHealth adoption. Thus, the term "antecedent" as used by Venkatesh et al. (2003) for technology adoption is used when referring to preceding factors potentially influencing diabetes app use for self-management.

5.2   The Relevance of Studies Looking into Antecedents of mHealth Use

The relevance of knowledge about antecedents for understanding diabetes app adoption and use processes can be demonstrated by looking into previous diabetes app use effect studies from an "outputs" perspective as described in Chapter 4.2.2. It can be argued that a lack of consulting theory on antecedents of diabetes app use when designing diabetes apps, might result in weak apps regarding their fit for the target users. For example, a diabetes app designed for a target user market with no experience in app use is unlikely to be adopted if experience as an antecedent is not considered when designing the app (e.g., by using a simple design for inexperienced users). A resulting lack of app adoption and usage due to an insufficiently designed diabetes app can then be reflected in effects studies not showing provable app effectiveness (compare Chapter 4.2.2 on effects studies). Unfortunately, in general it is rare that scientific foundation is considered when designing (diabetes) mHealth tools as shown before (compare Riley et al., 2011). Thus, it is not common to build diabetes apps based on knowledge about underlying processes and antecedents for successful usage. The missing consideration of antecedents and processes of adoption when designing diabetes apps might provide one potential explanation as to why the number of significant positive outcomes in diabetes app usage effect studies in comparison to non-significant effects or no effects is low, and not delivering convincing results on diabetes app use effectiveness (e.g., see Table 16 in Appendix, and Chapter 4.2.2). Effect studies based on weakly designed diabetes apps are less likely to show evidence for usage effects.

The lack of provable usage effects seems to be a common problem in mHealth research. Similar results on lacking or limited evidence on usage effects have previously been reported for both text-message interventions (Bloomfield et al., 2014; Free et al., 2013; Hall et al., 2015; K. R. Jones et al., 2014), and health apps in various mHealth usage effects study reviews, including diabetes (J. Baron, McBain, & Newman, 2012; El-Gayar et al., 2013; Fu et al., 2017; Kitsiou, Paré, Jaana, & Gerber, 2017; Wang, Xue, Huang, Huang, & Zhang, 2017). However, apart from pointing out study weaknesses (Wang et al., 2017), no research has comprehensively explained the lack of provable mHealth usage effects. It is argued here that lack of knowledge of antecedents of mHealth use might provide an additional explanation for lacking provable mHealth effectiveness. K. R. Jones et al. (2014) state that "many variables of interest are never identified, collected, and analyzed in the studies of mobile phone technology" (p. 85). A comprehensive and systematic understanding of antecedents of mHealth (app) use is therefore necessary.

5.3   Previous Studies Looking into Antecedents of mHealth Use

Few mHealth studies have considered anteceding factors of mHealth use as well as the theoretical background for adoption mechanisms to solve the black box problem behind mHealth use (Danaher et al., 2015). A small number of studies paid particular attention to anteceding factors of mHealth (app) use in the context of (chronic) disease self-management.

Based on the Technology Acceptance Model, Zhu et al. (2017) conducted a survey with 279 potential mobile chronic disease management system users in China, and found that perceived usefulness, perceived ease of use, perceived disease threat, and initial trust had a positive impact on the mHealth adoption intention, while the impact of perceived risk was negative. Technology anxiety had a negative impact on perceived ease of use. Furthermore, they found that there were age differences in perceptions, as well as differences between family members and chronically ill participants. Azhar and Dhillon (2016) systematically reviewed factors influencing mHealth app use for self-care from existing studies, and identified 68 factors related to app use for self-care. The most frequently cited factors were perceived usefulness, perceived ease of use, behavioral intention, social influence, self-efficacy, perceived privacy risk and attitude.

Apart from specific research on factors influencing app use for (chronic) disease self-management, there is more general research available examining underlying factors and processes of health app adoption and use (Woldeyohannes & Ngwenyama, 2017), as well as of mHealth adoption and use not only looking into health apps (Deng, 2013; Dwivedi, Shareef, Simintiras, Lal, & Weerakkody, 2016; Hoque & Sorwar, 2017; Lin, 2011; Rai et al., 2013). Moreover, there is a broad research field on antecedents of technology adoption and use (Agarwal & Prasad, 1998).

5.4   Antecedents of the Unified Theory of Acceptance and Use of Technology

Most studies of antecedents of the mHealth (app) use (Chapter 5.3) follow a classic technology adoption paradigm (in contrast to an appropriation paradigm, Wirth et al., 2008). This paradigm is generally dominant in mHealth research, as explained in Chapter 4.1 on the definition of mHealth "use". Within the technology adoption paradigm most studies are based on a limited number of theories that display factors influencing technology adoption and use. One of the most recent and most comprehensive technology adoption theories, used as a foundation for many mHealth studies (e.g., the studies in Chapter 5.3) and considering antecedents of mHealth use, is the Unified Theory of Acceptance and Use of Technology (UTAUT) developed by Venkatesh et al. (2003). The UTAUT is a validated and recognized model which provides a theoretical foundation for explaining technology use. It is based on eight previous theoretical models (J. Lee & Rho, 2013), including the Theory of Reasoned Action (TRA), Technology Acceptance Model (TAM), the Motivational Model (MM), the Theory of Planned Behavior (TPB), combined TAM and TPB, the Model of PC Utilization (MPCU), the Innovation Diffusion Theory (IDT), and Social Cognitive Theory (SCT). Thus, the UTAUT integrates "the fragmented theory and research on individual acceptance of information technology into a unified theoretical model that captures the essential elements of eight previously established models" (Venkatesh et al., 2003, p. 467). As a summary of the previous models, the UTAUT theorizes that the four factors performance expectancy, effort expectancy, social influence, and facilitating conditions are direct determinants of user acceptance and usage behaviors (Figure 1). Usage is understood as the dependent variable, and usage intention is used as a predictor of the actual usage behavior (Venkatesh et al., 2003). Performance expectancy is the degree to which an individual believes that using the technology will help attaining gains in behavioral performance. It influences the intention to use technology, similarly to the effort expectancy which is the perceived degree of ease of use of the technology. The intention to use technology is moreover influenced by social influence defined as the degree to which the individual perceives that important others believe he/she should use the technology. Facilitating conditions – as the degree to which the individual believes that an infrastructure exists to support the use of the technology – are theorized to be direct antecedents of usage behaviors instead of influencing an intention to use the technology only (Venkatesh et al., 2003). Moreover, the UTAUT theorizes that gender, age, experience with the new technology, and voluntariness (the degree to which the technology use is perceived as being of free will) are key moderating variables of the relationships between the influencing factors and acceptance and use of the technology (Venkatesh et al., 2003) (Figure 1).

Table 2 summarizes all factors mentioned by the UTAUT as influencing factors of technology adoption and use.

Translated from definitions by Venkatesh et al. (2003) for diabetes app use, performance expectancy is the degree to which the diabetes patient believes that using diabetes apps for self-management will help him/her to attain gains in self-management. According to the authors, this relates to perceived usefulness of an app, extrinsic motivation for its use, advantage from using the app, and outcome expectation from the app use. Effort expectancy is the degree of ease associated with the use of diabetes apps. This includes the perceived ease of use, the actual ease of use, and the complexity of usage. Social influence is the degree to which an individual perceives that others believe he or she should use the app for diabetes management. According to the authors, subjective norm, social factors, and image relate to social influence. Facilitating conditions is the degree to which the diabetes patient believes that an organizational and technical infrastructure exists to support the use of an app for self-management (e.g., inclusion in a diabetes care program). This includes perceived behavioral control and (technological) compatibility. The moderating variable experience refers to experience with a new technology (user experience), while voluntariness is described as the degree to which use of a diabetes app is perceived as being voluntary.

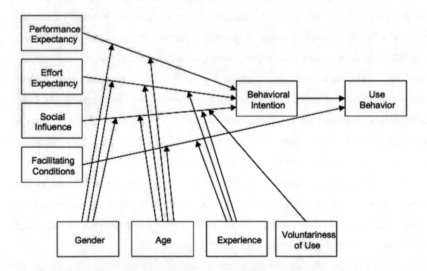

Figure 1. The Unified Theory of Acceptance and Use of Technology by Venkatesh et al. (2003).

Table 2. Factors Influencing Technology Use from the Unified Theory of Acceptance and Use of Technology

Factor	Explanation/definition	Original factors from previous models (root constructs)	Examples
Performance expectancy	Defined as the degree to which an individual believes that using the system will help him or her to attain gains in job performance	The five constructs from the different models that pertain to performance expectancy are perceived usefulness (TAM/TAM2 and C-TAM-TPB), extrinsic motivation (MM), job-fit (MPCU), relative advantage (IDT), and outcome expectations (SCT).	Productivity, usefulness in job
Effort expectancy	Defined as the degree of ease associated with the use of the system.	Three constructs from the existing models capture the concept of effort expectancy: perceived ease of use (TAM/TAM2), complexity (MPCU), and ease of use (IDT).	Ease of use
Social influence	Defined as the degree to which an individual perceives that important others believe he or she should use the new system.	The three constructs related to social influence: subjective norm (TRA, TAM2, TPB/DTPB, and C-TAM-TPB), social factors (MPCU), and image (IDT).	Opinion of others on use
Facilitating conditions	Defined as the degree to which an individual believes that an organizational and technical infrastructure exists to support use of the system.	This definition captures concepts embodied by three different constructs: perceived behavioral control (TPB/DTPB, C-TAM-TPB), facilitating conditions (MPCU), and compatibility (IDT).	Resources, knowledge, etc.
Demographics	-	-	Age, gender, etc.
Experience	Experience with a new technology (user experience).	-	Previous technology usage experience
Voluntariness	"The degree to which use of the innovation is perceived as being voluntary, or of free will" (Moore and Benbasat 1991, p. 195).	-	Use is voluntary

Notes. Based on the UTAUT by Venkatesh et al. (2003); definitions of the constructs are taken from Venkatesh et al. (2003), with abbreviations as commonly used for the theories.

5.5   Shortcomings of the Unified Theory of Acceptance and Use

The UTAUT has been criticized for a number of limitations:

First, the UTAUT has been criticized for its innovation positivism in previous research (e.g., Bagozzi, 2007). The UTAUT only pays attention to adoption, but fails to include usage barriers explaining not just adoption but also rejection, and thus non-use. When investigating diabetes app use, it is necessary to understand rejection of apps and non-use as a counterpart of adoption and maintained use. Only in this way, a comprehensive understanding of processes behind diabetes app use can be achieved.

According to Cenfetelli (2004) "inhibiting perceptions can add to our understanding of the antecedents of usage or outright rejection" (p. 472). He adds that research doesn't consider inhibiting factors in a comprehensive way, and that theoretical models of usage partly lack these aspects. Although the UTAUT doesn't include technology rejection and non-use, these aspects can be found in the models the UTAUT is based on. As part of attitudinal beliefs, the Theory of Planned Behavior (TPB) includes an appraisal of both positive and negative aspects of a behavior, and thus also considers usage barriers to some extent (Ajzen, 1991). Similarly to TPB and in more detail, the Mobile Phone Appropriation Model, short MPA (Wirth et al., 2008), includes "restriction evaluations" for mobile phone appropriation, looking at financial, technical, temporal, and cognitive barriers towards mobile phone appropriation (also compare Rossmann et al., 2019). Following the MPA authors, the restriction evaluations concern technological compatibility (technical), complexity of technology (perceived as complicated, cognitive), cost (financial), and time-efficiency (time-consuming, temporal). Yet, the MPA doesn't follow an adoption paradigm but an appropriation paradigm instead, and thus is of limited use due to the differing underlying understanding of technology use. In contrast to the adoption paradigm building on innovation diffusion, the appropriation paradigm follows cultural studies and frame analysis (Wirth et al., 2008).

Second, following Al-Mamary, Al-Nashmi, Hassan, and Shamsuddin (2016), research has argued that included UTAUT factors might be insufficient predictors of technology acceptance and usage. As analyzed by Venkatesh et al. (2016) a number of studies have suggested UTAUT extensions, including new exogenous and endogenous mechanisms, new moderation mechanisms, and new outcome mechanisms. The UTAUT doesn't include individual factors that can help explain technology acceptance and use (Al-Mamary et al., 2016). User performance or individual impact could be added as an indicator for technology acceptance and usage (Al-Mamary et al., 2016). Moreover, other factors like information quality (e.g., app quality) or computer/technology self-efficacy are needed as factors (Al-Mamary et al., 2016). Venkatesh et al. (2003) excluded computer self-efficacy from the UTAUT, hypothesizing that computer self-efficacy had no significant influence on behavioral intention. This hypothesis was confirmed in their study, finding that self-efficacy, anxiety, and attitude did not have any direct effect on intention. However, looking at the actual behavior and not just at behavioral intention, other theories like the Social Cognitive Theory (Bandura, 1977, 2002) showed that self-efficacy is a relevant variable influencing behaviors. "Perceived self-efficacy affects every phase of personal change" (Bandura, 1997; 2002, p. 288). As a result, San Martín and Herrero (2012) suggest that future research should explore other relevant antecedents of technology acceptance and use. Following these authors, it is argued here that especially intrinsic and extrinsic motivational antecedents are lacking in the UTAUT when using the UTAUT to explain technology adoption and usage in a disease self-management context. In the process of the UTAUT development, Venkatesh et al. (2003) differentiate extrinsic from intrinsic motivation in the context of the information system domain. Previously, Davis, Bagozzi, and Warshaw (1992) investigated intrinsic and extrinsic motivational determinants for the intention to use computers in the workplace, and thus used the motivational model to explain technology use. Similarly, Venkatesh et al. (2003) distinguish extrinsic and intrinsic motivation as two factors, and as part of a list of factors predicting intention for technology use (see Tables 5 to 7 in Venkatesh et al., 2003). Venkatesh et al. (2003) previously argued that the seven factors extrinsic motivation, intrinsic motivation, attitude toward using technology, perceived usefulness, job-fit, relative advantage, and outcome expectations from eight previous models "appeared to be significant direct determinants of intention or usage in one or more of the individual models" (Venkatesh et al., 2003, p. 446). From there, the authors combined the seven factors into the four factors *performance expectancy*, *effort expectancy*, *social influence*, and *facilitating conditions* (for details see the UTAUT factors and original factors from other models in Table 2). As a result, extrinsic motivation was represented only as part of the factor *performance expectancy*, while intrinsic motivation was only represented as part of the factor *attitude* towards technology use (Brew-Sam & Chib, 2020; see Table 2). In the following, the authors excluded attitude to using technology from the UTAUT, as attitude to using technology did not have a significant influence on intention to use technology (supported hypothesis 5c in Venkatesh et al., 2003). This means that intrinsic motivation is not part of the final UTAUT, and extrinsic motivation is just part of the related construct performance expectancy in the UTAUT. Social influence could be considered an extrinsic motivational factor as well, but the UTAUT includes only *perceived* social influence and thus "primarily [targets]… at the individual level…, thereby precluding the impact of socially enriched environments" (Graf-Vlachy, Buhtz, & König, 2018, p. 37). To conclude, the UTAUT does not sufficiently include intrinsic and extrinsic motivational factors as influencing factors of the intention to adopt and to use technology[5]. The relevance of both intrinsic and extrinsic motivation for technology adoption and use has been emphasized by motivational approaches in previous research (like Davis et al., 1992). Moreover, in Chapter 2.3, it was shown that motivation is of high relevance for disease self-management. A sufficient level of motivation is needed for desired self-management behaviors to be carried out. A lack in motivation on the other hand can be a major barrier to self-management (Ahola & Groop, 2013; Booth, Lewis, Dean, Hunter, & McKinley, 2013; Glasgow et al., 2001). Thus, additional motivational antecedents explaining technology adoption and usage are needed in a disease self-management context when using technology adoption theory like the UTAUT.

Third, the antecedent UTAUT factors contribute to behavioral intention instead of the behavior (Chang, 2012). There is a gap between intention and actual behavior as shown by recent studies (e.g., James, Perry, Gallagher, & Lowe, 2016). Thus, actual influences not just on usage intention but on the behavior itself have to be investigated. Considering these UTAUT limitations, one could argue that the UTAUT is not the best model to choose for research on diabetes app use due to the presented shortcomings. However, within the adoption paradigm other available models are not necessarily more suitable, with some not being specific for technology adoption and use (e.g., Theory of Reasoned Action, Social Cognitive Theory, Motivational Model), and some which are very similar or closely related to the UTAUT showing similar shortcomings (e.g., Technology Acceptance Model, Model of PC Utilization). Thus, within an adoption paradigm the UTAUT as a summary of eight previous models is still the most

---

[5] In the UTAUT2 as a further development of the UTAUT hedonic motivation appears as an additional influencing factor (Venkatesh, Thong, & Xu, 2012). However, other types of motivation are still lacking in UTAUT2.

technology-specific and comprehensive option. As previously shown, this thesis follows an adoption paradigm, and thus models with underlying different paradigms are not suitable due to differing underlying understandings of mHealth use (compare e.g., appropriation paradigm).

In the following, research gaps regarding theory are summarized from the previous chapters, and empowerment is suggested as a motivational approach that addresses the outlined research gaps.

6 Summarizing mHealth Research Gaps I: Alternative Theory is Needed

First, it has been elaborated that mHealth research generally lacks theory and that theoretical approaches are needed that go beyond traditional behavior change theories, especially in an mHealth context for self-management (Chapter 4.2.2).

Second, theory is needed that is suitable to study antecedents of mHealth app use for self-management, in view of the lack of research on underlying mechanisms of mHealth app usage (Chapter 5.2).

Third, theory is needed that can complement previous technology adoption models, accepting an adoption paradigm as a necessary foundation (Chapter 4.1).

Fourth, in Chapter 5.5 it was argued that technology adoption models like the UTAUT suggest antecedents for technology adoption, but show several shortcomings when applied to an mHealth self-management context. Thus, theory is needed that sufficiently addresses the shortcomings regarding antecedent factors in these models. Specifically, theory needs to not only be able to predict behavioral intention (as found in the UTAUT) but mHealth use as a self-management behavior itself. An intention to execute a behavior does not necessarily predict the behavior as shown in the previous chapter (James et al., 2016). Moreover, theory is needed that addresses individual aspects like self-efficacy to predict technology use instead of an intention to use technology only. Social cognitive theory showed that self-efficacy is a relevant variable predicting behaviors (Bandura, 1997, 2002). Computer self-efficacy was excluded from technology adoption models like the UTAUT (Venkatesh et al., 2003). Additionally, the lack of inclusion of intrinsic and extrinsic motivational factors in models like the UTAUT requires attention. Motivational factors have shown to be most fundamental for the execution of behaviors, especially in a self-management context (see Chapter 2.3). Thus, intrinsic and extrinsic motivational theory is needed to address a lack of intrinsic and extrinsic motivational antecedents in technology adoption models (Chapter 5.5).

Fifth, theory is needed that is of particular relevance for a disease self-management context and that accounts for a duality of both psychological self-management and social influence aspects (respective intrinsic and extrinsic motivational aspects) in di

abetes care as described in Chapters 2.2 and 2.3 on self-management and on influencing factors, and also in Chapter 3.3 on diabetes app reviews.

7 Empowerment as an Antecedent of Diabetes App Use

To close these theoretical (mHealth) research gaps, a theoretical empowerment approach is suggested in the following chapters because (1) it adds an alternative theoretical approach to mHealth that goes beyond traditional behavior change and technology adoption models, (2) it is suitable to study additional anteceding factors of (diabetes) app use (3) to replenish technology adoption factors from previous models in a self-management context, (4) it combines and distinguishes intrinsic and extrinsic motivational dimensions (psychological and social influence dimensions), (5) it addresses aspects of self-efficacy, (6) it is suitable to directly predict self-management behaviors and thus (7) it is of high relevance for diabetes self-management..

In the following chapters these aspects will be laid out in detail when empowerment with its dimensions is defined. It is explained why empowerment is a motivational approach with intrinsic and extrinsic dimensions, how it differs from traditional motivational approaches (Chapter 7.1), and why it is especially relevant for diabetes self-management (Chapter 7.2). Subsequently, previous research on empowerment and mobile technology use is described (Chapter 7.3). Finally, empowerment is suggested as a motivational anteceding factor of diabetes app use (Chapter 7.3), and related research gaps are outlined (Chapter 8) before summarizing the research interest and introducing research questions and hypotheses (Chapters 9 and 10).

7.1 The Empowerment Approach in Psychology and Management Research

A variety of interpretations in a large number of diverse empowerment studies and publications leaves an unclear understanding of empowerment (Asimakopoulou, Gilbert, Newton, & Scambler, 2012). Asimakopoulou et al. (2012) pointed towards some difficulties of the concept regarding its understanding and its necessary requirements for successful implementation. Differing yet sometimes overlapping empowerment approaches can be drawn from distinct disciplines. Amongst others, a conceptualization of empowerment is provided in psychology (e.g., community psychology, Rappaport, 1987), in management research with close relation to psychology (Thomas & Velthouse, 1990), in diabetes research with relation to clinical practice, behavioral medicine, or social psychiatry (e.g., Funnell et al., 1991), and in development studies (e.g., Ibrahim & Alkire, 2007).

Rappaport thought of a general definition of empowerment in the 1980s, embedded in a community psychology approach (Rappaport, 1987). This early definition describes empowerment as a multilevel construct, and comprises "both a psychological sense of personal control or influence and a concern with actual social influence" (Rappaport, 1987, p. 121). Rappaport emphasized that the construct pays attention to individuals in context, instead of individuals only (e.g., ecological perspective in community psychology). Empowerment can arise only if there is an authority holding power and subsequently shifting this power to the individual. Transferred to a health context, the healthcare professional as the authority is able to shift power to the patient. Thus, the early approach pointed out the relevance of understanding empowerment as a combination of psychological empowerment in the individual and social influence from others.

For reasons of simplicity, and to follow previous research (Logan & Ganster, 2007), the psychological component is referred to as "psychological empowerment" here, whereas the social influence component is called "behavioral empowerment" (or "role empowerment" in Logan & Ganster, 2007). Behavioral empowerment is not called "extrinsic empowerment" in contrast to "intrinsic (psychological) empowerment", to avoid confusion with intrinsic and extrinsic motivation. Previous empowerment research did not use the labels intrinsic and extrinsic empowerment, and the use of intrinsic/extrinsic empowerment would confuse rather than clarify when differentiating empowerment from motivation (see Chapter 7.1.3).

Management research played a significant role in the development of empowerment approaches. From management literature, both approaches on psychological and behavioral empowerment are available. Some authors in management research explored psychological empowerment as described in the following Chapter 7.1.1, closely related to psychological approaches. Thomas and Velthouse (1990) developed a theoretical empowerment model for management based on a psychological theory background. The psychological empowerment approach by Thomas and Velthouse (1990) is valuable because it was operationalized (Spreitzer, 1995), adapted to the health context (e.g., Menon, 2002), and used in health communication in mHealth projects on diabetes later in time (Mantwill, Fiordelli, Ludolph, & Schulz, 2015).

Other approaches from management literature highlighted the relevance of social influence (behavioral empowerment) as part of empowerment, like Logan and Ganster (2007). Chapter 7.1.2 explains behavioral empowerment in detail. In a health context "this vision takes on a relational (e.g., doctor-patient) dimension – emphasizing the need for more egalitarian structures and a more equitable distribution of power between practitioners and patients" (Schulz & Nakamoto, 2013, p. 4).

The idea of empowerment necessarily has to include both psychological and behavioral components; one is the behavior of the supervisor or health professional who empowers the subordinate or patient, and the other is the psychological state or feeling of the patient/subordinate. Chapter 7.1.2 will elaborate why both the psychological and the behavioral aspects of empowerment are relevant in a context of diabetes self-management.

In a health context, according to Schulz and Nakamoto (2013), empowerment is frequently referred to as *patient empowerment*, even if it is not necessarily limited to patients, for example in preventive approaches. "Generally, patient empowerment is conceived as the patient's participation as an autonomous actor taking increased responsibility for and a more active role in decision making regarding his or her health" (p. 5).

In diabetes research, there is a related yet differing approach towards empowerment (e.g., Funnell et al., 1991). Mainly, the diabetes empowerment approach focuses on aspects of psychological empowerment with a more applied study focus. Theoretical background is limited, and practical operationalization of empowerment is at the center of interest, e.g., in the form of the Diabetes Empowerment Scale (compare Study 3 methodology in Chapter 14.1.1). Here, psychological empowerment is defined and operationalized as diabetes-related psychosocial self-efficacy (R. M. Anderson, Fitzgerald, Gruppen, Funnell, & Oh, 2003; R. M. Anderson et al., 1995; R. M. Anderson, Funnell, Fitzgerald, & Marrero, 2000). Self-efficacy refers to expectations of personal efficacy (Bandura, 1977), or the "belief in one's agentive capabilities, that one can produce given levels of attainment" (Bandura, 1997, p. 382), which could be explained as perceived competence to perform an action. However, self-efficacy cannot be used synonymously for the overall empowerment concept. Some authors argue that defining psychological empowerment in terms of self-efficacy does not go far enough (Thomas & Velthouse, 1990). Moreover, "self-efficacy lacks the behavioural aspect of empowerment and cannot substitute for empowerment" (M. Lee & Koh, 2001, p. 689). M. Lee and Koh (2001) argue that self-efficacy can be increased without empowerment by the HCP, and thus the empowering behavior of the HCP or supervisor is not conclusively necessary. Measuring psychological empowerment merely with self-efficacy scales such as the General Self-efficacy Scale (Schwarzer & Jerusalem, 1999), or operationalizing psychological empowerment as self-efficacy as found e.g., in the Diabetes Empowerment Scale (R. M. Anderson et al., 2000) therefore should be discussed critically – disregarding other dimensions of empowerment. As a result, the empowerment approach as used in diabetes research was not focused on in this thesis.[6] To summarize, psychological and management literature was mainly used here, to be able to conceptualize empowerment for diabetes self-management, including both psychological and behavioral empowerment components. In the following chapters, both are described in greater depth.

7.1.1   Psychological Empowerment

The management literature plays an important role in the development of a psychological empowerment approach, with a large number of research results on psychological empowerment coming from the field of management research. Here, psychological empowerment refers to the feeling of being empowered (Schulz & Nakamoto, 2013). Some early approaches in management research comprehend *psychological* empow-

---

[6] Similarly, empowerment approaches from other research fields were not used, as they lacked applicability for a diabetes self-management context. For example, empowerment previously has been linked to mobile technological solutions with a developmental study focus (Hoan, Chib, & Mahalingham, 2016; Kleine, 2010; United Nations, 2005) (not necessarily focused on health). From a developmental perspective, empowerment is mainly defined by using arguments around *agency* (Alsop & Heinsohn, 2005; Ibrahim & Alkire, 2007), with *agency* being defined as freedom to set and pursue goals (Sen, 1999). However, some authors argue that empowerment and agency should not be used synonymously (Ibrahim & Alkire, 2007). This developmental approach focuses on a meso- or macro-perspective (groups, or societies) rather than a micro-perspective (individual) and is only of limited applicability to the field of diabetes management.

erment as the one-dimensional and motivational concept of self-efficacy (Conger & Kanungo, 1988), similar to the definition of empowerment as self-efficacy in diabetes research literature described in the previous chapter (R. M. Anderson et al., 2003; R. M. Anderson et al., 1995; R. M. Anderson et al., 2000). Thomas and Velthouse (1990) critically comment on a one-dimensional definition of psychological empowerment, and recommend a multi-dimensional approach instead (also see Brew-Sam & Chib, 2020). They argue that psychological empowerment includes more than self-efficacy. They suggest a four-dimensional cognitive model of psychological empowerment, with psychological empowerment including the four indicators[7]: perceived meaningfulness (relevance), perceived competence (self-efficacy), self-determination (choice), and perceived impact. "Psychological empowerment is defined as a motivational construct manifested in four cognitions: meaning, competence, self-determination, and impact" (Spreitzer, 1995, p. 1444).

Thomas and Velthouse (1990) explain that perceived meaningfulness represents an "individual's intrinsic caring about a given task" (p. 672) or the perceived relevance of an action, while perceived competence represents an effort-performance expectancy, perceived choice a perceived opportunity for a self-determined decision, and perceived impact a performance-outcome expectancy.

Translated to a health context (Schulz and Nakamoto, 2013), the psychological empowerment indicator perceived *relevance* (or *meaningfulness*) relates to the patient's perception if performed health behaviors are of relevance and thus worth investing energy and time in. If the experience is positive, this can lead to increased involvement and commitment. Perceived *competence* (or *self-efficacy*) describes confidence in the ability to manage one's own health condition. According to the authors perceived competence has been proven to have positive effects on health behaviors and outcomes. For example, if a patient experiences competence in dealing with a chronic condition, the interest in executing self-management behaviors is likely to be stronger. The two terms perceived competence and self-efficacy are used synonymously by the

---

[7] Dimensions of empowerment are categorized as psychological and behavioral, while indicators are subdimensions of these two (indicators are also called factors when examined as antecendent factors of diabetes app use).

authors, and are used as such here. Thus, self-efficacy is understood as one indicator of psychological empowerment in this empowerment approach. There are no convincing arguments as to why psychological empowerment should be defined using self-efficacy only, dropping the other three indicators. *Self-determination* (or perceived *choice*) indicates the possibility of actions initiated by the patients themselves, and finally, perceived *impact* is the feeling about making a difference in health outcomes, for example, exercises that result in weight loss (Schulz & Nakamoto, 2013; also compare Brew-Sam & Chib, 2020).

This psychological empowerment approach based on the four-dimensional model by Thomas and Velthouse (1990) is widely accepted and frequently cited in literature (e.g., Gagné, Senécal, & Koestner, 1997; Huang, 2017; Kirk et al., 2015; Kirkman & Rosen, 1999; Spreitzer, 1996), delivers a comprehensive understanding of psychological empowerment, and was thus considered suitable for the research on mHealth for diabetes self-management. An operationalization of the four psychological empowerment indicators in the context of management is available in Spreitzer (1995), and thus the four-dimensional psychological empowerment approach is also suitable for empirical research.

Research based on the four-dimensional psychological empowerment approach can be found in chronic disease management literature (e.g., Deng, Khuntia, & Ghosh, 2013). Eyuboglu and Schulz (2016) or Camerini and Schulz (2012) found that psychological empowerment indicators affected self-care behaviors and health outcomes. Apart from patient empowerment, the four-dimensional psychological empowerment approach was also used to look into psychological empowerment of nurses (Browning, 2013; Kennedy, Hardiker, & Staniland, 2015; Knol & van Linge, 2009; Ozbas & Tel, 2016). General applications of the multi-dimensional psychological empowerment model to a health context can be found in Menon (2002). He operationalized psychological empowerment as an individual's feelings of empowerment with regards to health and healthcare (pleading for a three-dimensional health empowerment model by dropping the empowerment indicator perceived impact).

Apart from the multi-dimensional empowerment approach, in various publications psychological empowerment was operationalized as self-efficacy (as criticized earlier), for example in a study on hemodialysis patients by Moattari, Ebrahimi, Sharifi, and Rouzbeh (2012). Moreover, there are literature reviews on patient empowerment in the field of pain management, as found in Te Boveldt et al. (2014). In their literature search they defined the role of the patient, the role of the professional, resources, self-efficacy, active coping, and shared decision-making as elements of empowerment. However, this paper does not explicitly distinguish between psychological dimensions and social influence dimensions (behavioral empowerment). Overall, disease self-management literature is very non-uniform about the concept of psychological empowerment.

7.1.2 Behavioral Empowerment

As described in the previous chapter, psychological empowerment covers the psychological part of empowerment, which is the inner feeling on an individual level. However, the uniqueness of empowerment approach derives from the idea that empowerment is not only an individual feeling but additionally requires empowerment of a subordinate (e.g., patient) by a superordinate (e.g., physician) on an interpersonal level (Asimakopoulou et al., 2012; M. Lee & Koh, 2001). Empowerment comprises an individual intrinsic feeling of being empowered, as well as an extrinsic behavioral influence by others who empower, because "people are both actors and acted upon" (Hewson, 2010, p. 13). Behavioral empowerment refers to someone empowering someone else by showing specific behaviors. It does not refer to the behavior of the empowered person him- or herself. Looking at the role a subordinate (patient) takes in his her or relation to the (super)ordinate (e.g., doctor) it can also be called "role empowerment" (Logan and Ganster, 2007). Thus, behavioral empowerment includes an extrinsic behavioral aspect coming from other individuals (e.g., a doctor). Due to the behavioral component, empowerment cannot happen only within the individual ("I empower myself") (Brew-Sam & Chib, 2020). The term "em-power-ment" itself states the extrinsic influence by literally meaning to "give (someone) the authority or power to do something" (Oxford Dictionaries, 2016). The empowering support by others (behavioral/role empowerment) has been shown to influence the feeling of empowerment (psychological empowerment) (Logan & Ganster, 2007; Spreitzer, 1996).

In management research one can find a differentiation of both psychological and behavioral empowerment as explained above (e.g., Logan & Ganster, 2007). In contrast to other authors who just focus on one of the two components (Schulz & Nakamoto, 2013; Spreitzer, 1995; Thomas & Velthouse, 1990), M. Lee and Koh (2001) provide an empowerment definition that includes both a psychological and a behavioral component.

> We would suggest that a proper definition of empowerment has to integrate aspects of both behaviour and perception. Thus, we define empowerment as the psychological state of a subordinate perceiving four dimensions of meaningfulness, competence[,] self-determination and impact, which is affected by empowering behaviours of the supervisor. (p. 686)

Similar to this definition, a much stronger focus on both empowerment components is necessary in research, including a clearer differentiation between both psychological and behavioral empowerment. In contrast to psychological empowerment, the behavioral or role component of empowerment is still underexposed in empowerment research literature, or is covered but not specifically pointed out (e.g., in Zoffmann & Kirkevold, 2012). Zoffmann and Kirkevold (2012) for example studied health decision-making and problem-solving methods called Guided Self-Determination (GSD) that focus on HCPs advocating empowerment in patient care. However, they did not explicitly subsume this aspect of empowerment under role or behavioral empowerment. A similar focus can be found in Burson and Moran (2015).

In nursing literature, Knol and van Linge (2009) distinguish psychological empowerment from structural empowerment. They define structural empowerment as "power based on the employee's position in the organization" (p. 359). They found that both structural and psychological empowerment were predictors of behavior, and that psychological empowerment was a mediator between structural empowerment and (innovative) behavior. However, structural empowerment differs from role or behavioral empowerment, looking at organizational positions instead of supervisors' behaviors.

Menon (2002) argues for psychological empowerment taking place in a context of individual (patient) communities, health service providers (hospital, physicians, pharmacies, etc.), and health policy and health systems (regulatory policies and laws regarding health, budgetary and policy making bodies, medical education institutions and systems, health insurance systems, etc.). Te Boveldt et al. (2014) for example mention the role of the professional, and shared decision-making as elements of empowerment.

Behavioral empowerment at least to some degree takes place within a doctor-patient relationship, with the doctor frequently being the first source of professional medical support for patients. As described in Chapter 1.1, this is especially relevant in the context of the changes from medical paternalism to collaborative doctor-patient interaction (Chin, 2002). Looking at doctor-patient interaction, Emanuel and Emanuel (1992) developed the four models *paternalistic, informative, interpretive,* and *deliberative* model, describing the doctor-patient relationship with a variance in decision-making styles of the doctors.

Decision-making is "defined as the propensity of physicians to involve patients in treatment decisions" (Heisler, Bouknight, Hayward, Smith, & Kerr, 2002, p. 246). In their approach, the paternalistic model considers the doctor as the patient's guardian taking the final medical decisions, while the deliberative model treats the doctor as the patient's friend, taking decisions in a shared way. The informative model considers the doctor the purveyor of technical expertise, while the patient is making final decisions. The additional interpretive model in Emanuel and Emanuel (1992) is a mixed form in-between the other models. Overall, Emanuel and Emanuel (1992) suggest the deliberative model as the preferred one. According to them it reflects the idea of shared decision-making in the most suitable way, embodies the authors' ideal of autonomy, is not a disguised form of paternalism, and recognizes the relevance of physicians' and patients' values in the process of shared decision-making. An empowering doctor-patient relationship encompasses neither the exclusive control of the doctor ("paternalistic" model) nor the absolute autonomy of the patient ("informative" model), but a collaborative process of joint decision-making with an active contribution of both (deliberative model, Emanuel & Emanuel, 1992). If the doctor uses shared decision-making and a participatory consultation style, his or her behavior can empower the patient (Brew-Sam & Chib, 2020), with the definition conceiving patient empowerment "as the patient's participation as an autonomous actor taking increased responsibility for and a more active role in decision making regarding his or her health" (Schulz & Nakamoto, 2013, p. 5). Thus, shared decision-making styles by the doctor can be considered an aspect of behavioral empowerment. This is especially relevant for the operationalization of behavioral empowerment.

In relation to behavioral empowerment by the doctor, doctor-patient communication has to be taken into account as part of decision-making style and as part of doctor-patient interaction (Roter & Hall, 1989). (Verbal) communication can reflect the doctor's decision-making style, for example during consultations. Thus, communication styles should be considered another indicator of behavioral empowerment. For example, the more medical information is willingly shared with the patient in doctor-patient communication, the more a shared decision-making style is supported, and the more empowering the doctor's communication behavior can be considered.

Apart from doctors, other healthcare professionals (HCPs) can be sources of behavioral empowerment (e.g., diabetes educators, Burke, Sherr, & Lipman, 2014). The empowerment definition by the World Health Organization (WHO) specifically doesn't speak of doctors but of health-care providers to include other HCPs in addition to doctors (World Health Organization, 2009). However, there is still a special focus on the doctor as the main medical supervisor, for example in HCP-patient interaction literature (e.g., Roter & Hall, 1989). In this thesis, all HCPs are considered when discussing behavioral empowerment, but the main focus is put on the doctor as the main medical advisor.

Apart from HCPs, it has to be further investigated if other individuals additionally could be sources of behavioral empowerment, including private social networks of diabetes patients (e.g., peer patients, family, friends). The definition of empowerment by M. Lee and Koh (2001) limits behavioral empowerment to the "'behaviour of a supervisor' who empowers his/her subordinates" (p. 685), thus implying a hierarchy between empowering and empowered individuals, as well as a difference in professionalism. However, with a change towards shared decision-making approaches this hierarchy loses at least some of its relevance (Chin, 2002). HCPs take the role of advisors, and medical information is received from other additional sources increasingly gaining relevance for diabetes patients to be able to make self-responsible health decisions (e.g., eHealth, mHealth, self-management training and support groups, etc.). U. Isaksson, Hajdarevic, Abramsson, Stenvall, and Hornsten (2015) previously showed that higher psychological diabetes empowerment was not just associated with support from HCPs but also with support from relatives. The relevance of social support by peers, family, and other members of private social networks for self-management has been widely investigated in both older and recent diabetes studies (Armour, Norris, Jack, Zhang, & Fisher, 2005; Bennich et al., 2017; Grant & Schmittdiel, 2013; Heisler, Vijan, Makki, & Piette, 2010; Helgeson, Mascatelli, Seltman, Korytkowski, & Hausmann, 2016; U. Isaksson et al., 2015; Kaselitz, Shah, Choi, & Heisler, 2018; Kowitt et al., 2017; A. G. Ramirez & Turner, 2010; Shao, Liang, Shi, Wan, & Yu, 2017; Strom & Egede, 2012; van Dam et al., 2005; Wallace et al., 2018; Whitehead, Jacob, Towell, Abu-Qamar, & Cole-Heath, 2018), and has also been compared to professional HCP support (Heisler et al., 2010; Rosland et al., 2008). "Evidence suggests that higher levels of social support are associated with improved clinical outcomes, ...and the adaptation of beneficial lifestyle activities" (Strom & Egede, 2012, abstract). In summary, social support by private social networks has been found to be an important factor influencing diabetes management outcomes.

In the context of (mobile) online media, an equally large body of computer-mediated communication literature supports the relevance of online social support for disease self-management (e.g., Batenburg & Das, 2015; Gomez-Galvez, Suarez Mejias, & Fernandez-Luque, 2015; Litchman, Rothwell, & Edelman, 2018; Maki & O'Mally, 2018; Oh & Lee, 2012; van Uden-Kraan, Drossaert, Taal, Seydel, & van de Laar, 2009; White, 2001; Wright, Rains, & Banas, 2010).

Fewer studies looked into the relation of empowerment and social (online) support by private networks in the context of diabetes (Gomez-Galvez et al., 2015; Oh & Lee, 2012) or in other health contexts (van Uden-Kraan et al., 2009). In a Korean study, Oh and Lee (2012) presented significant positive relationships between diabetes patients' online social support, the sense of empowerment (psychological empowerment), and the intention to develop active doctor-patient communication. They found that perceived social support significantly predicted an intention to communicate actively with the doctor through a sense of empowerment. Psychological empowerment was confirmed to be a valid underlying mechanism explaining how perceived social online support influenced the intention for active doctor-patient communication.

Other studies do not mention the concept of empowerment but relate social support by private social networks to aspects of empowerment. Shao et al. (2017) for example found that social support was positively associated with patient self-efficacy in diabetes management, and that self-efficacy mediated the relationship between social support and glycemic control. Self-efficacy is not synonymous with psychological empowerment as shown in Chapter 7.1. However, self-efficacy can be considered one indicator of psychological empowerment as previously explained (perceived competence, Table 3). Overall, previous studies showed that social support by private social networks can lead to a feeling of empowerment. Overall, the empowering support by others (behavioral empowerment) has been shown to influence the feeling of empowerment (psychological empowerment) (Logan & Ganster, 2007; Spreitzer, 1996).

With the relevance of support from private social networks for diabetes self-management, diabetes outcomes, as well as its relation to feelings of empowerment (psychological empowerment), social networks should be considered another indicator of behavioral empowerment in addition to HCP support. A review of previous literature indicates that more research is still needed to relate social support by private social networks specifically to the theoretical behavioral empowerment component.

To summarize, the empowerment approach as used here includes psychological and behavioral dimensions, with perceived relevance, perceived competence, self-determination, and perceived impact being indicators of psychological empowerment, and HCP decision-making, HCP-patient communication, and support by private social patient networks being indicators of behavioral empowerment. Table 3 summarizes all empowerment dimensions, and respective definitions as used as a foundation for this research.

Table 3. Empowerment Dimensions

Dimensions	Indicators		Definitions
Psychological empowerment			"'Psychological empowerment', refers to … subjective feelings of empowerment."[a]
	Perceived relevance		"Meaningfulness is about the individual experiencing the feeling that what he or she does is meaningful and worth investing energy in."[a]
	Perceived competence		"Self-efficacy is the belief in one's capabilities to produce desired results by one's actions."[a]
	Self-determination		"Self-determination (or choice) refers to a decision that is characterized by autonomous initiation and is self-determined. It presupposes a distinction between an intentional behavior where people want to act in a way that would yield certain outcomes and a kind of behavior that is pressured and coerced by intra-psychic or environmental forces."[a]
	Perceived impact		"Impact means that the accomplishment of a task is perceived to make a difference in the scheme of things…. The more impact individuals believe they have, the more internal motivation they should feel."[a]
Behavioral empowerment			"'Behaviour of a supervisor' who empowers his/her subordinates."[b]
	HCP support		"Empowering behaviours of the [medical] supervisor[s]"[b] (doctors and other HCPs, like nurses, dieticians, etc.)
		HCP decision-making	"Defined as the propensity of physicians [and other HCPs] to involve patients in treatment decisions."[c]
		HCP-patient communication	"Satisfaction with provider communication about… illness and treatment."[c]
	Social support by private social networks		"Social support refers to the various types of support (i.e., assistance/help) that people receive from others."[d]

Notes. Definitions on [a]psychological empowerment by Schulz and Nakamoto (2013, pp. 5-6), on [b]behavioral empowerment by M. Lee and Koh (2001, p. 685), on [c]HCP decision-making and HCP patient communication by Heisler et al. (2002, p. 246), and on [d]social support by Seeman (2008).

Now that the basic definitions of psychological and behavioral empowerment have been formulated, the following chapter argues why empowerment is a motivational approach.

7.1.3   Empowerment as a Motivational Approach

Scientific literature agrees that empowerment is a *motivational* construct (Menon, 2001; Schulz & Nakamoto, 2013; Spreitzer, 1995; Thomas & Velthouse, 1990). Schulz and Nakamoto (2013) call patient empowerment a motivational construct because there has to be willingness of the patient to participate in health decision-making. Despite the fact that the authors relate empowerment to motivation, Brew-Sam & Chib (2020) argue that it is quite unclear how the two concepts relate to one another. The mentioned literature states that empowerment is motivational, but does not clarify the distinction between the constructs or the relationship of one to the other. Other literature uses both terms synonymously (e.g., Kamphoff, Hutson, Amundsen, & Atwood, 2016).

As explained in previous chapters, empowerment combines psychological aspects (the feeling of empowerment) with behavioral aspects (support by others) in one approach. There is a certain similarity of psychological and behavioral empowerment to the concepts of intrinsic and extrinsic motivation (for definitions of intrinsic and extrinsic motivation see Chapter 2.3) that has not been explicitly discussed by previous research. The distinction between empowerment and motivation is necessary to avoid the claim that it is "old wine in new bottles" (Lincoln, Travers, Ackers, & Wilkinson, 2002), that empowerment is just a new term for existing concepts, and thus superfluous with the concept of motivation sufficiently explaining the same ideas regarding successful disease self-management (Brew-Sam & Chib, 2020). M. Lee and Koh (2001) discuss the relationship between empowerment and motivation on a general level (not separately for psychological and behavioral empowerment). They argue that motivation and empowerment are not synonymous concepts, and that empowerment contains specific characteristics that make it unique. According to them, the difference between empowerment and motivation is that at a first glance motivation is a broader concept than empowerment. They call empowerment one method of motivation. They state that individuals who are motivated are not necessarily empowered, with other methods of motivation available. However, their argumentation can be criticized with "method" being an inappropriate term because it fits for extrinsic motivation but not for intrinsic motivation. There are extrinsic motivational methods (e.g., providing incentives), but no intrinsic motivational methods, with intrinsic motivation solely being inherent in the individual. A feeling (of being empowered) cannot be called a method. Despite the term "method" being problematic, relationships between empowerment and motivation were found in previous studies, hinting towards empowerment being an antecedent of motivation. Regarding psychological empowerment, Fook, Brinten, Sidhu, and Fooi (2011) found in a study on work motivation that all indicators of psychological empowerment significantly correlated with intrinsic work motivation. In a study investigating relationships between job characteristic, psychological empowerment and motivation, Gagné et al. (1997) reported that "aspects of empowerment differentially affected intrinsic motivation" (p. 1222). They summarize that intrinsic motivation is "the resulting will and energy that drives behavior, whereas the feelings of competence and the like that precede it are cognitive evaluations of the context and of oneself" (p. 1224). In a similar way, Thomas and Velthouse (1990) call the four-dimensional psychological empowerment a "proximal cause of intrinsic task motivation" (p. 668). Representing behavioral empowerment, other studies showed that social support (behavioral empowerment) provides (extrinsic) motivation (e.g., G. Isaksson, Lexell, & Skär, 2007). However, other studies found that social support significantly influenced not just extrinsic, but also intrinsic motivation (Vatankhah & Tanbakooei, 2014).

Thus, it could be concluded that motivation can be considered the result of empowerment. Psychological empowerment could evoke intrinsic motivation (Thomas & Velthouse, 1990), but is not the only source of it. Intrinsic motivation can result from more than the feeling of empowerment. Oftedal et al. (2011) for example mention health beliefs as another source of intrinsic motivation. Similarly, it could be argued that behavioral empowerment by other individuals can especially result in extrinsic motivation. Again, other sources of extrinsic motivation are available besides empowering and supporting behaviors by others, like providing incentives (Deci, Koestner, & Ryan, 1999).

However, it is also insufficient to consider motivation merely a result or an outcome of empowerment. If empowerment is merely an antecedent of motivation (Gagné et al., 1997), motivation is not a necessary result (also compare the discussion of "anteced-

ent" in Chapter 5.1). Yet, M. Lee and Koh (2001) argue that individuals who are empowered are always motivated, thus the concept of empowerment includes aspects of
motivation, and does not merely lead to them. They conclude that the relationship
cannot be simplified, and that empowerment has to be considered a new paradigm
instead of considered part of traditional motivation theory.

> The concept of empowerment is really a new paradigm shifted from the tradi-
> tional motivation approach (Thomas and Velthouse, 1990). We call it a para-
> digm shift, as the concept of empowerment has been brought in as a solution
> for the motivation issues that could not be settled with old theories. This is why
> we cannot simply say that motivation is 'wider' than empowerment. We cannot
> substitute empowerment with motivation. (M. Lee & Koh, 2001, p. 688)

Similarly, Bainbridge Frymier (1994) wrote that empowerment is an "expanded and
more inclusive conceptualization of motivation" (p. 184). Empowerment is unique in
a way that it incorporates specific intrinsic and extrinsic motivational aspects in one
approach. Empowerment adds and combines specific concepts in a unique way, and
thus adds value to existing motivational theories. Empowerment is a unique approach
in itself that cannot be substituted for by similar concepts such as authority, delegation,
motivation, self-efficacy, autonomy, self-determination, self-management, self-control,
self-influence, self-leadership, high-involvement, or participative management (M.
Lee & Koh, 2001).

7.1.4   Empowerment and Self-Determination

Wehmeyer (2004) connects empowerment to self-determination by stating that "the
route to 'enablement' [i.e., empowerment] is by providing opportunities and supports
that promote and enhance the self-determination of people" (p. 23). As such, promoting self-determination is a way to achieve empowerment (Wehmeyer, 2004). Confirming previous argumentation, self-determination can be called an aspect of empowerment, and as an indicator of psychological empowerment in the multi-dimensional
empowerment model (see Chapter 7.1.1).

When the empowerment approach and the Self-determination Theory (SDT) are compared, the similarities of both theoretical approaches stand out. In SDT, a satisfaction of three basic needs facilitates people's autonomous motivation, whereas thwarting the needs promotes extrinsic motivation (i.e., feeling pressured to behave in particular ways) or being unmotivated (Deci & Ryan, 2008). "Self-determination theory proposes that competence, autonomy and relatedness are essential for one to be intrinsically motivated towards a goal" (Sundar, Bellur, & Jia, 2012, p. 114). Following Sundar et al. (2012), autonomy is the degree to which an individual feels volitional or as the initiator of his or her own behavior, whereas competence is the degree to which the individual feels able to achieve set goals, and relatedness is the feeling of connection to a group.

SDT is similar to empowerment, especially concerning its similar main focus on motivation. Like empowerment, SDT has been used to study behavior change and influencing factors in relation to diabetes (e.g., Austin, Senécal, Guay, & Nouwen, 2011; Hill & Sibthorp, 2006; Williams, McGregor, Zeldman, Freedman, & Deci, 2004). According to Brooks and Young (2011), "the construct of empowerment is built upon SDT principals" (p. 50) and "the… primary [psychological] empowerment factors overlay quite neatly with the basic human needs as delineated by Deci and Ryan (2002)" (p. 50). The concept of competence appears in both SDT and empowerment, and autonomy in SDT resembles the empowerment indicator self-determination/choice. Some diabetes studies even do not explicitly distinguish between empowerment and self-determination concepts, leading to confusion regarding the two approaches (e.g., Zoffmann & Kirkevold, 2012).

Despite their similarity, neither approach is exchangeable, with differences in assumptions and included concepts. For example, SDT focuses on needs that have to be satisfied, while psychological empowerment lacks this consideration of needs. Perceived relevance of an action is not a need that has to be satisfied but rather an evaluation of an action. SDT does not focus on perceived impact and perceived relevance, but uses relatedness in addition to perceived competence and perceived autonomy. Moreover, SDT focuses on relatedness as a need that has to be satisfied, instead of focusing on actual social influences. In contrast, empowerment as conceptualized here includes a component of actual social influence (behavioral empowerment) as discussed in Chapter 7.1.2, but lacks an inclusion of perceived relatedness. Overall, despite their similarity, SDT and empowerment display some considerable differences that should prevent the synonymous use of both approaches.

7.2 Empowerment and its Relevance for Diabetes Self-Management

Empowerment as a motivational approach is essential for diabetes self-management. By now, a large body of literature is available that explains the relevance of empowerment for diabetes self-management (Asimakopoulou et al., 2012; Cinar & Schou, 2014; Di Iorio, Carinci, & Massi, 2015; Funnell & Anderson, 2004; Graffy, 2013; Meer, 2015; Scambler, Newton, & Asimakopoulou, 2014; Sigurdardottir & Jonsdottir, 2008; Yang, Hsue, & Lou, 2015). In a search for the term empowerment in 2010 Asimakopoulou et al. (2012) found at least 353 papers on Scopus that covered the topic of empowerment in diabetes (term empowerment in title, abstract or keywords). Generally, according to Gutschoven and van den Bulck (2006), "empowerment is expected to enhance the capacity for self-management and to promote the adoption of healthier lifestyle" (p. 7).

A number of studies has shown that both psychological and behavioral empowerment are predictors of (diabetes) self-management behaviors, as well as of health outcomes. For psychological empowerment, a cross-sectional study by Yang et al. (2015) with 885 diabetes patients in China proved that perceived diabetes empowerment was a predictor of self-care behavior and HbA1c in the included T2DM patients. They used linear regression to show that perceived empowerment significantly predicted self-care behaviors even after controlling for age, gender, marital status, educational level, and diabetes duration. A similar study was conducted by Kleier and Dittman (2014) with an African American sample of diabetes patients. Eyuboglu and Schulz (2016) found that *impact* and *self-determination* (psychological empowerment indicators) predicted the frequency of self-reported self-care behaviors in a Turkish study with 167 Turkish diabetes patients. In a different chronic disease context, a cross-sectional study with 209 patients by Camerini, Schulz, and Nakamoto (2012) indicated that three psychological empowerment indicators positively influenced health outcomes. Moreover, in an experimental study with 165 patients, the results indicated that the psychological empowerment indicators *perceived relevance* and *perceived impact* affected health outcomes (Camerini & Schulz, 2012). Tol, Alhani, Shojaeazadeh, Sharifirad, and Moazam (2015) argue that "one of the key concepts in [psychological] empowerment is self-efficacy", relating to the psychological empowerment indicator perceived competence in the multi-dimensional approach, and that "self-efficacy is the most important precondition for behavior change" (Tol et al., 2015, p. 6). From the diverse study results it can be summarized that psychological empowerment was found to be a predictor of diabetes self-management behaviors and outcomes (compare Brew-Sam & Chib, 2020).

Similarly, regarding behavioral empowerment, plenty of studies proved the impact of social support by HCPs, peers, and family on diabetes-related behavioral and health outcomes (Bennich et al., 2017; Grant & Schmittdiel, 2013; Rosland et al., 2008; Shao et al., 2017; Strom & Egede, 2012; van Dam et al., 2005). In a systematic review of 37 studies, Strom and Egede (2012) published that "higher levels of social support are often associated with better glycemic control, increased knowledge, enhanced treatment adherence, and improved quality of life…. Conversely, lack of social support has been associated with increased mortality and diabetes-related complications" (Strom & Egede, 2012, see their chapter "social support and diabetes"). This also includes a lack in support related to lacking understanding, nagging behaviors, expressions of pity, and negative instead of supporting behaviors by others (e.g., Bennich et al., 2017; Carter-Edwards, Skelly, Cagle, & Apple, 2004; Grant & Schmittdiel, 2013; Sanjari, Peyrovi, & Mehrdad, 2015). Evidence from studies suggests that higher levels of social support influence more positive clinical and psychosocial outcomes, as well as positive behavior change outcomes in study participants (e.g., Strom & Egede, 2012).

To summarize, previous research displays that empowerment with its psychological and behavioral dimensions has predictive value for health behaviors (R. M. Anderson et al., 2000; Yang et al., 2015) and that empowerment can lead to successful diabetes self-management (Tol et al., 2015). Therefore, it also has to be considered an antecedent factor of diabetes self-management (Funnell & Anderson, 2003; Tol et al., 2015; also compare Brew-Sam & Chib, 2020). Conversely, a lack of psychological and behavioral empowerment can hinder self-management behaviors, for example when patients do not experience relevance in their dutiful actions as one indicator of empowerment they become disengaged (Schulz & Nakamoto, 2013). Following Glasgow et al. (2001), "although high levels of self-efficacy and social support are generally facilitative of self-management, low levels of these factors can be considered as barriers" (p. 33).

The cited studies focus on single aspects of empowerment (e.g., psychological empowerment only) instead of looking into the combination of psychological empowerment and social influence (behavioral empowerment). However, both psychological and behavioral empowerment are simultaneously relevant for diabetes self-management to comprehensively address intrinsic and extrinsic motivation relevant for successful self-management (Chapter 7.1.3). "The management of diabetes appears to operate on multiple levels: first, internally, in terms of personal identity and self, but also externally, in terms of… intersubjective realities of medical consultations" (Gomersall et al., 2011, p. 854). Diabetes self-management requires a certain degree of intrinsic self-motivation as one of its most important psychological determinants (Martinez et al., 2016). Empirical studies show that intrinsically motivated individuals are more successful in weight-loss/-management and diabetes management programs than those whose behaviors are solely controlled by external factors (Sundar et al., 2012). However, for a change towards more favorable and effective diabetes self-management, the interpersonal process between the healthcare professional and the diabetes patient is additionally important (Gomersall et al., 2011). As suggested here, the empowerment approach including both psychological and behavioral empowerment comprehensively addresses empowerment as a predictor for self-management.

After the explanation of the relevance of (psychological and behavioral) empowerment for diabetes self-management in general, the following chapter looks into empowerment in relation to technology-supported diabetes self-management.

7.3 Empowerment and Diabetes App Use

7.3.1 Research on Empowerment and Diabetes App Use: Outcome Perspectives

Previous literature on the combination of a theoretical empowerment approach and mHealth research is hardly available (Anshari & Almunawar, 2015). Moreover, empowerment is frequently not explained sufficiently in an mHealth context (Bradway, Arsand, & Grottland, 2015; Cumming, Strnadová, Knox, & Parmenter, 2014). Most (diabetes-related) mHealth projects focusing on empowerment are of applied character and do not consider a theoretical empowerment approach (e.g., Park, Burford, Lee, & Toy, 2016). Anshari and Almunawar (2015) dedicate a short chapter on a theoretical empowerment approach and mHealth research, but point out that "research that specifically discusses the issue of empowerment in the domain of mHealth is still very limited" (p. 529).

Krošel, Švegl, Vidmar, and Dinevski (2016) are among the few authors addressing empowerment of diabetes patients with mobile health technologies and explaining empowerment from a theoretical point of view (Brew-Sam & Chib, 2020). However, their paper has shortcomings. According to the authors, in diabetes care patient empowerment replaced concepts of compliance and adherence, referring to the shifts from paternalistic care approaches to collaborative approaches (Chapter 1.1). Empowerment is explained as a result of (technology-supported) self-management in Krošel et al. (2016). "Mobile health technologies are already offering different means for introduction of the concept of empowerment into patients' everyday life" (p. 35). The authors do not directly explain how mHealth introduces empowerment, but the reader can understand from their argumentation that mHealth offers tools for education, self-management, and shared decision-making, and through the use of these tools empowerment can be promoted. mHealth technologies include "mobile phones, patient monitoring devices, tablets, personal digital assistants, other wireless devices, and numerous apps" (p. 31). Empowerment as an outcome of mHealth use is argued to promote active patient involvement. The difference between self-management and active involvement is not explained by the authors, and is not clear. According to the authors, empowerment promotes active involvement of the patient, and "can be achieved through education, self-management, and shared decision making" (p. 34). If both self-management and active involvement are the same, a circular relationship between empowerment and self-management is described in their paper. Empowerment is described as a result of (mHealth supported) self-management, that leads to active patient involvement. The authors do not explain relationships between their concepts in detail, and a more detailed look into relationships between mHealth use, empowerment, and self-management processes is necessary. The authors conclude that mHealth still plays a minor role in diabetes management, with shortcomings of diabetes apps, and lack of perceived benefit and ease of use of diabetes apps (Krošel et al., 2016).

Similar to Krošel et al. (2016), most previous research looking into empowerment in the context of mHealth use focused on empowerment as an outcome of mHealth use (Bradway et al., 2015; Chib & Jiang, 2014; Cumming et al., 2014; Mantwill et al., 2015; Park, Burford, Hanlen, et al., 2016). Unfortunately, empowerment is frequently mentioned as an outcome of mHealth but not explained in this context at all (e.g., Bradway et al., 2015; Cumming et al., 2014). As one of the few papers, Park, Burford, Hanlen, et al. (2016) go into further detail when talking about empowerment as an outcome of mHealth use for diabetes self-management. Park, Burford, Hanlen, et al. (2016) describe how mobile devices can be tools for compelled self-management and tools for patient empowerment for type 2 diabetes patients. From their understanding, patient empowerment can result from mHealth use and aims at enhancing autonomous self-management. "The general consensus was that active information seeking, communication, self-reflection, and education can empower patients to engage in sustainable self-management activities" (Park, Burford, Hanlen, et al., 2016, p. 27). They found that empowerment could occur when diabetes patients share information or receive social support using mobile devices, when patients realize the outcomes of their mHealth supported activities, or when the mobile devices are used for better activity or support planning. "The mHealth program can enable patients to exercise 'autonomy with their health and be more proactive, which will help us (staff) tend better to the patients' (Kira)" (Park, Burford, Hanlen, et al., 2016, p. 29). Their results suggested that devices might be more empowering when activities go beyond "simple day-today self-management" (p. 27), by adding educational activities, customized management, reflective activities etc. (Park, Burford, Hanlen, et al., 2016).

To add to the explanations by Krošel et al. (2016) and Park, Burford, Hanlen, et al. (2016) and to go further into detail, a differentiation between psychological and behavioral empowerment is needed when looking at empowerment as an outcome of mHealth use, to account for intrinsic and extrinsic motivational aspects related to mHealth use. A short description of potential relationships is added which then is substantiated with existing literature.

It can be expected that successful diabetes app use can potentially influence psychological empowerment in the patient indirectly by improving self-management processes. For example, a blood glucose (BG) diary/logbook app might provide a useful tool to improve regular blood sugar checking and recording. A diary app provides the opportunity to record daily blood sugar values and delivers an overview of blood sugar developments over time, e.g., by automatically created graphs. Through this app, blood sugar monitoring might improve due to the structured recording and monitoring guidance from the app. Reminders of the diary app can prevent diabetes patients from forgetting blood sugar checks, and can improve recording adherence. With successful app use, improvements of the perceived overall competence to manage the disease (as one psychological empowerment indicator) are possible as a result. An improved monitoring might also affect blood sugar values positively (health outcomes), which might strengthen the perceived impact of technology-supported self-management for diabetes outcomes. In this way, one or several indicators of psychological empowerment in the diabetes patient might improve indirectly through the app use. Behavioral empowerment might improve through app use when the app provides structures that enhance social support, e.g., by HCP feedback or feedback by other peer users. Apart from a potential indirect influence of app use on psychological empowerment (through improved self-management), it is unclear if the app use could influence empowerment not only indirectly but directly as well.

Most examples of the available but scarce empirical research on empowerment in an mHealth context look into empowerment as an outcome of mHealth use and focus on psychological empowerment. For example, Deng, Khuntia, and Ghosh (2013) proposed an examination of the relationship between situation interpretation and psychological empowerment as an outcome, mediated by digital integration (technology use). Mantwill et al. (2015) used the four-dimensional psychological empowerment concept to study the support of empowerment by a web and mobile based platform for diabetes patients. Similarly, Li, Owen, Thimbleby, Sun, and Rau (2013) examined whether the use of mHealth features affected empowerment (self-efficacy) and health outcomes. They hypothesized that tagging features (annotating mHealth readings, representing user perceptions of the readings) encourage patients to be more active in self-management, and that confidence in measurement features (summarizing and visualizing tagging data) encourages self-responsibility. Published results of these three studies were not available (yet). A study by Husted, Weis, Teilmann, & Castensoe-Seidenfaden (2018) explored the influence of diabetes app use on empowerment-related aspects in young T1DM patients' self-management. Study participants for example reported (increased) perceived competence by sharing experiences and knowledge with others through the app.

In a different mHealth context, Lin et al. (2018) investigated the effectiveness of a cognitive behavioral therapy based health app for smoking cessation, and proved that the app use psychologically empowered the users which was key for smoking cessation: "A one-unit increase on a 7-point Likert scale in the app's ability to empower smokers in their daily lives led to a reduction of cigarettes smoked per day of 53%" (p. e10024).

Another study by Signorelli et al. (2018) investigated the feasibility of a nurse-led eHealth intervention aiming at engaging cancer survivors in cancer-related follow-ups. The primary outcome investigated was health-related self-efficacy (empowerment) measured at several points in time. Other outcomes measured included health behaviors, beliefs, engagement in healthcare, information needs and emotional well-being. The study is ongoing, and study results have not been published yet. Other studies examined psychological empowerment as an outcome of the use of eHealth systems in healthcare organizations (Anshari, Almunawar, Low, & Al-Mudimigh, 2012; Anshari & Almunawar, 2016). Results for example showed that online health education programs (eHealth) improved patients' confidence in self-management and health services (Anshari & Almunawar, 2016). Overall, research results on psychological empowerment outcomes after mHealth use are not widely published, and further research is needed.

Only occasionally, papers add aspects of behavioral empowerment to psychological empowerment aspects when looking at empowerment as an outcome of mHealth use, and these papers frequently do not refer to the distinct dimensions of empowerment or the theoretical empowerment concept (e.g., Chib & Jiang, 2014).

Other literature focusing on social support (behavioral empowerment) outcomes by using mHealth or eHealth tools mostly do not specifically refer to empowerment. There are very few papers investigating outcomes or effects of mHealth use for non-professional social support or the support by the private social patient network (e.g., family, friends). Mayberry et al. (2016) for example found that when T2DM patients and support persons received mHealth text messages, both groups reported that the mHealth messages improved communication about diabetes. With a similar focus but in a different study context, Wittenberg, Xu, Goldsmith, and Mendoza (2019) developed an app which aimed at supporting informal caregiver communication (family, friends) about cancer. However, their study is a feasibility and technology development study, and does not report actual effects of the app use on communication outcomes between patients and their informal caregivers.

Looking at effects of mHealth use on professional healthcare support, there is a large body of literature investigating effects of patient eHealth/mHealth use for the physician-patient relationship. Already in 2003, Murray et al. found in a survey with 1.050 physicians on the use of online health information in patients prior to the consultation with their physician that "the physician's feeling that the patient was challenging his or her authority was the most consistent predictor of a perceived deterioration in the physician-patient relationship". Other studies reported positive effects of online health information seeking for the physician-patient relationship (e.g., Tan & Goonawardene, 2017).

It has to be noted that the majority of the available studies do not look into social support outcomes specifically of mHealth use. If they focus on mHealth only, mostly studies look at social support delivered through mHealth influencing health and self-management outcomes. For example, Burner et al. (2018) state that "mHealth is a feasible, acceptable, and promising avenue to improve social support and diabetes outcomes" (p. 39). Yet, they mainly looked into the latter, with patients who received family and friends network support in the mHealth program improving HbA1c, glucose self-monitoring, and physical activity in contrast to control groups showing less beneficial outcomes.

7.3.2   Understanding the Overall Process of Empowerment and Diabetes App Use

Apart from investigating psychological and behavioral empowerment as outcomes of mHealth app use and thus considering it a state that occurs after an app use, it has to be acknowledged that empowerment is a process rather than a state (Rappaport, 1987). The process perspective suggests that there is a pre-existing level of psychological empowerment in the patient that can constantly change, and that psychological empowerment develops in the course of a patient's self-management process. Spreitzer (1995) and M. Lee and Koh (2001) describe empowerment as a continuous variable: "Subordinates will be considered more or less empowered, rather than empowered or not empowered" (M. Lee & Koh, 2001). After initial education to provide the patient with necessary knowledge and skills for self-management (Funnell & Anderson, 2003), psychological empowerment as a feeling of empowerment can develop with ongoing psychosocial and behavioral self-management support (R. M. Anderson & Funnell, 2010). Transferred to diabetes app use for self-management, this means that a pre-existing level of psychological empowerment can change in the course of the app use, and in combination with behavioral empowerment by others (Brew-Sam & Chib, 2020).

To understand empowerment as a process, Rappaport (1987) recommends looking at empowerment in a longitudinal way to understand its development in individuals and in their life contexts. Previous mHealth research frequently lacks process perspectives, with the majority of studies using rather short-term study designs (K. R. Jones et al., 2014). Previous reviews on mHealth effects criticized mHealth study designs that lacked longitudinal research perspectives especially relevant for diabetes (B. Holtz & Lauckner, 2012; K. R. Jones et al., 2014).

Very few publications looked into the process of empowerment in relation to eHealth or mHealth by using pretest-posttest designs with empowerment being one of the variables. Camerini and Schulz (2012) looked at psychological empowerment as a mediating factor by testing whether psychological empowerment mediated a possible relationship between the availability of interactive features on an eHealth application and fibromyalgia syndrome patients' health outcomes. Using a pretest-posttest design, they looked at both empowerment before and after the use of different versions of an eHealth application. They hypothesized that knowledge and empowerment mediated the effect of interactivity of an eHealth application on health outcomes. They could not find any significant impact of functional interactivity on empowerment or on knowledge. Generally, they found that the empowerment indicators' relevance and impact positively affected health outcomes. They did not specifically focus on empowerment processes, but rather on the role of interactivity in eHealth applications.

In another pretest-posttest study, L. M. S. Miller et al. (2017) examined the effects of eHealth-based food label-reading training on perceptions of empowerment (psychological empowerment). They compared healthful food-choice empowerment before and after eHealth label-reading sessions. They found improvements in empowerment after the web-based label-reading training. The food-choice empowerment scores were about 7.5% higher on average after the training ($p < .001$). Despite looking at empowerment from a process perspective, due to the intervention design neither study looked into empowerment affecting eHealth use.

For behavioral empowerment (social influence) it was found that most research studies looked either at social influence as an outcome of mHealth use (Chapter 7.3.1), or at mHealth as means of delivering social support, while examining its usage impact on health and self-management outcomes. A few studies applied process perspectives. Fortuna et al. (2018) for example examined preliminary effects of a peer-delivered and technology-supported self-management intervention for older people in a pretest-posttest study. Their findings delivered preliminary evidence for the feasibility and acceptability of peer-delivered technology-supported intervention, and associated it with enhanced self-management and empowerment.

According to Brew-Sam and Chib (2020), focusing only on empowerment as an outcome of diabetes app use leads to a neglection of the fact that that empowerment is a process. Thus, a step back from outcome research is required, to look into empowerment as an antecedent of diabetes app use in order to understand the overall empowerment process in relation to diabetes app use. Regarding diabetes app use, it has to be investigated if pre-existing psychological empowerment levels and social influence (behavioral empowerment) are affecting diabetes app adoption and use before a successful app use can even influence empowerment levels. For empirical research this means that instruments are needed that are able to measure levels of empowerment in the patient and social support at various points in time, which can be the level of empowerment before an app use, or as an outcome in between or after the use.

7.3.3   Empowerment as an Antecedent of Diabetes App Use

Looking into empowerment as an antecedent of diabetes app use, a diabetes patient brings along a certain level of empowerment before adopting and using apps for self-management. A low psychological empowerment level, and low behavioral HCP support for self-management can be expected to result in insufficient patient initiative for self-management behaviors, including a lack of motivation for the use of diabetes apps for self-management. Following explanations in Chapter 7.1, psychological empowerment can deliver intrinsic motivation for app use, influenced by extrinsic motivation by empowering support by diabetes supervisors or other individuals.

Specifically looking at the psychological empowerment indicators *relevance*, *competence*, *self-determination* and *impact* (Schulz & Nakamoto, 2013), and as argued in Brew-Sam and Chib (2020), it means that all psychological empowerment indicators are likely to influence diabetes app use. For perceived relevance, the diabetes patient for example has to experience the diabetes app use as a relevant activity for his or her overall self-management to develop the motivation to start and maintain using an app. When patients do not consider a diabetes app relevant for themselves, long-term app use will be less likely. If a patient feels competent to use apps for diabetes self-management (e.g., perceived technological competence), app use is more likely than when there is a lack of perceived competence. Looking at self-determination, the app use is influenced by the voluntariness of this behavior. An app use is expected to be less likely if the use is obligatory. This supports ideas of intrinsic motivation with voluntary actions being more efficient than forced action (Deci, 1975; Leasure & Jones, 2008). Concerning the psychological empowerment indicator impact, if the patient has the feeling that he or she can influence self-management or health outcomes by using a diabetes app, app use will become more likely. In addition to the psychological empowerment dimension, the behavioral empowerment by supervisors, such as the support from HCPs to use a diabetes app, is also likely to influence app use for self-management. HCP support regarding app use can possibly influence app adoption, e.g., positively when recommending the use of an app, or giving regular feedback on the app use. For example, if a patient perceives the relevance of a diabetes logbook app as high for him- or herself e.g., because he/she perceives it as useful for improving blood sugar monitoring, feels competent to use the app as part of the overall diabetes self-management, feels free to adopt or to reject the app, expects the impact of the logbook use for the overall self-management outcomes or the health outcomes as high, and is at the same time supported by supervising HCPs to use the app, then it can be expected that the patient is likely to adopt and to use the logbook app as part of his/her diabetes self-management if other anteceding factors are not preventing the adoption and use.

Looking for further confirmation of empowerment as an antecedent of mHealth use in previous literature, no publication could be found that specifically looked into psychological empowerment as an antecedent of mHealth use, and influencing mHealth adoption and use. Regarding behavioral empowerment, Talukder and Quazi (2011) examined the impact of peer and social network influences on attitudes toward innovation and the impact of that attitude on individuals adopting innovation. They found "that social network impacts significantly on attitudes toward an innovation which, in turn, affects the innovation adoption behavior of employees. Furthermore, social network has been found to directly influence the innovation adoption process" (p. 111). Davis (1985) and Davis, Bagozzi, and Warshaw (1989) state that it is difficult to distinguish if the user's own attitude causes a certain behavior, or if this behavior is caused by the influence of others on the user's intention. Here, behavioral empowerment looks at social influence instead of internalized perceptions about social influence. In contrast, social influence as one of four influencing factors on technology adoption in the UTAUT refers to perceptions of the individual about others believing that she or he should use the technology. This differs from actual social influence in the form of behaviors of others (e.g., other patients using specific diabetes apps, HCPs recommending diabetes apps, diabetes apps as part of diabetes programs, etc.). In a different context, Bozan, Davey, and Parker (2015) examined "the social forces that influence patient portal use behavior among the elderly" (p. 517). Based on institutional theory and the UTAUT, they conducted a study with 117 older people in the US. Their findings suggested that "older people follow their providers' advice and follow the behavior of a respected, higher-status peer from their network. Normative pressure was found to be an insignificant force, which indicated that older people do not follow the bandwagon effect" (p. 517). Thus, the study was able to confirm that social influence had effects on eHealth or mHealth use in older people. In another study, Hao, Padman, Sun, and Telang (2014) were interested in studying the social influence on physicians' (sustained) information technology use behavior and conducted a study in the US. They found that technology users undergo "psychological changes in response to social influence at different stages of technology adoption and use. Therefore, this brings up a practical policy implication regarding how to leverage this change and what type of social influence should be considered to leverage during the technology implementation stage, for promoting early adoption or for encouraging sustained use" (p. 2751).

Other available studies did not look into social support influencing mHealth use, but looked at social support delivered through mHealth influencing health and self-management outcomes. For example, Omboni, Caserini, and Coronetti (2016) showed that the use of blood pressure telemonitoring through eHealth or mHealth for hypertension management has been found to result in blood pressure reduction in several randomized studies. Moreover, they showed that "additional benefits are observed when BPT [blood pressure telemonitoring] is offered under the supervision of a team of healthcare professionals, including a community pharmacist" (p. 187).

Most studies looking into social support influencing mHealth or technology adoption and use do not refer to (behavioral) empowerment specifically. More research is still specifically needed on HCP influences, and private social network influences as part of behavioral empowerment on diabetes app use.

8 Summarizing mHealth Research Gaps II: Empowerment and Diabetes App Use

8.1 Empowerment as a Multi-Dimensional Antecedent of Diabetes App Use

Chapter 7.3 outlined how empowerment has been related to mHealth research in only a limited number of studies (Anshari & Almunawar, 2015), and frequently a theoretical perspective on empowerment is missing, with the concept left unexplained (Bradway et al., 2015; Cumming et al., 2014). As shown in the previous chapters, psychological empowerment has been investigated in relation to mHealth research in a small number of studies (Camerini & Schulz, 2012; Lamprinos et al., 2016; Mantwill et al., 2015), and social support (behavioral empowerment) has been studied in relation to eHealth or mHealth use without specifically referring to empowerment (Barak, Boniel-Nissim, & Suler, 2008; Litchman et al., 2018; Maki & O'Mally, 2018; Oh & Lee, 2012; van Uden-Kraan et al., 2009).

Despite very few studies combining research on psychological and behavioral empowerment in relation to mHealth, it has been shown that there is a relationship between psychological and behavioral empowerment with empowering support by others influencing the feeling of empowerment (Logan & Ganster, 2007; Spreitzer, 1996). U. Isaksson et al. (2015) showed that social support was associated with higher psychological diabetes empowerment. Shao et al. (2017) found that social support was positively associated with patient self-efficacy, and that self-efficacy mediated the relationship between social support and glycemic control. In an mHealth/eHealth context, Oh and Lee (2012) found that perceived online social support significantly predicted an intention to communicate actively with the doctor through a sense of empowerment (psychological empowerment). There is still a gap in mHealth research using a holistic theoretical empowerment concept, and there is further need to study the combination of psychological and behavioral empowerment in relation to mHealth to understand both intrinsic and extrinsic motivational antecedents of mHealth use.

Moreover, in Chapter 7.3 it could be shown that most mHealth research looked at empowerment as an outcome of mHealth use, and research is needed that expands the

N. Brew-Sam, *App Use and Patient Empowerment in Diabetes Self-Management*, https://doi.org/10.1007/978_3_658_29357_4_8

view towards empowerment as an antecedent factor of mHealth use to satisfy empowerment process perspectives, especially in context of disease self-management.

The aim of this research is to close both research gaps by using a multi-dimensional and theoretical empowerment approach including both psychological and behavioral facets for empirically studying empowerment as an antecedent of diabetes app use for self-management.

8.2   Two Research Perspectives on Empowerment as an Antecedent of Diabetes App Use

When empowerment is examined as an antecedent of diabetes app use, two research perspectives are needed, looking at empowerment in relation to (1) diabetes apps and their characteristics (app perspective), and (2) diabetes app (non-) users and their perspectives on diabetes apps for self-management (user perspective). From both perspectives, adoption/use as well as rejection/non-use aspects need to be considered, as previously outlined (e.g., in Chapter 5.5. addressing UTAUT shortcomings with a focus on technology rejection missing).

(1) The first perspective is needed because characteristics of apps have been shown to influence diabetes app adoption/rejection and maintained app use, as well as other self-management behaviors. Sundar et al. (2012) state "that certain structural features of the technology can be leveraged to build intrinsic motivation among users" (p. 113). Structural features in an app are for example digital photography features, interactive features (chat functions, gaming elements), etc. (Sundar et al., 2012). Smith, Frost, Albayrak, and Sudhakar (2007) for example showed in two studies that digital photography features that were added to a glucometer encouraged users through visualization to monitor and regulate their diet. The adherence to regular BG recording is insufficient in some patients, yet crucial for good self-care (Parkin & Davidson, 2009). By providing e.g., monitoring features, the patient has a tool at hand that can help with structured and regular BG recording (e.g., using reminders). Depending on user preferences, attitudes and user characteristics (see user perspective), the availability of certain app features can influence the adoption/rejection and (maintained) use or non-

use of an app for diabetes self-management. Moreover, as outlined in Chapter 3.3 studies showed that app quality influences app usage intentions (Dutta et al., 2010), and app adoption and maintained app use (Henze, Pielot, Poppinga, Schinke, & Boll, 2011, maintained app use is also called app "stickiness", see Furner et al., 2016). Learning from previous app quality studies (Kamel Boulos et al., 2014; Schoeppe et al., 2017; Sunyaev, Dehling, Taylor, & Mandl, 2015), low app quality can hinder an app adoption and use.

Research that combines diabetes app analyses and reviews with the concept of empowerment is lacking although a decent number of studies on diabetes apps is already available (see Chapters 3.2 and 3.3). Previous research on diabetes apps for self-management (e.g., app reviews) have not used theoretical empowerment approaches to study characteristics of mobile diabetes tools for self-management, apart from the mentioned study by Camerini and Schulz (2012) who tested whether psychological empowerment mediated a possible relationship between the availability of interactive features on an eHealth application and patients' health outcomes, and found no impact of functional interactivity on empowerment dimensions. No other mHealth research could be found that had previously studied characteristics of mHealth tools in relation to a theoretical empowerment approach. Nor did app reviews separate features for patient self-management (corresponding to psychological empowerment), from features for social influence by others (corresponding to behavioral empowerment) as described in Chapter 3.2. Thus, the own research focuses on diabetes apps and their characteristics in relation to empowerment when investigating the relation between empowerment and app (non-) use (diabetes app perspective).

(2) The second perspective needs to focus on diabetes patients' psychological empowerment levels, and social influence from others (behavioral empowerment) in relation to previous app (non-) use and the (non-) users' perceptions of diabetes apps for self-management (user perspective[8]). As argued before in Chapter 7.3, only very few studies have related a theoretical empowerment approach to mHealth or eHealth use, and

---

[8] It could be argued that a doctor or HCP perspective is necessary to receive information about patient empowerment from a professional perspective. However, it can also be argued that information received from the patients directly should be more accurate than an indirect assessment through health professionals.

research connecting theoretical empowerment to mHealth mainly focused on psychological empowerment. Chapter 7.3 already delivered an overview on previous research on empowerment in relation to usage perspectives. The own research investigates psychological and behavioral empowerment in relation to diabetes app (non-) use and includes both user and non-user perspectives when trying to understand antecedents of app use (based on Chapter 5.5).

To conclude, a comprehensive understanding of empowerment as an antecedent of diabetes app use can be achieved only by using both (1) diabetes app and (2) diabetes app (non-) user perspectives. Not only psychological empowerment in the diabetes patient, and behavioral empowerment by others potentially influence diabetes app use, but characteristics of the apps themselves can contribute to successful app adoption and use as well. Cenfetelli (2004) highlights that:

> Given that a core artifact of interest to IS [information systems] researchers is the design and functionality of a system, it follows that we should study those variables specific to the attributes of a system that encourage or discourage use.... Further, it is important to study a user's perceptions of those objective attributes. (p. 474/475)

9 Summarizing Model on Empowerment and Diabetes App Use

To summarize the previous Chapters 7.3 to 8, and to address the outlined research gaps, a graphical model (Figure 2) was used illustrating the overall expected processes between empowerment and diabetes app (non-) use. From the overall model, it is explained which parts of the model specifically were focused on in this research. From there, Chapter 10 introduces research questions and hypotheses.

In the previous Chapter 8.2, it was argued that both a diabetes app perspective and a diabetes (non-) user perspective are necessary in order to examine (psychological and behavioral) empowerment as an antecedent of diabetes app use. Figure 2 therefore addresses both perspectives with diabetes app characteristics possibly influencing diabetes app (non-) use in addition to psychological empowerment levels in the diabetes patients and behavioral empowerment by others.

In Chapter 7.2 both psychological and behavioral empowerment have been shown to be a precondition for behavior change and self-management behaviors (Figure 2, arrow 1). Similarly, psychological empowerment in the patient and behavioral empowerment by others (e.g., HCPs) can be expected to serve as antecedents of diabetes app use, with the app use being one self-management behavior among other behaviors (see Chapter 4.1). Higher psychological and behavioral empowerment can be expected to make an app use more likely, if the diabetes apps used are of sufficient quality and deliver adequate features (app characteristics, Figure 2, arrow 2), and if no other anteceding factors hinder the diabetes app use (Figure 2, arrow 3). Successful app adoption and use possibly influence other self-management behaviors (Figure 2, arrow 4). For example, the use of a blood glucose diary app potentially improves blood glucose monitoring due to assistance from the app. Improved self-management behaviors can then be reflected in improved health outcomes (e.g., better blood glucose values) (Figure 2, arrow 5). With perceived improvements in self-management and health outcomes, psychological empowerment is expected to improve in return (Figure 2, arrows 6 and 7). This is because the diabetes patient for example perceives the impact of his or her behaviors on health outcomes as higher, or perceives his or her self-management competence as higher than before using a diabetes app. Moreover, behavioral empowerment potentially changes as well due to changed self-management

N. Brew-Sam, *App Use and Patient Empowerment in Diabetes Self-Management,* https://doi.org/10.1007/978-3-658-29357-4_9

and health outcomes. For example, a doctor noticing improved self-management out-comes might react in more or less supportive ways (Figure 2, arrows 6 and 7).

Health outcomes possibly influence self-management behaviors directly, e.g., by the perceived seriousness of the condition (Figure 2, arrow 8), or influence self-management mediated by empowerment (Figure 2, arrows 6 and 1). For example, pos-itive health outcomes could affect psychological and/or behavioral empowerment pos-itively, and improved empowerment could lead to improved self-management in re-turn. Similarly, other self-management behaviors like blood sugar monitoring, diet, or exercise could influence diabetes app use through empowerment (Figure 2, arrows 7 and 2) or directly (Figure 2, arrow 9), e.g., if general self-management is poor, app adoption is expected to be less likely. In addition, diabetes app use potentially influ-ences psychological and behavioral empowerment directly rather than through other self-management behaviors (Figure 2, arrow 10). The overall process can be expected to be circular.

Focus of the Thesis and the Empirical Research

Within the described process between empowerment and diabetes app use, the thesis focuses on one specific aspect as a first step towards understanding the overall pro-cess: In contrast to previous research which mainly considered empowerment as an outcome of mHealth use (Figure 2, arrows 4-10), the focus of the research is on both psychological and behavioral empowerment as anteceding factors of diabetes app use from both a diabetes app and a diabetes app (non-) user perspective (Figure 2, arrow 2) and in addition to other existing factors from previous technology adoption and self-management research (Figure 2, arrow 3). Empowerment is expected to add value to previous factors from technology adoption models (UTAUT) in a diabetes self-management context as shown in Chapters 6 and 7. Self-management factors were shown to be generally relevant to diabetes self-management in Chapter 2.3, and thus have to be taken into consideration when looking into antecedents of diabetes app use.

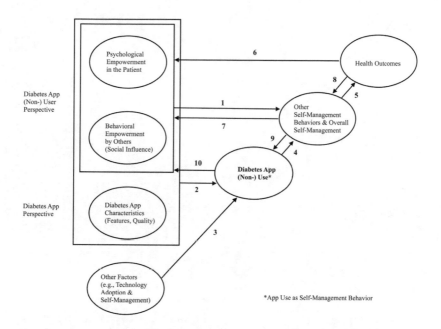

Figure 2. The process of empowerment and mHealth (app) use for diabetes self-management.

Notes. (1) Psychological and behavioral empowerment can improve self-management, and (2) can promote diabetes app use as a technology-supported self-management behavior, (3) influenced by other factors from technology adoption and self-management theory, as well as (2) by app characteristics. (4) Successful app use can support other self-management behaviors (e.g., improved monitoring), (5) can lead to improved health outcomes, and (6/7/10) can promote psychological and begavioral empowerment and (8/9) improved self-management in return (including app use). The described process is circular.

10 Research Questions and Hypotheses

The previous chapters were dedicated to theoretical implications and previous research. This research aims to complement previous mHealth research by addressing research gaps as outlined in Chapters 6 and 8 (e.g., shortcomings of previous technology adoption theories regarding an inclusion of motivational antecedents of technology use, main focus of mHealth research on empowerment as an outcome of mHealth use and lacking inclusion of psychological and behavioral dimensions). The main research gap that is addressed and that derives from the theoretical suggestions relates to the general lack of understanding of diabetes app use processes. To shed light on mechanisms behind diabetes app adoption and use or app rejection and non-use, antecedents of diabetes app use are examined, specifically addressing empowerment as an antecedent factor, as it has specific relevance for diabetes self-management (Chapter 7.2).

The resulting primary research aim is to investigate from both (1) a diabetes app and (2) an app (non-) user perspective *if empowerment with its psychological and behavioral dimensions is an antecedent of diabetes app use complementing other antecedents from technology adoption and self-management theory.* Thus, only specific processes displayed in the model in Figure 2 are focused on here (arrows 2 and 3).

(1) As a first step towards examining empowerment as an antecedent of app use from an app perspective (Figure 2), this research examines *how the technological diabetes app features correspond to theoretical indicators of psychological and behavioral empowerment (RQ 1a and RQ 1b)* to be able to evaluate the potential of diabetes apps for self-management (relevance of app characteristics for app use). This is based on the theoretical empowerment approach in Chapter 7.1, and based on the lack of mHealth (app) reviews looking into empowerment (Chapter 8.2). Previous research showed that app quality influences app usage intentions (Dutta et al., 2010), and thus *app quality is investigated as an additional app characteristic (RQ 1c)* to account for its relevance as highlighted in Chapter 3.3 (K. Anderson et al., 2016; Grundy et al., 2016; Hides et al., 2014; Singh et al., 2016; Stoyanov et al., 2015) For example, when an app for diabetes self-management crashes frequently indicating that the app quality

© The Editor(s) (if applicable) and The Author(s), under exclusive license
to Springer Fachmedien Wiesbaden GmbH, part of Springer Nature 2020
N. Brew-Sam, *App Use and Patient Empowerment in Diabetes
Self-Management*, https://doi.org/10.1007/978-3-658-29357-4_10

is poor, it is unlikely that the diabetes patient will continue to use the app even if it provides promising potential with features corresponding to empowerment indicators. Finally, based on the analysis of diabetes app features against the theoretical psychological and behavioral empowerment background, and by assessing the diabetes app quality, the potential of diabetes apps for empowered self-management is interpreted and discussed.

This analysis of diabetes app characteristics delivers an update on available diabetes apps compared with previous research on app features and app types, and provides a foundation for the following diabetes app (non-) user perspective.

In (2) the diabetes (non-) user perspective, the level of psychological empowerment in the patient, and the behavioral empowerment derived from support by HCPs and private social patient networks are investigated in relation to previous diabetes app (non-) use. Here, both qualitative and quantitative research methods are used to shed light on empowerment as an antecedent of diabetes app use.

Using a diabetes app user and non-user typology in a first step, exploratory research investigates *how diabetes app users and non-users differ in psychological (RQ 2a) and behavioral empowerment (RQ 2b)*. To examine empowerment in relation to other influencing factors, *app (non-) user differences regarding factors from technology adoption theory (RQ 2c) and from self-management research are investigated (RQ 2d,* Table 4). This serves as an exploratory foundation to draw conclusions about the relevance of empowerment as an influencing factor on app use in relation to other factors. The exploratory (non-) user perspective furthermore delivers general information about both diabetes app use and non-use (attitudes) relevant for understanding the adoption and use of diabetes apps.

Based on this exploratory research as well as on theory, specific hypotheses are tested in a second step. Hypotheses deriving from theory relate to the general research interest (Table 4; more specific hypotheses derive from the exploratory Study 2 results introduced in Chapter 13.2.4.2):

In Chapter 4.1 it was argued that the use of diabetes apps for self-management (e.g., recording blood sugar values in a diary app) is a technology-supported self-management behavior that can be considered an additional behavior complementing other traditional self-management behaviors, like pricking the finger for blood sugar checks, or like counting carbohydrates. Moreover, in Chapter 7.2 it was argued that a positive relationship has been proven between empowerment and health behaviors or self-management behaviors in previous literature (Funnell & Anderson, 2003; Tol et al., 2015), and empowerment has been shown to be a precondition for health behaviors (Tol et al., 2015).

From the two presumptions that diabetes app use is a self-management behavior, and that empowerment is an antecedent of self-management behaviors, *a positive relationship between empowerment and diabetes app use is hypothesized (H I), as well as that empowerment is a motivational antecedent of diabetes app use (H II) complementing other antecedents from previous technology adoption and self-management theory (H III)* (Table 4).

Table 4 summarizes the research questions and hypotheses as introduced here. The research questions and hypotheses build on one another, from the more general to the specific and as a foundation for the Studies 1 to 3.

Table 4. Research Questions and Hypotheses

	No.	Research Question or Hypothesis	Study
Diabetes app perspective	RQ 1	How do diabetes app features correspond with indicators of empowerment, and what is the level of diabetes app quality? a) How do diabetes app features correspond with indicators of psychological empowerment and ... b) ... behavioral empowerment? c) What is the level of app quality in diabetes apps for self-management?	Study 1
Diabetes app user perspective	RQ 2	What can diabetes app user and non-user group differences (types of non-/users) tell about empowerment as a factor influencing diabetes app use for self-management in addition to other factors? a) How do diabetes patients differ in their diabetes app use regarding psychological empowerment and ... b) ... behavioral empowerment? c) How do diabetes patients differ in their diabetes app use regarding technology adoption factors and ... d) ... self-management factors?	Study 2 & Study 3
	H I	Psychological and behavioral empowerment are positively related to diabetes app use.	Study 3
	H II	Psychological and behavioral empowerment are antecedents of diabetes app use for self-management.	Study 3
	H III	Empowerment as a motivational antecedent of diabetes app use is complementing other anteceding factors from technology adoption and self-management theory.	Study 3 (/Study 2)

11 Overview of the Research Design

This research is one of the first insights into empowerment as an antecedent of diabetes app use for self-management. Three studies were conducted to investigate empowerment as an anteceding factor of diabetes app usage in addition to other factors.

Study 1 examined diabetes apps in an app feature and app quality analysis (diabetes app perspective), while Studies 2 and 3 investigated empowerment and app use from a diabetes (non-) user perspective in semi-structured face-to-face interviews (Study 2) and in a standardized online survey (Study 3). In the following, an overview over the empirical research is given, before Chapters 12 to 14 introduce the three studies in detail.

11.1 mHealth Research on Diabetes App Use in Singapore

The empirical research was conducted in Singapore for two reasons. First, Singapore shows high diabetes prevalence (Singapore Government, 2015), and second it shows outstanding mobile tech-affinity (Sleigh, Chng, Mayberry, & Ryan, 2012). According to the International Diabetes Federation IDF, thirteen percent of adults in Singapore suffered from diabetes in 2014 (International Diabetes Federation, 2015b). Worldwide this was the second highest proportion of diabetes among developed nations at that point in time (only the US showed higher prevalence rates in the latest report by IDF) (Singapore Government, 2015). New approaches for technology-supported diabetes treatment and management are thus of high relevance for Singaporean society. Moreover, following Sleigh et al. (2012) "the Southeast Asia region… shows a stronger interest in new online services than the global audience" (p. 9), and "in today[']s digital world, Southeast Asians place more emphasis on digital connection and sharing than the global norm" (p. 21). The Consumer Barometer by Google reports that Singapore showed the highest smartphone penetration in the world in 2014 (Consumer Barometer, 2014). It reports that 91% of people used a smartphone in Singapore in 2016 (Consumer Barometer, 2017). In December 2016 the mobile penetration rate in

Singapore was at 150% (Infocomm Media Development Authority Singapore, 2017)[9].
To conclude, these characteristics provided the opportunity to conduct research in a
pioneer country for smartphone use which at the same time stressed the urgent need
for further research on diabetes care.

11.2 Research Procedure

In Study 1, one hundred twenty-one available diabetes apps for self-management were
investigated from an app perspective, by assessing how their features corresponded to
indicators of empowerment, as well as app quality, in order to assess their potential
for self-management (diabetes app review, Brew-Sam & Chib, 2019). Although previous diabetes app reviews were available (Arnhold et al., 2014; Chomutare, Fernandez-Luque, Årsand, & Hartvigsen, 2011; Rossi & Bigi, 2017), a specific update on
diabetes apps in Singapore was needed. Moreover, previous reviews did not examine
diabetes apps for self-management against the theoretical empowerment background.
App feature and content analytical procedures were used based on previous research.
From Study 1, a diabetes app for self-management was chosen for Study 2, so that app
use could be discussed with interview participants while they were shown an exemplary app.

Similar to the procedure used by Weymann, Harter, and Dirmaier (2016), who conducted semi-structured interviews with diabetes patients followed by a self-assessment
questionnaire based on the interview results, semi-structured interviews with 21 diabetes patients were conducted in Study 2. The interviews delivered first exploratory results on diabetes patients' app use for self-management, on psychological and behavioral patient empowerment levels, and on basic ideas about a potential relationship
between empowerment and diabetes app use. A patient typology helped to examine
differences in app user and non-user groups regarding psychological and behavioral
empowerment and other factors likely influencing diabetes app use. In this way, em-

---

[9] The smartphone penetration rate was at 73% in 2016 (Statista, 2017).

powerment could be investigated in relation to diabetes app use from a qualitative perspective.

From Study 2 interview results, specific hypotheses were derived that were statistically tested in a larger sample in Study 3. Study 3 included a standardized self-assessment online questionnaire that was developed based on the results of the Study 2 interviews, and administered to a sample of 65 diabetes patients (after exclusion of incomplete questionnaires; a larger sample could not be achieved, see Chapter 13.4). Cluster analysis was used to test the Study 2 user and non-user typology, as well as binary logistic regression to examine the strength of empowerment and other influencing factors on diabetes app use. In this way, the relationship between empowerment, other factors, and diabetes app use was investigated following a quantitative research approach.

Detailed information on the three study procedures is provided in Chapters 12 to 14.

12 Study 1 – Diabetes App Features Corresponding to Indicators of Empowerment: An App Feature and Quality Analysis

Previous results from available diabetes app reviews were introduced in Chapter 3, showing that most diabetes apps included few features (Arnhold et al., 2014; Brzan et al., 2016), and offered limited potential especially for specific target groups (J. A. Rodriguez & Singh, 2018), had usability problems (Fu et al., 2017), and sometimes showed insufficient app quality (Basilico et al., 2016; Brzan et al., 2016; Chavez et al., 2017). Despite a large number of studies on diabetes apps, empowerment was found to be still underinvestigated in mHealth research in relation to diabetes apps (Chapter 7.3), despite their relevance for diabetes self-management (Chapter 7.2). Based on this research background, the purpose of Study 1 for the overall research project was threefold:

First, Study 1 aimed to bring the two research perspectives on diabetes app reviews and on empowerment research together, to advance the inclusion of theoretical approaches in mHealth app reviews (mHealth as an applied research field generally lacks theoretical foundation, Chapter 7.3.1). Empowerment as a theoretical approach is of high relevance especially for technology-supported diabetes self-management (Chapter 7.2). Second, as explained in the previous chapters, Study 1 added an app perspective to the following patient (non-) user perspective in studies 2 and 3 (Figure 2). The extent to which diabetes app features supported theoretical indicators of psychological (*RQ 1a*) and behavioral empowerment (*RQ 1b*) was examined, and an app quality assessment was added (*RQ 1c*, Table 4) to enable discussion of the app potential for empowered self-management. Third, the app review was a general foundation for studies 2 and 3 in terms of knowledge on types and features of available diabetes apps in Singapore in contrast to previous reviews (Arnhold et al., 2014; Chomutare et al., 2011; Demidowich et al., 2012; Research2guidance, 2014b).

12.1 Method

12.1.1 Operationalization

As outlined in Brew-Sam & Chib (2019), an exploratory and interpretive approach was taken as a first step towards understanding diabetes apps, as well as to what extent their features supported indicators of psychological and behavioral empowerment. To collect information about diabetes app types and their features (*RQ 1a* and *RQ 1b*), the app coding scheme by Arnhold et al. (2014) was used as a starting point to create a coding scheme for an app (content) analysis (codebook see Chapter 1.4 in Appendix). Existing instruments from survey research were used to inform operationalization where no operationalization from app content analysis was available. The collected available features of apps were then investigated against the theoretical psychological and behavioral indicators of empowerment (as described in Chapters 7.1.1 and 7.1.2), by preliminarily assigning the features to the theoretical empowerment indicators, and by comparing this assignment with prior research results. At this stage, the procedure resembled a qualitative procedure with an open assignment of app features to theoretical indicators of empowerment. Considering app quality as a factor influencing app use (*RQ 1c*), the potential of diabetes apps for empowered self-management was interpreted and discussed from the results (interpretive and exploratory approach).

For psychological empowerment (*RQ 1a*) app features were searched for that corresponded to the theoretical indicators of psychological empowerment perceived relevance, perceived competence, perceived self-determination, and perceived impact. Translated from the psychological empowerment descriptions as described by Schulz and Nakamoto (2013) in Chapter 7.1.1, features supporting perceived *relevance* of self-management behaviors increase the chance that a diabetes patient experiences the feeling that a specific behavior (app use, other self-management behaviors) is worth investing energy in. Features supporting perceived *competence* increase the chance that the patient believes in his or her capabilities to produce desired results by the app use. Features supporting perceived *self-determination* promote the choice to make autonomous decisions about self-management behaviors. Features supporting the perceived *impact* enhance the feeling that the executed behaviors (e.g., app use) have an impact on self-management outcomes.

For behavioral empowerment (*RQ 1b*) app features were searched for corresponding to the theoretical indicators of shared decision-making between HCPs and patients, and respective HCP-patient communication. The more relevant information is willingly shared with the patient through the app (HCP-patient communication), and the more feedback is given by the HCP using the app, the more empowering the communication can be considered, based on the idea of shared decision-making as described in Chapter 7.1.2 (Emanuel & Emanuel, 1992). Thus, features supporting shared decision-making styles and respective HCP-patient communication were collected following the theoretical understanding of behavioral empowerment by HCPs. Features to communicate with HCPs were expected to deliver a channel for HCP-patient communication and HCP support.

In addition to behavioral empowerment by the HCPs, and following the theoretical argumentation in Chapter 7.1.2, features supporting behavioral empowerment by the patient's private social networks were collected from the data. A patient's social networks can be a source of behavioral empowerment (family, other patients, friends, etc.) as argued in Chapter 7.1.2. Thus, options in the app to communicate with other individuals suffering from diabetes, or with family members, were expected to provide a channel for social support by the private social user network.

For an app quality assessment (*RQ 1c*) an adapted version of the Mobile App Rating Scale (MARS) by Hides et al. (2014) was used. At the time of data collection, only few published tools for measuring app quality in a systematic and comprehensive way were available. Based on 372 criteria for assessing app quality from 25 published papers, conference proceedings, and online resources (Hides et al., 2014), the MARS was the most comprehensive available tool for rating app quality. It had shown good internal consistency with $\alpha = .90$, and inter-rater reliability of ICC = .79 in Hides et al. (2014), and had been used in several studies to measure app quality (Bardus, van Beurden, Smith, & Abraham, 2016; Bohme, von Osthoff, Frey, & Hubner, 2017; Chavez et al., 2017; Larco, Diaz, Yanez, & Luján-Mora, 2018; Masterson Creber et al., 2016; Schoeppe et al., 2017; Thornton et al., 2017). The MARS includes an engagement score, a functionality score, an aesthetic score, an information score, and a subjective quality score (Table 5).

Only the most relevant ten MARS items were included for reasons of parsimony (Table 5) and a 5-point Likert scale was used, with one displaying the lowest quality and five the highest. From the MARS, all items of the app subjective quality score (MARS, section E) were included to have the full subjective quality score at disposal, as well as one or two items from each the engagement score (section A), the functionality score (section B), the aesthetics score (section C), and the information score (section D) that best represented the respective score and were most relevant for the respective score, and were best suitable and most relevant for the analysis of diabetes apps (details see Chapter 1 in Appendix). In this way all sections were taken into consideration while shortening the MARS considerably. Due to its length the MARS could not be included in the analysis in full. Section E as an additional MARS part looking at perceived app impact was excluded due to irrelevance to this research (similar in Chavez et al., 2017). The five quality aspects *app availability*, *user impression*, *professionalism*, *comprehensiveness*, and *app profit orientation* were added to the analysis as these aspects had been found relevant for a quality assessment throughout the app review (Table 5). User impression and availability appear in MARS in the general app classification. Table 5 displays the operationalization of app quality in the diabetes app analysis.

The final codebook contained 1) detailed information on the search procedure to detect apps, 2) the background app information from the respective app store, 3) the app feature assessment, 4) the app user target group assessment, and 5) the app quality assessment (see Chapter 1.4 in Appendix, Brew-Sam & Chib, 2019).

12.1.2   App Collection Procedure

An Android and iOS app search was conducted (at the end of October/the beginning of November, 2015) on English free-to-download diabetes apps that were frequently downloaded and used by Singaporean end-users in 2015 (Statista, 2015), using the keywords *diabetes*, *blood sugar*, and *glucose*. The focus was on English apps, as English was the most spoken language in Singaporean homes at the time the study was conducted (Department of Statistics Singapore, 2015).

Table 5. App Quality Assessment (Study 1)

Subcategory/scale	Items	Description	Source
MARS scale – A: Engagement	Entertainment	Is the app fun to use?	MARS item 1 (Hides et al., 2014)
MARS scale – B: Functionality	Performance Ease of use	How accurately/fast do the app features and components work? How easy is it to learn how to use the app; how clear are the menu labels/icons and instructions?	MARS items 6 and 7 (Hides et al., 2014)
MARS scale – C: Aesthetics	Visual appeal	How good does the app look?	MARS item 12 (Hides et al., 2014)
MARS scale – D: Information	Accuracy of app description Correctness of app content	Does app contain what is described? Is app content correct, well written, and relevant to the goal/topic of the app?	MARS items 13 and 15 (Hides et al., 2014)
MARS scale – E: Subjective App Quality	App recommendation App use frequency Willingness to pay Overall star rating	Subjective app quality rating by coder	MARS items 20 to 23 (Hides et al., 2014)
Availability	Platform availability	System availability	MARS app classification (Hides et al., 2014)
	Technical aspects (app features)	Assessing what features app offers	Adapted from MARS app classification Hides et al. (2014)
Comprehensiveness	Connectivity to external devices, availability of websites, desktop versions, Facebook pages, related apps	Quality aspects that relate to app comprehensiveness	Added
Professionalism	Privacy policy, app certification	Quality aspects that relate to app professionalism	Added
Profit Orientation	Advertising, in-app purchases	Quality aspects that relate to app profit	Added
User Impression	User ratings, rating numbers	User ratings, user impression	MARS app classification (Hides et al., 2014)
	Download numbers	Numbers of downloads	Added

Note. Due to the length of the MARS scale only the most relevant items regarding diabetes apps were selected.

The focus was on free-to-download apps for two reasons: First, the majority of app users were found to download mainly apps that are free-to-download (Statista, 2015). Viennot, Garcia, and Nieh (2014) previously reported that paid apps accounted for only .05% of app downloads. Second, a first check of the app stores showed that the vast majority of the apps were free-to-download, aiming to attract app users and using in-app purchases instead (apps free-to-download with in-app purchases were included in the analysis).

Only apps from the two operating systems Android and iOS were included, comprising almost the entire global market share with 97% (International Data Corporation, 2015). Due to a lack of established criteria, the app store ranking was used as an indicator for usage frequency (further information on this aspect see Appendix Chapter 1.1 on the app store characteristics and the app store search). The app search was conducted by a trained researcher through the Apple App Store and Google Play on two mobile Android and iOS devices from 29th of October to 7th of November, 2015.

The search results in the app stores varied depending on the country of the registered accounts, or the country device settings. A previous comparison of app searches from devices with different country account settings had shown highly varying search results. This confirmed previous findings on country differences in app reviews (Grundy et al., 2016). An iPad was set back to default settings and was registered anew with a Singaporean dummy account, to assure iOS search results were shown for Singapore (this was not relevant for Android). An iPad was chosen for the iOS search because the iPad displayed further category and ranking settings that were not shown on an iPhone. The devices used for the app search (iPad mini model ME276GP/A with iOS 9.1 and Samsung Galaxy S4 with Android Version 4.3) contained the latest operating systems to make sure the latest apps could be found and run on the devices.

Similar to the app review by Arnhold et al. (2014), only diabetes specific apps were searched for (excluding apps like general calorie counters that were not specifically designed for people with diabetes). In the search for diabetes apps for self-management there was no limitation on the type of diabetes to be analyzed or which type of diabetes patients the included apps targeted.

To ensure a sufficient number of apps on the one hand, and to limit the overall number of apps on the other, the first 50 free-to-download apps were selected for each search term (diabetes, blood sugar, glucose) in each app store (for more information on Study 1 methodology see Appendix). The number of included apps in previous app reviews was shown to vary widely (see Table 2 in Appendix). A study by Grundy et al. (2016) showed that the number of apps included in 91 app review studies varied from sample sizes of six to 3727 apps. In an analysis of the Google Play app store, Viennot et al. (2014) found that the top 10% of most downloaded apps accounted for over 96% of the total downloads, and the top one percent for over 78%. A study by Dogruel et al. (2015) and Henke, Joeckel, and Dogruel (2018) reported that users searching for apps tended to pick the apps shown in the top positions of the app stores. Thus, the first 50 apps were expected to be the ones most frequently downloaded by users. A potential bias caused by selecting only the first 50 apps in each store for each search term is discussed in Chapter 12.4 on study limitations.

After removal of duplicate apps and apps that did not follow inclusion criteria by the main researcher (Table 6), the final app list contained 121 diabetes apps for Android and iOS, with 24 iPad-specific apps, 51 iPhone apps, and 46 Android apps for diabetes self-management (Table 7) that were fully coded using the developed codebook (Chapter 1.4 in the Appendix; Brew-Sam & Chib, 2019). iPad & iPhone apps were treated as duplicates if the app names and the provider names were identical and if the apps showed identical content. Additionally, 22 diabetes apps that included diabetes recipes, magazines, and journals were available. Due to their static character and similarity to an electronic book these apps were recognized but not used for further coding of features, with no features being available (Table 7).

12.1.3   Pretesting and Coding Procedure

Coders were trained on the codebook and the procedure before the pretest and main coding took place (Brew-Sam & Chib, 2019). The pretest contained several steps, included 45 apps and was run with three academic coders, to ensure that the information provided in the codebook was understood the same way by all coders. The average coding time for one app was 28 minutes at the beginning of the pretest. The coding time improved, and the coding proved more coherent after additional coder training. As a following step, an inter-coder reliability test was conducted to check for reliability in the coding procedure. Here, the coders coded 30 apps to cover 10% of the original number of 301 found apps as a standard procedure (DeSwert, 2012). Forty-seven variables were included in the codebook version of the third pretest. The Holsti formula (Holsti, 1969) was used to calculate the total actual agreement across all variables in the three coders in 30 apps, as well as the agreement for each variable.

Table 6. Diabetes App Inclusion Criteria (Study 1)

	Criteria
App store	Apps found in specified app stores: 1. Google Play Store (accessed through an Android phone or tablet) 2. Apple App Store (accessed through an iPad)
Keywords (app search)	Apps found through specified keywords: 1. Diabetes 2. Blood sugar 3. Glucose
App language	Apps available in English
App download	Apps that can be downloaded for free (despite potential in-app purchases)
App purpose	Apps designed specifically for diabetes self-management, e.g., glucose monitoring, diabetes nutrition, diabetes diary, etc. (apps that are not diabetes specific are e.g., apps for measuring general blood pressure)

Table 7. Diabetes App Collection Procedure Results (Study 1)

Apple App Store – iPad only	Apple App Store – iPhone only	Google Play Store
any age group, sorted by relevance	any age group, sorted by relevance	search in apps only (category)
142	150	150
442 free-to-download apps in English 141 duplicates removed (same app name and provider name in same app store) 301 apps		
61	112	128
30 excluded: 6 duplicates 12 not diabetes specific 3 not available anymore 2 not free to download (paid) 0 prank apps[a] 3 require specific devices 3 technical failure 1 other reason	57 excluded: 2 duplicates 40 not diabetes specific 3 not available anymore 1 not free to download (paid) 0 prank apps[a] 1 requires specific devices 9 technical failure 1 other reason	71 excluded: 0 duplicates 10 not diabetes specific 6 not available anymore 1 not free to download (paid) 49 prank apps[a] 0 require specific devices 3 technical failure 2 other reasons
31	55	57
7 not coded (features) due to static character:	4 not coded (features) due to static character:	11 not coded (features) due to static character:
3 diab. journal/magazine 4 diab. recipe apps	1 diab. journal/magazine 3 diab. recipe apps	3 diab. journal/magazine 8 diab. recipe apps
24 iPad	51 iPhone	46 Android
121 apps coded (features)		

Note. Reprint/replicate from Brew-Sam & Chib, 2019 [a] Prank apps are apps that just pretend to deliver a certain service (e.g., fake blood pressure measurement through the device screen)

Only codes that were fully identical were accepted as agreement, which meant that all codes, as well as missing data, should occur equally in each coder. The overall result showed an average agreement percentage of 66% across all variables ($M = .66$, $SD = .100$) with a range of Min = .43 and Max = .87. Four variables showed an agreement of $M \geq .80$, fourteen variables an agreement of $M \geq .70$, eighteen variables an agreement of $M \geq .60$, nine variables an agreement of $M \geq .50$, and two variables an agreement of $M \geq .40$.

The relatively low agreement values potentially could be explained with the interactivity of mobile smart device apps. Krippendorff (1980) suggests an agreement value of .80 as an acceptable intercoder agreement with an acceptable minimum of $\alpha = .60$ to $\alpha = .67$ (DeSwert, 2012). Depending on the devices used, device settings, tailoring options of the devices and the apps themselves, the content displayed differently. The interactivity and dynamic of online apps had to be considered. After a round of final training, a check was made for improvement in inter-coder reliability (six apps). The score using Holsti method was $M = .82$ ($SD = .190$; Min = .33; Max = 1.00) this time (43 variables included, few variables changed after pretest 3). Sixteen variables showed full agreement of $M = 1.00$, fifteen variables an agreement of $M = .83$, eight variables an agreement of $M = .67$, one variable an agreement of $M = .50$, and 3 variables an agreement of $M = .33$. The low agreement in few variables again mainly derived from the interactivity of the apps and features, as well as some differences in understanding of features. To remove these low agreement values an additional coder training was undertaken. Inter-coder reliability improved after this additional training, resulting in an acceptable agreement.

After pretesting, the app coding (2nd to 29th of February, 2016) was conducted by three trained academic coders, using an Android smartphone, an iPad, and iPhones (with the latest operating systems for coding; Coder 1: Mi4, Android 5.0; Coder 2: Apple iPad Air Wi-Fi-16GB iOS 9.2.6 and iPhone 6 iOS 9.2.1, Coder 3: iPhone 6, iOS 8.2).

The coding unit was the single information delivered in the app (e.g. app feature). The unit of analysis was the respective app. The unit of context was additionally information on the related app store or related websites (e.g., release date).

Overall, the app review did not intend to provide a full coverage of all available apps in 2015/2016 due to a dynamic app market. It had to be acknowledged that app data gets outdated quickly. However, the situation on the app market for diabetes self-management has not drastically changed since the data analysis in 2016 (a check for new apps was conducted 2018).

12.1.4 Data Analysis

Numeric and text variables were defined, and coder comments were entered where additional information on the coded data was available. Ninety-nine was defined as missing data ("don't know" category). An overall shortened-MARS score was calculated (mean score from ten items). For analytical purposes, it was assumed that an app quality score below two denoted poor app quality, while a score above four denoted good quality (5-point scales used). Quantitative data analysis was undertaken in IBM SPSS version 25.

12.2 Results

12.2.1 Features and Types of Diabetes Apps

As outlined in Brew-Sam & Chib (2019), the majority (62%) of the analyzed 121 apps comprised diabetes or health data logbooks for diabetes data monitoring (diabetes trackers/diaries, Figure 3). These mainly included logbooks to record and to analyze BG values over time. A smaller percentage included learning tools and information apps to educate the user, for example through educational videos (12%). In addition, the app sample contained blood glucose or other conversion calculators (7%, e.g., calculators to convert BG values measured in mmol/l to mg/dl) and diabetes community apps (3%, e.g., forum/chat apps). Marginal diabetes app categories comprised nutrition apps (e.g., databases for carbohydrate content in food), exercise apps, and specific diabetes apps for kids (logbooks for kids) or gaming/quiz apps (diabetes quiz) (Table 8).

In addition to the mentioned types of the 121 included apps, 22 diabetes recipe apps and diabetes journals, eBooks, magazines, and audiobooks were found. These were not included for coding of features due to their static character (no features available to code) (Table 7). Overall, the majority of diabetes apps aimed to provide a tool to support data tracking and to guide self-management. For example, instead of writing down BG values by hand, the (logbook/diary) apps offered direct health data input, sometimes in combination with other features.

Despite the main focus on diabetes apps for diabetes patients, three percent of the apps were targeted at HCPs in the context of diabetes self-management procedures. These were not excluded in the app search procedure. Ninety-four percent of all apps were clearly designed for adult diabetes patients, with a mere one percent aimed at children with diabetes. Eighty-five percent of the diabetes apps were designed for use by all diabetes patients without targeting a specific type of diabetes patient (Table 8).

12.2.2 App Features Corresponding to Psychological Empowerment Indicators

Specific app features (Table 8) corresponded specifically with theoretical indicators of empowerment (see Table 9 for link, see Brew-Sam & Chib, 2019). App features such as customization, rewards, and interactivity were assigned to the psychological empowerment indicators of (1) perceived relevance. Educational and data monitoring features (including reminders) were assigned to (2) perceived competence while analytical and graphic features were assigned to (4) perceived impact (*RQ 1a*). Features supporting (3) perceived choice could not be found.

(1) Tailoring/customization features were of importance for the empowerment indicator of *perceived relevance* by providing an opportunity to individualize and adapt an app for individual needs. The majority of the analyzed apps failed to tailor services to specific patient subgroups with differing needs (e.g., young versus older people). Eighty-five percent did not target any specific type of diabetes patient, but were meant for general use by all individuals with diabetes (Table 8). Only 13% of the analyzed apps specifically targeted T2DM patients, and an equal 13% targeted T1DM patients. A marginal percentage of apps had specific functionality for other forms of diabetes

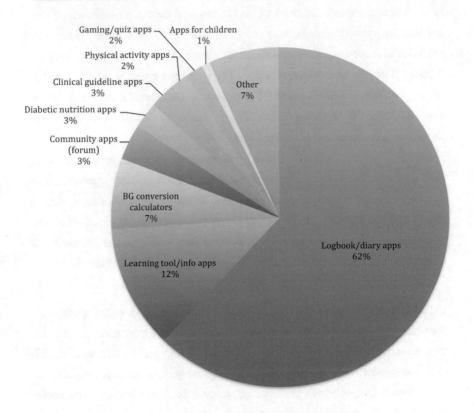

Figure 3. Types of diabetes apps in the sample (Study 1)

Notes. Reprint/replicate from Brew-Sam & Chib (2019), *N* = 121.

(8%) or for pre-diabetes patients (5%). Ninety-four percent of all apps were designed for adult diabetes patients, with one percent aimed at children with diabetes (Table 8). Furthermore, there was hardly any tailoring for disease characteristics, such as length of the disease since diagnosis, or for demographic categories such as age (in 14% of the apps, Table 8), or gender. It is acknowledged that this analysis focused on app features and did not consider the content of messages in the apps, for example the text content.

Table 8. Diabetes App Features and Characteristics (Study 1)

Variable	Characteristics	% of N
App Type	Logbook or tracker or diary for data monitoring	62.2
	Learning tool/info app/guide (e.g., educational videos)	11.8
	BG conversion calculator	6.7
	Community app/patient forum	3.4
	Diabetes nutrition app	2.5
	Clinical guidelines	2.5
	Exercise/physical activity app	1.7
	Gaming/quiz app	1.7
	Kids app for diabetes	.8
	Unspecific/others	6.7
App Features	Documentation function (monitoring)	69.2
	Analysis function	59.2
	Feedback to app provider	45.8
	Login	39.2
	Export function	32.5
	In-app purchases	31.1
	Registration mandatory	30.8
	Data forwarding	29.2
	Reminder/Notifications	25.8
	Learning function	25.0
	Advertising	24.4
	Connection to external devices	17.8
	Registration optional	15.0
	Comm. with app users	10.8
	Recipe suggestions	9.4
	Comm. with personal network	9.2
	Pictures/videos	9.2
	Reward features	6.7
	Gaming	5.0
	Advisory function/therapy support	3.3
	Inclusion therapy/care program	2.5
Other App Characteristics	iOS availability	73.1
	Android availability	65.0
	App website(s) available	55.8
	Privacy policy available	36.7
	App social media page available	27.5
	Advertising in app	24.4
	Desktop version available	18.5
	Quality criteria available	7.6
	Tailoring for demographics	14.2
	Tailoring for disease	9.2
	Tailoring for other	0
Target Groups	Patients (adults)	94.2
	Other users	7.5
	Physicians/qualified health personnel	5.8
	Children/adolescents	.8
	Not specified diabetes type	85.1
	T2DM	13.3
	T1DM	12.5
	Other diabetes types (e.g., gestational)	7.6
	Pre-diabetes	5.0

Notes. Table based on Brew-Sam & Chib (2019), $N = 121$, the values do not sum up to 100% because of partly mixed forms of apps.

Therefore, no conclusions could be drawn for the current analysis in relation to appropriateness of written content for users, and whether the content enhanced the perceived relevance of an app use, as well as of other self-management activities.

Few other app features aligned with the perceived relevance of diabetes apps, such as reward features (7%), for example, bonus point systems for regular app use as part of a self-management regimen. These also included interactive features like gaming elements (5%), which could enhance the individual relevance for specific target groups, such as adolescents.

(2) *Perceived competence* for self-management was supported by app learning features that potentially enhanced diabetes knowledge. Improved knowledge could strengthen perceived self-management competence. A quarter of the apps (25%) were found to provide features supporting learning processes and diabetes-specific knowledge through educational text or video content (Table 8). It was concluded that diabetes education was not the primary aim of most diabetes apps in the sample.

Facilitated data input through structured self-monitoring was also assigned to the empowerment indicator perceived competence for self-management. Features for structuring BG documentation could promote improved diabetes monitoring, in turn leading to perceived competence. The available app features confirmed typical characteristics of diabetes logbooks in a majority of the app sample, with 69% of the apps supporting structured documentation of health data, like the storage of regularly measured BG values (Table 8). Documentation options included automatic data upload from the BG meter to the app via Bluetooth, taking pictures of the meter screen, or using the device keyboard to type BG and health data. Eighteen percent of the apps allowed a connection to external devices (e.g., BG meter, Table 8). Another quarter of the apps included reminders or automatic notifications (26%), such as reminders to test BG values, that could support structured self-monitoring.

(3) Features corresponding to *perceived choice* (self-determination) in self-management could not be found, such as information on various treatment alternatives, insulin options, or oral medication differences. Choice could provide a foundation for the patient to feel better informed and better able to make his/her own decisions. Regarding perceived choice, no information was found on voluntary or obligatory use of

apps as part of specific programs (e.g., DAFNE, Dose Adjustment For Normal Eating program, http://www.dafneonline.co.uk). An obligatory use of diabetes apps could potentially hinder perceived choice regarding the feeling of self-determined technology-supported self-management. On the other hand, an obligatory app use might deliver extrinsic motivation to regularize an app use for self-management, and thus create the feeling of necessity to use the app as part of an overall diabetes program.

(4) Data monitoring features were frequently accompanied by data analysis options, as well as options of graphic data outputs (59%). Graphic data outputs and data analysis features bear the potential to promote the *perceived impact* of self-management activities. The analytical features facilitate health data interpretation by the user and provide overviews over outcomes of health behavior changes. An app displaying improvements in the BG values might directly communicate the effectiveness of the self-monitoring to the patient. Thus, graphic and output features can be expected to enhance the perceived impact of the app use (Brew-Sam & Chib, 2019).

12.2.3   App Features Corresponding to Behavioral Empowerment Indicators

As outlined in Brew-Sam and Chib (2019), app features were investigated that linked with behavioral empowerment indicators by allowing for shared decision-making with HCPs and supportive HCP-patient communication, as well as social support from private social patient networks (*RQ 1b*). Features that included apps in ongoing diabetes programs (including automatic data access for HCPs), forwarding and export features to provide HCPs with health and lifestyle data, and HCP contact opportunities were assigned to behavioral empowerment (HCP-patient relationship), as were features to communicate with other users and the individual social patient networks (social support by the private network). The results indicated that only a small percentage of the apps (3%) were part of a larger therapeutic program for diabetes care (Table 8). With almost two thirds of apps being logbooks for data monitoring (62%) (Figure 3), one third of all apps were found to provide export features (33%) or data forwarding features (29%).

Table 9. App Features Corresponding to Empowerment Dimensions (Study 1)

Empowerment dimensions	Indicators	App features	Description
Empowerment – psychological	1) Perceived relevance	Tailoring features for specific patients' needs (disease background, demographics, other), reward systems, gaming/interactive features	Features supporting perceived relevance
	2) Perceived competence	Diabetes education & learning functions, data monitoring, reminders	Features supporting perceived competence
	3) Self-determination/perceived choice	Features on treatment alternatives & voluntariness of use	Features supporting perceived choice and own initiative
	4) Perceived impact	Data analysis functions, graphic output	Features supporting perceived impact
Empowerment – behavioral	1) HCP-patient relationship (shared decision-making) & communication	Advisory functions, data export & forwarding, registration & login, part of therapy program, feedback to developer	Features supporting HCP-patient relationship and communication
	2) Support by private social networks	Communication with private social networks, communication with other app users	Features relating to the support by private social networks

Note. Reprint/replicate from Brew-Sam & Chib (2019)

These features allowed the app user to provide HCPs with app patient data, e.g., via email or print (Table 8). Most apps did not enable automatic access to mobile patient data for the HCPs, and thus user-friendliness of the data download and export options was likely to influence the usefulness of such features.

The functionality of registration and login options made continuous data tracking and automatic data access more complicated. Registration (mandatory 31%, optional 15%) and login options (39%, Table 8) were partly available for communication and data storage. Only three percent of the apps included some sort of direct contact to HCPs for therapy support or for advisory purposes (Table 8), for example direct online feedback from HCPs through chat. One app (Glyco by Holmusk, https://glycoleap.com) provided a chat function allowing direct contact to dieticians. Overall, the diabetes apps failed to enable direct and improved contact to HCPs, in order to empower the patient through direct feedback, information, or motivational support.

Social support by private patient networks has been presented as an essential aspect of behavioral empowerment, and it can be argued that features allowing information exchange with other diabetes patients, or with private patient networks, would promote online communication that could empower the user. However, only a tenth of diabetes apps included features to communicate either with other app users (11%), or with their own private social user networks (9%, Table 8). Thus, the idea of support by private patient networks was not promoted comprehensively in the apps of the sample.

In contrast to the few features promoting social support (HCPs, private networks), feedback to app providers was possible in almost half the apps (46%, frequently through email), and an additional analysis revealed that more than half the apps had an accompanying website connecting the user to the app provider (56%), while one third had a Facebook page that could deliver additional company information (28%).

In summary, only a limited range of app features could be found that supported the theoretical dimensions of psychological and behavioral empowerment in the majority of the examined apps. Features frequently were limited to sub-sections of the apps, and innovative features were almost completely absent (Brew-Sam & Chib, 2019).

12.2.4 Diabetes App Quality Assessment

App quality was described as influencing the use of diabetes apps, as well as their potential for self-management. Overall, the apps performed relatively poorly in terms of subjective quality assessment (*RQ 1c*, subjective quality score, Table 10, MARS section E) with $M = 2.82$ ($SD = 1.16$, 5-point scale), with coders rating the average subjective app quality lower than the medium range 3.00 (Table 10). A closer examination of subjective app quality distribution revealed that 33% of the analyzed apps were rated low subjective quality (≤ 2.00). Only 15% were rated high subjective quality (values ≥ 4.00). Similar to subjective app quality, the app engagement score was lower than the medium range 3.00 (fun/entertainment of app, Table 10, section A). The functionality score (app performance and ease of use), the aesthetics score (app visual appeal), and the information score (app accuracy) showed slightly better results with values somewhat above medium range (Table 10, sections B to D).

Using MARS, few apps exhibited very good app quality, with seven apps rated above a total MARS score of 4.50, including the MySugr Apps, Tactio Health Logbook, or the Diabetes Tracker (Table 11). For example, the MySugr Junior App ranked high due to the quality of the app content, accuracy, visual appeal, ease of use, performance and entertainment.

In addition to the MARS items, app availability, professionalism and comprehensiveness, profit orientation, and user impression were examined, with the MARS and the analysis in this research hinting at relevance of these aspects to understanding app quality in greater detail (Table 5). Regarding app availability, seventy-three percent of the apps were available for iOS, while 65% were available for Android (Table 8).

Table 10. Diabetes App Quality Scores from Adapted MARS (Study 1)

Items/scores	M	SE	Median	Mode	SD	R	Min	Max
A. Engagement score (1 item)	2.52	.089	2.00	2.00	.979	4.00	1.00	5.00
Fun/entertainment (1[b])	2.52	.089	2.00	2.00	.979	4.00	1.00	5.00
B. Functionality score (2 items)	3.47	.080	3.50	4.00	.862	4.00	1.00	5.00
Performance of app features (6[b])	3.34	.096	4.00	4.00	1.035	4.00	1.00	5.00
Ease of use (7[b])	3.60	.081	4.00	4.00	.883	4.00	1.00	5.00
C. Aesthetics score (1 item)	3.14	.088	3.00	3.00[a]	.964	4.00	1.00	5.00
Visual appeal (12[b])	3.14	.088	3.00	3.00[a]	.964	4.00	1.00	5.00
D. Information score (2 items)	3.42	.082	3.50	3.00	.891	4.00	1.00	5.00
Accuracy of app description (13[b])	3.49	.084	4.00	4.00	.917	4.00	1.00	5.00
Correctness of app content (15[b])	3.34	.092	3.00	4.00	1.004	4.00	1.00	5.00
E. Subjective app quality (4 items)	2.82	.107	2.75	1.75	1.157	4.00	1.00	5.00
Recommendation of app (20[b])	2.94	.117	3.00	3.00	1.285	4.00	1.00	5.00
App use frequency (21[b])	3.02	.117	3.00	3.00	1.283	4.00	1.00	5.00
Willingness to pay for app (22[b])	2.28	.113	2.00	1.00	1.238	4.00	1.00	5.00
Overall star rating (23[b])	3.09	.107	3.00	4.00	1.152	4.00	1.00	5.00
MARS total score (10 items)	3.06	.084	3.00	3.90	.898	3.60	1.30	4.90

Notes. N = 113-120, 5-point scales with higher values displaying more positive quality results.
[a] Multiple modes exist, so the smallest value is shown
[b] Item numbering from MARS (Hides et al., 2014; Stoyanov et al., 2015)

An examination of aspects of app professionalism demonstrated that only 37% of the apps provided a privacy policy, and less than 10% provided criteria for third-party accreditation (e.g., certificates) (Table 8). A minority of the apps offered inclusion in associated therapy/prevention programs that might stand as a proxy for high quality standards. In terms of app comprehensiveness, only around a fifth of the apps offered a desktop versions for the computer (19%), or could be connected to external devices like blood glucose meters (18%). As mentioned before, only a part of the apps were accompanied by a website (56%) or by a Facebook page (28%) (Table 8). Registration and login options were partly available for communication and data storage. A quarter of the free-to-download apps were found to contain advertising (which did not even include all pop-ups during use), and around one third included in-app purchases (Table 8).

Table 11. Apps Rated Best in Quality – Overall Adapted MARS Score (Study 1)

App name	Provider name	MARS score
MySugr Junior	MySugr GmbH	4.90
Health2Sync- Diabetes Care & Blood Sugar Tracking	H2 Inc	4.80
MySugr Diabetes Diary	MySugr GmbH	4.70
Tactio Health: My Connected Health Logbook	Tactio Health Group	4.60
Diabetes Kit Blood Glucose Logbook	Diabetes Labs LLC	4.60
Diabetes Tracker	Mig Super	4.50
Diabetes in Check: Coach, Blood Glucose & Carb Tracker	Everyday Health Inc.	4.50

Notes. Apps with total MARS rating ≥ 4.50 (MARS scale from 1.00 lowest app quality to 5.00 highest app quality), 10 items from MARS scale by Stoyanov et al. (2015)

Table 12. App Downloads and User Ratings (Study 1)

	N	M	SD	Min	Max
User rating Android (1-5 stars)	46	4.13	.408	3.00	4.80
Number of Android user ratings	46	1256.83	2843.104	4.00	12015.00
Number of Android downloads	46	33923.91	77663.374	500.00	500000.00
User rating iOS current app version (1-5 stars)	19	4.03	.950	1.50	5.00
Number of user ratings iOS current app version	19	122.37	403.623	5.00	1775.00
User rating iOS all app versions (1-5 stars)	43	3.96	.687	2.00	5.00
Number of user ratings iOS all app versions	43	1519.67	7788.343	5.00	50959.00

Note. Codebook in Chapter 1.4 in Appendix; user ratings were available for both Android and iOS from 1 to 5 stars, with 5 stars displaying the best user rating; no download numbers were available for iOS apps

Despite some evidence of lacking app quality in the sample (e.g., MARS, privacy policy), the user impression analysis showed average medium to high ratings for both iOS apps (N = 75) and Android apps (N = 46), with both systems using a user rating scale from one to five stars (with five stars the best rating, Table 12). The availability of user ratings was limited for iOS apps (Table 12), and comparability between iOS and Android could not be proven due to potential underlying rating differences. Correlations between user ratings and MARS scores were weak and not significant (r = .258, p = .104, n = 41 for iOS user ratings on all app versions with MARS total score; r = .179, p = .245, n = 44 for Android user ratings with MARS total score from 10 items).These results indicated that a user rating analysis might be of limited suitability for assessing app quality from a professional perspective. Further research should examine discrepancies between user ratings and app quality assessment.

12.2.5 MySugr App Series Chosen for Study 2

From the diabetes app quality assessments and the feature analysis, the diabetes app with the highest app quality in the sample (MARS score) and a high variety in provided app features was chosen for further use in Study 2 interviews. Table 11 displays that the MySugr App (https://mysugr.com/) rated highest in app quality. MySugr is not a single app but a series of diabetes apps for self-management, including a blood sugar logbook for adults (MySugr Diabetes Diary/Tracker/Logbook), a logbook app for children (MySugr Junior), a learning app providing educational content (MySugr Academy/Diabetes Training), a fun app (MySugr Monster Selfie), a scanner app to transfer BG values from the BG meter to the app using the device camera (MySugr Scanner/Importer), and a quiz app (Diabetes Quiz by MySugr, see Figure 4, access 2016/2017). Five of these six apps appeared in the app search and were part of the app sample (see list of included apps in Table 3 in Appendix). Only the MySugr Monster Selfie App did not appear in the sample[10].

Due to the combination of six apps, the MySugr App Series provided a large range of features that could be combined individually. Features assigned to all empowerment dimensions were available, like tailoring options (e.g., specific app for children, Junior App), (graphic) analysis features (Logbook App), gaming features (Quiz App), educational content (Academy App), feedback functions (Logbook App), or synchronization functions (Scanner App). In addition, MySugr provided an additional desktop version (https://hello.mysugr.com/app/login/#login), and used social media for addi-

---

[10] An advanced graphic analysis web tool was added for analyzing BG developments (*MySugr Analyse*, access date 03/01/2018), as a well as a web tool for importing data into the app (*MySugr Importer*) and a coaching option for feedback from certified diabetes educators. However, at the time of the diabetes app analysis these tools were not available yet. The *Junior App*, the *Monster App* and the *Quiz App* could not be found in 2018 anymore, and probably were removed from the app market due to low user numbers.

tional information (e.g., Facebook, https://www.facebook.com/mySugr/). In this way, MySugr was the most innovative and advanced diabetes app option in the app sample. The app quality was rated high for the MySugr Apps (two apps among the apps with highest quality in the sample, Table 11). As a result, the six apps of the MySugr Series (Logbook, Junior, Scanner, Monster, Academy, Quiz App) were chosen as exemplary app series for discussion of diabetes apps with patients in Study 2 interviews.

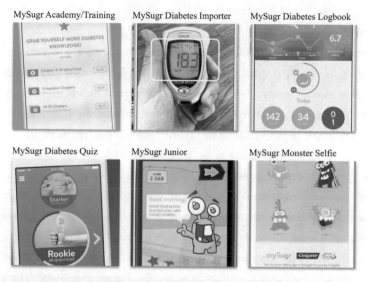

Figure 4. MySugr app series (2016/2017).

The MySugr App Series previously had been evaluated or analyzed in a couple of publications (Biller Krauskopf, 2017; A. S. Miller, Cafazzo, & Seto, 2016; Rose, König, & Wiesbauer, 2013). Rose et al. (2013) used the MySugr management system in a trial and found that the retention of use was 88% over 12 weeks, and 70% over 28 weeks. Moreover, "self-reported clinical outcomes included a reduction of HbA1c blood results" (p. 1). Thus, previous studies confirmed the high quality of the MySugr App Series found here.

12.3 Discussion

When the results of this research and previous literature and research findings were compared, conclusions could be drawn about the previous assignment of diabetes app features to indicators of empowerment. The analytical review of features revealed that the potential of the analyzed diabetes apps for empowerment was far from being realized. Features corresponding to indicators of empowerment were limited to a small set of infrequently applied features (e.g., limited tailoring).

Psychological Empowerment

(1) As shown in Brew-Sam and Chib (2019), previous research on app features assigned to indicators of psychological empowerment showed that tailoring (as a means for *perceived relevance*) could enhance individual message relevance (Kreuter & Wray, 2003). Indeed, diabetes research frequently demonstrated the differences in self-management requirements in T1DM or T2DM patients (American Diabetes Association, 2010). Likewise, differences in age groups require diverse tailoring strategies for age specific content (e.g., addressing children versus older people). The diabetes apps studies and developers need to tailor information more specifically to the type of diabetes and other demographic characteristics of specific patient groups (Thabrew, Stasiak, Garcia-Hoyos, & Merry, 2016). In particular, the lack of children as an app target group in the sample (Table 8) suggested that app developers failed to realize the potential of technology for young "digital native" target groups highlighted by previous studies (Lau, Lau, Wong, & Ransdell, 2011). A case for stronger inclusion of interactive elements (assigned to perceived relevance) for selected target groups can be made on the basis of prior mHealth studies on the effects of gamification (S. C. Boyle, Earle, LaBrie, & Smith, 2017; Johnson et al., 2016; Lister, West, Cannon, Sax, & Brodegard, 2014), such as reward systems implemented in mobile games (e.g., bonus points) (Lewis, Swartz, & Lyons, 2016).

(2)/(3) The *perceived competence* component of psychological empowerment suggests that app features comprising educational elements and for structured self-monitoring are important. Previous studies found significant relationships between knowledge and perceived competence (e.g., Glajchen & Bookbinder, 2001), demonstrating that structured patient training can improve both perceived and actual (glycemic) control (Debussche et al., 2018; Howorka et al., 2000), and that knowledge can be promoted by interactive features (Cook, Levinson, & Garside, 2010). According to Cook et al. (2010) "studies revealed that audio narration, video clips, interactive models, and... facilitate higher knowledge and/or satisfaction" (p. 755). However, it is also possible that educational content might not just promote but also reduce perceived competence, e.g., when a person is educated on something too complex to understand. Existing research is unclear whether structuring self-monitoring elements can enhance perceived self-management competence, yet shows that these elements can potentially improve perceived control (Debussche et al., 2018; Howorka et al., 2000). Perceived control is used synonymously with the empowerment indicator *self-determination/choice* (Gutschoven & van den Bulck, 2006; Menon, 2002).

(4) Prior studies confirmed that graphic elements influence *perceived impact* and health-related behavioral intentions (Villanti, Cantrell, Pearson, Vallone, & Rath, 2014), as well as data interpretation (Jansen, McCaffery, Hayen, Ma, & Reddel, 2012). The Study 1 sample reiterated existing research findings showing that analytical and graphic output features frequently went along with self-monitoring features in the sample (assigned to *perceived impact* of a diabetes app use).

Behavioral Empowerment

Regarding indicators of behavioral empowerment, and features supporting *HCP-patient interaction* and *support by private social user networks*, the literature is quite established (Brew-Sam & Chib, 2019). The relevance of both HCP support and peer or family support has previously been proven for diabetes self-management (Armour et al., 2005; U. Isaksson et al., 2015; Litchman et al., 2018; A. G. Ramirez & Turner, 2010; Wallace et al., 2018; Whitehead et al., 2018). Research suggests that mobile health applications are not efficient as stand-alone means for self-management support, but have to be included into the *HCP-patient relationship* or into larger care programs to guarantee long-term use and effectiveness by HCP support (Katz, Mesfin, & Barr, 2012). Apps need to be officially approved for inclusion in diabetes care (e.g., apps promoted by the government) (Kwong, 2015). Inclusion of apps in diabetes programs provides synergetic effects, with a stronger motivation for app use due to program inclusion, app selection and informed app use, as well as technology supported HCP-patient cooperation, time-saving feedback procedures, improved data monitoring (adherence), and improved patient data collection (K. H. Miller, Ziegler, Greenberg, Patel, & Carter, 2012). Moreover, diabetes apps should provide features to enable support by private social patient networks (other patients, family, etc.), with (online) support by private social networks having been proven effective for self-management motivation (Barak et al., 2008; Barrera, 2006; Bartlett & Coulson, 2011; Batenburg & Das, 2015; Gallant, 2003; Gomez-Galvez et al., 2015; Litchman et al., 2018; Maki & O'Mally, 2018; Oh & Lee, 2012; van Uden-Kraan et al., 2009; White, 2001; Wright et al., 2010). Despite these previous study results, the Study 1 sample hardly included any features supporting HCP support or an inclusion of private social networks in patient self-management.

Potential of Diabetes Apps for Self-Management

Interpreting an app potential for empowered self-management from the results could only be summarized as sobering, as there were only limited features that corresponded to the theoretical empowerment dimensions, as well as limited app quality causing concern, and dissatisfactory quality of standards (e.g., lack of privacy policies). The subjective quality results indicated that app quality left a lot to be desired, and that the majority of the apps needed improvement to satisfy higher quality standards. The results confirmed previous study findings, concluding that:

> There is a great need for high quality tools that can be prescribed by physicians and whose use can be monitored by a health care team.... If we are to engage patients in self-management, we need to provide them with more sophisticated tools within the context of the patient-physician relationship that ensures that patients have the guidance they need to succeed in their own care on all disease dimensions, not just one or two. (Brahmbhatt et al., 2017, p. 52)

The analysis also led to certain interpretive conclusions on the likelihood of maintained long-term use of the provided diabetes apps, also referred to as app "stickiness", (Furner et al., 2016). The feature analysis revealed few strategies by app providers to gain sustained users by including reward systems, gaming elements, or entertainment features. These features have been proven effective in previous research yet were found in fewer than 10% of the apps (DeShazo, Harris, Turner, & Pratt, 2010; Kato, 2012). Studies also started to consider the possibility of prescription of diabetes apps as an effective strategy, similar to prescribing medication (Berkowitz, Zullig, Koontz, & Smith, 2017; Martin, Vicente, Vicente, Ballesteros, & Maynar, 2014; Osmani, Forti, Mayora, & Conforti, 2017).

The reasons for non-inclusion of these features need to be discussed, including the awareness of app developers of the relevance of certain features for self-management as stated by research results, or if the exclusion of certain features was intentional as they were considered not to be attractive to consumers (e.g., an exclusion of communication features in diabetes apps might be explained by the fact that patients use other apps for communication with peer patients).

Further obstacles hindering sustained app use included frequent technical app failure (Table 7), required in-app purchases (in 31% of the apps), frequent advertising in the apps (in 25% of the apps) and an unstable market dynamic preventing the apps from being reliable and trustworthy tools for diabetes self-management. Fifteen apps had been excluded from the coding procedure due to persistent technical failure (Table 7). A further 12 apps had been excluded due to the dynamic of the app market, and were no longer available between app collection and app coding.

Overall, strategies to motivate diabetes patients to maintain the app use over time should be advanced (Thabrew et al., 2016) and more sophisticated mobile tools within the context of the HCP-patient relationship are needed (Brahmbhatt et al., 2017; Zaires et al., 2017). However, advanced and innovative diabetes apps cannot be designed by simply adding multiple features to an app to satisfy theoretical concepts or target group requirements. This would lead to a laundry list of must-have app features (Brew-Sam & Chib, 2019). From a technical perspective this is not a feasible nor practical approach, as multiple features would make a diabetes app unwieldy, and hard to use for less tech-savvy user groups (Brew-Sam & Chib, 2019). Instead of including a variety of features at once, other strategies have to be thought of to improve the diabetes app potential. Features have to be carefully selected for specific needs of specific target audiences, and ways of giving target audiences choices in feature selection have to be found. App series or app "packages" provide an opportunity, offering several apps that can be individually selected and combined by the user (e.g., MySugr app series, https://mysugr.com/). Moreover, the idea of combined apps has to be taken one step further by providing a choice to patients in selecting the app features individually that are relevant to them, to enhance app usage and the potential of diabetes apps for self-management (Brew-Sam & Chib, 2019). Moreover, addressing data protection issues might increase trust in diabetes apps, with data protection issues not solved yet (Huckvale, Prieto, Tilney, Benghozi, & Car, 2015; Sunyaev et al., 2015). Health data is usually sensitive, and concern about health data protection might be one potential reason for lacking app use.

12.4 Study Limitations

There was general concern about reliability and comparability of coding throughout the app analysis due to the interactivity and dynamic of diabetes apps. Compared with computers mobile smart devices are more problematic regarding this aspect as these devices differ considerably in size, display, and settings. To achieve acceptable intercoder reliability, appropriate strategies have to be found.

Accessibility of app features and functions varied considerably, as well as displayed app content, and app functionality. For example, some features of an app showed only after specific input, with algorithms altering the display of app content considerably. Similarly, the device's operating system possibly influences app functionality in a way that some features or add-ons do not appear. Looking at app accessibility, some apps were free with all functions (full version), while some were free with limited available functions and features (lite versions), and some versions were accessible with all functions but for a limited period of time (trial versions). These differences were hard to distinguish in the coding but mattered greatly, depending on the app version used. Functions and features of apps to be coded needed to be specified very clearly to achieve acceptable intercoder reliability. Similarly, similarity in app names caused confusion for coders who were looking for an app with a specific name. Specific additional information had to be given to identify a specific app (also see Brew-Sam and Chib, 2019).

Some difficulties related to the definition of the unit of analysis occurred in the course of the app analysis. The apps usually were not independent from other online sources, but connected to additional websites, forums, online platforms, etc.. Online mobile diabetes tools are changing into cloud-platforms that can be accessed through various mobile and non-mobile devices.

The dynamic of the app market was a general problem for app selection and has to be addressed in future research (4% of apps had been removed from the app store between the collection of the apps and the main coding).

Concerning inclusion criteria, only free-to-download apps for diabetes self-management were examined. Further research is needed that evaluates if pay-to-download apps are more theoretically relevant than free-to-download apps, and if bias could be caused by a one-sided selection. It could be argued that apps that have to be paid for might deliver products higher in quality than free apps, or might include more features supporting behavioral empowerment (contact to HCPs, inclusion in diabetes programs). However, the vast majority of apps in the sample offered in-app purchases instead of pay-to-download. Thus, only a small number of pay-to-download apps were excluded from the analysis (apps that were free-to-download containing in-app purchases were included, see Table 6).

Similarly, including the 50 apps appearing at the top of the app stores might cause a certain bias regarding the app evaluation. It is likely that apps frequently downloaded appear at the top of the stores. However, ranking algorithms were non-transparent especially for the Apple App Store, and other apps outstandingly supporting empowerment or relevant in other aspects might be missed.

Overall, most coding challenges just appeared in the coding process itself due to the interactivity of contents. The development of the codebook therefore required more time than in a traditional content analysis, with several pretesting steps necessary. From a communication scholar's perspective, solutions for dealing with communication content becoming more and more dynamic and interactive have to be found. The traditional approach to understanding content analysis in communication studies as a "research technique for the objective, systematic and quantitative description of the manifest content of communication" (Berelson, 1952, p. 18) is facing problems when it comes to interactive online content. It is questionable if there is still "manifest content of communication" at all when looking at app content (study limitations of Study 1 also see in Brew-Sam & Chib, 2019).

12.5 Conclusion

To summarize, Study 1 revealed that the diabetes mHealth apps field is at a nascent stage of development, with current implementation failing to live up to the potential (Brew-Sam & Chib, 2019). In addition to partly insufficient app quality, only a narrow set of app features supported psychological and behavioral empowerment dimensions in the majority of the examined diabetes apps. This is contrasted with literature that points to the relevance of these app features for empowerment. Further research is required that examines app features corresponding to empowerment dimensions in greater depth (Brew-Sam & Chib, 2019).

Research that discusses what empowered self-management means for different users of diabetes apps is also needed. Thus, a diabetes (non-)user perspective was necessary after the app perspective as a next research step towards understanding empowerment as an antecedent of diabetes app use here. The app analysis showed that the technological status quo of diabetes apps needed improvement, yet could not deliver information on actual diabetes app use as part of empowered self-management, and thus interview and survey research was necessary to get a more detailed idea of user and non-user views. Despite the limitations of most diabetes apps, the MySugr app series providing an array of features and high quality could be chosen as an example for discussing app use in Study 2 interviews.

Due to the relevance of an app quality assessment – with (low) app quality interfering with maintained app use over time – the study suggests an initial criteria set for determining app quality, with a preliminary list of the top apps derived from this process (Table 11). The shortened MARS scale created and used in this research was proposed as an initial framework for gauging and communicating app quality. Further research is needed that tests a shortened version of the MARS scale for validity.

Future research should also look at empowerment in the sense of machine-based empowerment delivered through algorithms. Based on the definition of empowerment, machine-based empowerment was not included here. It has to be discussed if behavioral empowerment can also be delivered by apps using automatic algorithms. In this context, it has to be evaluated in what sense the empowerment by a machine is still "behavioral" (being understood as a behavior of another individual).

Moreover, future research should further relate app quality aspects to theoretical empowerment aspects. Quality dimensions for example could be related to decision-making styles of HCPs as part of behavioral empowerment. Quality could then be understood in a broader sense, asking to what extent an app supports e.g., participatory decision-making by HCPs (or paternalistic decision-making styles as the contrary).

13 Study 2 – Interviews on App Use for Diabetes Self-Management and the Relevance of Empowerment

After consideration of aspects of empowerment as an antecedent of diabetes app use from an app perspective in Study 1, studies 2 and 3 added a diabetes (non-) user perspective (*RQ 2*) as explained in Chapter 8.2 and as included in Figure 2. With a lack of basic research on underlying diabetes app adoption and usage processes (Chapter 4.2.3) as well as empowerment as a potential anteceding factor from this perspective (Chapter 7.3), Study 2 followed a qualitative research approach as a first step, before adding quantitative research in Study 3.

Study 2 was used to (1) receive basic information on diabetes app use as well as usage rejection from a diabetes (non-) user perspective to be able to understand underlying use processes in greater detail. as well as to (2) get a first insight into the relevance of empowerment as an anteceding factor of diabetes app use in addition to technology adoption and general self-management factors. To achieve the latter, the role of empowerment as a factor for explaining app user and non-user differences (*RQ 2a* and *RQ 2b*, Table 4) in addition to factors from technology adoption theory (*RQ 2c*) and from diabetes self-management (*RQ 2d*) was examined (Table 4). This exploratory procedure allowed first conclusions about differences between diabetes app (non-) user types regarding empowerment. This then delivered first information about the role of empowerment for diabetes app use.

13.1 Method

To answer the research questions (*RQ 2a-d*) and to get a first insight into the use of diabetes apps for self-management and empowerment as a potential antecedent, 21 semi-structured face-to-face interviews were conducted with diabetes patients in Singapore between December, 2015 and September, 2016.

The use of a semi-structured interview guide (see Chapter 2.1 in Appendix) enabled respondents to answer all interview questions, as well as to leave the interviews open for the patients' detailed contribution. To collect comprehensive data the participants were asked to contribute as much information as possible. To be able to answer *RQ 2* on diabetes app (non-) user differences regarding empowerment (Table 4), the interview guide contained (1) questions on psychological and behavioral empowerment presented in the form of general questions on the diabetes condition, the treatment, and the self-management, (2) questions on previous diabetes app use, perceived app utility, and app preferences, and (3) questions relating empowerment aspects to app use.

To receive further detailed information on technology adoption and self-management background factors (*RQ 2c* and *RQ 2d*, Table 4), as well as to be able to use additional scales on empowerment (*RQ 2a* and *RQ 2b*), a background information questionnaire (paper-and-pencil, see Chapter 2.2 in Appendix) collected further details not asked in the interviews, as well as relevant scale scores for each participant. This prevented the researcher from presenting a number of scales in the interviews. The scale results were needed to help distinguish diabetes app (non-) user types regarding empowerment (*RQ 2*).

The background information questionnaire included (1) demographic information, (2) diabetes background information (type, length of disease, medication, check-ups, other diseases, diabetes education, support group participation, perceived difficulty of diabetes), (3) a scale summarizing self-management activities (SDSCA, Toobert, Hampson, & Glasgow, 2000), (4) previous eHealth and mHealth use (specific websites and apps used), (5) a psychological empowerment scale (Mantwill et al., 2015) and a second scale for comparison (R. M. Anderson et al., 2003), (7) two behavioral empowerment scales on HCP decision-making and HCP-patient communication (PDMstyle and PCOM, Heisler et al., 2002), and information on social support by private patient networks. Information on the included scales can be found in Chapter 3.3 in the Appendix. The questionnaire was considered useful to be able to draw back to additional information for explanatory and analytical purposes. The operationalization is explained in detail in the following chapter.

13.1.1 Operationalization

Operationalization of Empowerment

The operationalization of empowerment in Study 1 was based on the theoretical approach described in Chapter 7.1. Psychological empowerment was examined using open interview questions on all four psychological empowerment indicators *perceived relevance, perceived competence, self-determination, and perceived impact* in the interview guide (direct and indirect questions), and the psychological empowerment scale of the EMPOWER project by Mantwill et al. (2015) in the background information questionnaire ($M = 4.62$, $SD = .14$, $\alpha = .943$).

The EMPOWER project scale (Mantwill et al., 2015) measuring psychological empowerment was chosen because it captures all four indicators of psychological empowerment in a health context. The scale can be adapted for specific diseases by updating disease information accordingly. The EMPOWER project specifically used the scale in context of diabetes. The scale is an adaption of the management empowerment scale by Spreitzer (1995), which is based on the empowerment model by Thomas and Velthouse (1990). Based on the model by Thomas and Velthouse (1990), Schulz and Nakamoto (2013) developed what is called the "Health Empowerment Model" in Trentini et al. (2015). Based on the Health Empowerment Model, the same research team adapted Spreitzer's (1995) scale to the health context, and used the resulting scale in the context of the EMPOWER project on diabetes (Mantwill et al., 2015). The scale measures perceived relevance, perceived competence, self-determination and perceived impact, for example by assessing the level of agreement with "dealing with my diabetes is very important to me" (perceived relevance).

A validation of the specific EMPOWER project scale has not been published within the EMPOWER project yet. However, several validations are available and these were considered sufficient proof for the validity of the psychological empowerment scale by Mantwill et al. (2015). First, a validation of Spreitzer's empowerment scale can be found in Spreitzer (1995). Second, a validation of the Health Empowerment Model can be found in Trentini et al. (2015). Third, as part of the EMPOWER project Lamprinos et al. (2016) validated the ICT-based patient empowerment framework. Fourth, the homogeneity of interview results regarding empowerment and the EMPOWER project scale results delivered additional proof of scale validity. For information on the scale also see Chapter 3.3 in the Appendix.

Behavioral empowerment was measured using open direct and indirect questions on empowering behaviors of the interviewees' supervising HCPs and private social networks. Chapter 7.1.2 showed that HCP decision-making styles and HCP-patient communication can be considered aspects of behavioral empowerment by HCPs. Thus, the focus was especially put on decision-making and communication when assessing behavioral empowerment by HCPs. The Provider Participatory Decision-making Style Scale (PDMstyle, $M = 3.69$, $SD = .29$, $\alpha = .947$) and the Provider Communication Scale (PCOM, $M = 3.51$, $SD = .71$, $\alpha = .880$) by Heisler et al. (2002) were included in the background questionnaire to measure HCP decision-making and HCP-patient communication as aspects of behavioral empowerment (also see Chapter 3.3 in the Appendix for scale information and validity). The PDMstyle scale for example asks how often the HCPs took patient preferences into account when making treatment decisions. The PCOM for example asks the participant to rate how the HCPs who took care of the patient were at explaining side effects of medication. Background information on all supervising HCPs and their relevance to diabetes care was collected from each patient. As described in the theoretical chapter on behavioral empowerment (7.1.2) a special focus was put on behavioral empowerment by the doctor as the patient's main medical supervisor.

Behavioral empowerment by private social patient networks was examined using questions adapted from the Diabetes Care Profile (Fitzgerald et al., 1996b) on social support in the interview guide and in the background information questionnaire (see Chapter 2 in Appendix).

Operationalization of Diabetes App Use and Influencing Factors

Following the definition of "app use" in Chapter 4.1, diabetes app use was investigated openly with all information collected about previous app use for diabetes self-management reported by the interview participants, in addition to general online use for diabetes self-care (websites, online health information seeking). For example, information was collected on reasons for starting a diabetes app use, and for maintaining it. Information on the types and the names of diabetes apps used, the length of the app use, and information sharing through the apps was collected (see Study 2 interview guide and background information questionnaire in Chapter 2 in Appendix).

The non-usage aspect, including app rejection and app usage barriers, was relevant for the study to be able to differentiate types of both diabetes app users and non-users. As described in Chapter 5.5 and to answer *RQ 2* (Table 4), it was necessary to understand rejection of apps and non-usage as a counterpart of use. Following theoretical suggestions in Chapter 5.5, inhibiting factors (usage barriers towards diabetes app use) were examined based on theoretical "restriction evaluations" from previous models (Wirth et al., 2008). Information was collected on reasons for stopping a diabetes app use, or on reasons for never using diabetes apps, as well as on general interest in the app use, and knowledge about diabetes apps.

Apart from empowerment, information supporting other factors from the UTAUT expected to influence diabetes app use (Table 2), as well as factors influencing successful diabetes self-management (Table 1) was collected using the interviews and the background information questionnaire. Apart from collecting all text extracts that represented the UTAUT and the self-management factors from the interviews, the background questionnaire added questions on personal factors including self-management and attitudes, demography, personal diabetes background, physical factors including type of diabetes, medication, length of disease, and other diseases, and provider and care access factors including diabetes education, and support group participation similar to the Diabetes Care Profile (DCP) (Fitzgerald et al., 1996b). An adapted version of the Summary of Diabetes Self-Care Activities (SDSCA, $M = 4.10$, $SD = .84$, $\alpha = .563$) (Toobert et al., 2000) was used to collect data on coping in the form of self-management behaviors. This scale evaluates previous self-management activities, for example by asking: "On how many of the last seven days did you eat five or more servings of fruits and vegetables?". Due to the low Cronbach's alpha value of this adapted SDSCA, the items of the scale were partly used as single items in data analysis. The low alpha probably derived from the changes made in the original SDSCA version (removal of items). Attitudes towards diabetes were collected with an item

about the perceived influence of diabetes on life. Chapter 13.2.3 and Table 16 introduce all Study 2 results on theoretical factors.

13.1.2   Sampling and Data Collection Procedure

Due to the exploratory character of Study 2, purposeful sampling was used to select
Study 2 participants (Singaporean diabetes patients). Twenty-one Singaporean patients suffering from diabetes were chosen for interview participation. Participants
were chosen in a way that a variety of demographic and disease characteristics were
available in the sample (age groups, gender, employment, type of diabetes, length of
diabetes, etc.). A variety of characteristics was relevant for the app (non-) user typology, to be able to identify different user and non-user subgroups based on usage differences and influencing factors. Both type 1 and type 2 diabetes patients were included
in the sample (one participant had pre-diabetes as a condition that can lead to T2DM).
Participants for the first 15 interviews were addressed and chosen through contacts in
the   diabetes   society   of   Singapore   support   group   (former   DSS,
http://www.diabetes.org.sg), as well as research contacts to the DAFNE group (Dose
Adjusting for Normal Eating) in Singapore (SingHealth, 2017). DAFNE is a specialized program teaching insulin injecting patients how to calculate carbohydrates to adjust the insulin injection accordingly. Participants for the rest of the interviews (16 to
21) were chosen through a cooperation with TOUCH Diabetes Support
(http://www.diabetessupport.org.sg). A potential bias caused by a certain degree of
self-selection and the participation in support groups due to the sampling method is
discussed in Chapter 13.4 on study limitations.

Before data collection, an IRB application (IRB-2016-01-012) was submitted to and
approved by the Nanyang Technological University Review Board for ethical approval of the interviews.

Despite the development of the interview instruments (interview guide, background
information questionnaire) based on theory and research questions, a dynamic qualitative data collection approach was followed, with data being collected and analyzed as
a part of the resulting narrative (Bryman, 2008a, Chapter 22). Thus, the interview
guide and the background information questionnaire were extended when interview

data delivered relevant information that was not included in the interview instruments. This procedure allowed the capture of missing relevant information that came up during conducted interviews.

The interviews were conducted with no other persons present except for the interviewer, to create a confidential atmosphere for the participant. Consent forms were signed by all interview participants. All interviews were conducted by the same interviewer (researcher) in English. As described in Chapter 12.2.5, from Study 1 diabetes app review results, the MySugr app series including six different apps was chosen to be shown to the interviewees as an exemplary diabetes self-management app. MySugr provided a range of six apps with interactive features and was found to be of high quality. In comparison with other apps, this app series was found to be one of the more advanced apps for diabetes self-management in 2016/2017. The six apps were shown to the participants and they were asked to comment on the app features, as well as to talk about their app usage, preferences regarding app usage, perceived usefulness of diabetes apps and other app related aspects. Moreover, the apps were used to introduce diabetes apps to participants who had never used apps for diabetes self-management before.

The background information questionnaire was filled in by each participant subsequent to the face-to-face interview. A 20 Singapore dollar gift voucher was offered as a compensation for participation in the approximately one hour interview after interview completion.

13.1.3 Data Analysis – Thematic Analysis

As a foundation for examining diabetes app (non-) user differences regarding empowerment and other influencing factors (*RQ 2*), thematic analysis was chosen for interview data analysis because there was a theoretical foundation available (empowerment approach, UTAUT, self-management), and the aim was to use a theory for data analysis rather than to develop a theory from the data[11]. Braun and Clarke (2006) de-

---

[11] Theory and the research questions stood at the beginning of the research, thus one of the approaches most frequently used for qualitative data analysis "the grounded theory approach" (Glaser & Strauss, 1967) did not

fine thematic analysis as "a method for identifying, analyzing, and reporting patterns (themes) within data" (p. 6) and state that "through its theoretical freedom, thematic analysis provides a flexible and useful research tool, which can potentially provide a rich and detailed, yet complex account of data" (p. 5). Other advantages of thematic analysis can be found in Braun and Clarke (2006). According to the authors, in thematic analysis themes or patterns are searched for across an entire data set, rather than just within one data item.

To fulfill quality criteria for thematic analysis, major issues and decisions had to be made transparent from the analysis. It had to be specified what was considered a theme and what "size" a theme needed to be (Braun & Clarke, 2006). In the analysis, a theme was considered a topic deriving from any numbers of statements containing the same or similar idea of content relevant in relation to the research questions. The key themes derived from theory (empowerment, UTAUT, MPA, self-management) and were divided into subthemes. Moreover, relevant interview content was additionally considered a theme if the same idea repeatedly occurred in several data sets.

The aim of the analysis was not to describe the overall data set to reflect its full content, but the focus was on the specific theoretical background and the research questions *RQ 2a* to *RQ 2d*. According to Braun and Clarke (2006), the analysis could be called "theoretical thematic analysis" because the themes derived (at least partly) from the theoretical background in contrast to an inductive approach. A semantic (essentialist/realist) approach (Braun & Clarke, 2006) was chosen in which the data was analyzed at an explicit level according to what had been said in the interviews, and the meaning of the said content was interpreted in a straightforward way. Both description and interpretation of the data in context of the theory was provided. In line with the described phases of thematic analysis by Braun and Clarke (2006, p. 35), the data analysis included several steps:

---

seem to be the most suitable one. This is because grounded theory aims at developing theory out of the collected data (Holloway & Todres, 2003) instead of using theory for looking into the data (see process in Bryman, 2008a, p. 545). In contrast to the selected thematic analysis approach here, the goal of a grounded theory analysis is described as "to generate a plausible – and useful – theory of the phenomena that is grounded in the data" (Braun & Clarke, 2006, p. 8; McLeod, 2001).

(1) The interviews were transcribed completely (full interviews) with all verbal information included by three research assistants (communication studies). Only explicit verbal communication was transcribed. The transcribers used common audio programs (Audacity, Quick Time Player, VLC Player) to transcribe the interviews manually. No program was used for automatic transcription. Each interview was listened to and compared with the transcript for accuracy. Especially accuracy of interpunction was checked, with meanings of sentences changing with differing interpunction.

(2) Following suggested procedures for thematic analysis (Braun & Clarke, 2006; Bryman, 2008b), preliminary categories were created following the research questions, the theoretical approaches, the interview guide, and the background information questionnaire. A matrix was created for these preliminary categories. The extracts from the interviews were filled into the categories and additional explanatory notes were added in brackets if needed. The matrix contained the categories and subcategories (dimensions from theory), the numbered questions from the interview guide and from the background information sheet, as well as the interview numbers and dates, and the interview content extracts. The matrix enabled an overview of the participants' answers in each category and subcategory. If important interview extracts didn't fit into existing categories, new categories were added.

(3) From the categories, larger themes were created where necessary, from the interview content and from grouping important extracts. The procedure of creating categories, and themes was dynamic and was constantly adapted in a process of learning from interview content.

(4) The themes were reviewed in relation to the data extracts and the entire data, and (5) results were analyzed (user and non-user typology), related back to the research questions and literature, summarized, and interpreted. The 15-point checklist found in Braun and Clarke (2006) was used for all relevant steps in thematic analysis[12].

---

[12] The checklist includes: "1. The data have been transcribed to an appropriate level of detail, and the transcripts have been checked against the tapes for 'accuracy'. 2. Each data item has been given equal attention in the coding process. 3. Themes have not been generated from a few vivid examples (an anecdotal approach), but instead the coding process has been thorough, inclusive and comprehensive. 4. All relevant extracts for all each theme have been collated. 5. Themes have been checked against each other and back to the original data set. 6. Themes are internally coherent, consistent, and distinctive. 7. Data have been analysed – interpreted, made sense of – rather than just paraphrased or described. 8. Analysis and data match each other – the extracts illustrate the

The additional information given in the background information questionnaire was given codes, and analyzed in IBM SPSS version 25. Mean scores were calculated from the included scales (empowerment scale, PDMstyle and PCOM scales). Scoring information on the empowerment scale had not been published in the EMPOWER project. However, sum scores were applied with higher values displaying higher levels of psychological empowerment (Trentini et al., 2015). The results from the scales were added to the thematic analysis results of the interviews for creating the diabetes app (non-) user typology.

13.1.4   Data Analysis – Diabetes App User Typology

To be able to answer *RQ 2* on (non-) user differences regarding empowerment and other factors from technology adoption and self-management theory (Table 4), and based on the categories derived from thematic analysis results, a diabetes app user and non-user typology was developed to understand the role of empowerment as an antecedent of diabetes app use by using an exploratory and qualitative approach.

Firstly, diabetes app users and non-users were grouped together based on the diabetes app (non-) usage characteristics *previous use and non-use*, including *reasons for the use or non-use, interest in and knowledge about diabetes apps* in non-users, the *length of usage* in users, *types and names of apps used*, and *information sharing through the apps*. Individuals with similar characteristics regarding these diabetes app (non-) usage aspects were grouped together until there was a maximum of homogeneity within a group, and a maximun of heterogeneity between the groups. This resulted in a typology of diabetes app users and non-users with a limited number of subgroups.

---

analytic claims. 9. Analysis tells a convincing and well-organised story about the data and topic. 10. A good balance between analytic narrative and illustrative extracts is provided. 11. Enough time has been allocated to complete all phases of the analysis adequately, without rushing a phase or giving it a once-over-lightly. 12. The assumptions about, and specific approach to, thematic analysis are clearly explicated. 13. There is a good fit between what you claim you do, and what you show you have done – i.e., described method and reported analysis are consistent. 14. The language and concepts used in the report are consistent with the epistemological position of the analysis. 15. The researcher is positioned as active in the research process; themes do not just 'emerge'" (Braun & Clarke, 2006, p. 36).

Secondly, the resulting types of app (non-) users were compared for psychological and behavioral empowerment, for other factors influencing technology use (based on the UTAUT for use, see Table 2, and based on technology rejection categories e.g., from MPA for non-use, see Chapter 5.5), and for factors influencing general self-management (see Table 1). Diabetes self-management factors were taken into consideration because interview data showed that general self-management factors were relevant to all self-management behaviors. Diabetes app use was described as one self-management behavior among others in Chapter 4.1. All factors from theory that were found to be of relevance and that were sufficiently supported by text paragraphs were extracted from the interview data (for results see Chapter 13.2.3).

Thirdly, further hypotheses were drawn from the typology results regarding the relationship between empowerment as an antecedent factor, other antecedent factors, and diabetes app use to be tested in Study 3 (hypotheses see Chapter 13.2.4.2).

13.2 Results

13.2.1 Sample Description

In total, 21 face-to-face interviews of approximately one hour each were available in English language, as well as 20 additional background questionnaires (one was missing, Ming). Half of the sample was female ($n = 10$), and half male ($n = 11$). The sample contained type 1 ($n = 9$) and type 2 ($n = 11$) diabetes patients (and one with pre-diabetes). Diabetes patients of all age groups were present in the sample: Five patients were younger than 30 years old, four patients were aged 35 to 50, three patients were in their 50s, and eight were older than 60. Both married and non-married patients were equally present, and education levels were medium (some high school) to high (undergraduate degree). Some participants were working full-time ($n = 8$), while some were working part-time, homemaker, student, or retired ($n = 3$ in each category). Apart from one person, all held Singaporean passports (one Malay). Table 13 delivers an overview of all interview participants (including age, type of diabetes, medication, and year of diagnosis), while Table 14 summarizes all main sample characteristics.

Diabetes Background

The length of diabetes since diagnosis ranged from four to 38 years (Table 14), with the sample majority having suffered from the condition for a long time ($n = 7$ less than ten years, $n = 4$ ten to twenty years, $n = 8$ more than twenty years). In terms of family history of diabetes, the sample showed that more than half of the participants ($n = 12$) explicitly mentioned a family history of diabetes (either type 1 or type 2). For example, Deng Li (age 68, T2DM) said: "I was expecting it because I got a diabetic line.... I used to give my dad injections, many years ago.... So I was expecting it, and I knew it was creeping up". Some participants didn't know whether one of their ancestors had diabetes, or were unsure about it. Regarding the health status of the interview participants, eight patients suffered from other diseases as well, like heart conditions, high blood pressure, high cholesterol, hypothyroidism, or breast cancer (Table 14).

The participants went for regular health checkups every two to six months, with an average of $M = 3.83$ months ($SD = 1.36$). Seventeen diabetes patients had received diabetes education at some point, and due to the sampling method 15 were part of a diabetes support group (Table 14). Two were part of the DAFNE diabetes program for type 1 diabetes patients (dose adjusting for normal eating, SingHealth, 2017).

Some differences between T1DM and T2DM patients were analyzed, and between patients injecting insulin and patients taking oral medication. Twelve patients injected insulin using a syringe, two used insulin pumps, and ten took oral diabetes medication (Table 13). All nine T1DM patients reported to inject insulin exclusively, while four T2DM participants used insulin injections and oral medication parallel, one injected insulin (but was supposed to use oral medication in addition; Bharat, age 66, T2DM), and six took oral medication only. The pre-diabetes patient (Kang, age 67) was not on any medication (Table 13). These results showed that insulin injection could not be assigned to T1DM only. Thus, the commonly used term "insulin-dependent diabetes" for T1DM is misleading (e.g., Roger, 1991).

For both T1DM and T2DM groups, healthy nutrition, exercise, foot and eye care, BG testing and recording, and regular checkups were mentioned as essential components of their self-management (similar for pre-diabetes). Self-management behaviors could not be assigned to one type of diabetes, and thus the self-management similarities in diabetes types rather than the differences were emphasized. For example, adherence to self-management behaviors and a rigorous regimen occurred in both groups, and were not necessarily related to the type of diabetes. Yet, it could be confirmed that T1DM participants in the sample were diagnosed earlier in life, and on average at a younger age ($M = 37.78$, $SD = 18.12$) than T2DM patients ($M = 56.00$, $SD = 11.66$). Four type 1 diabetes patients (Sona, Cheng, Kaiyan, and Navin) reported counting carbohydrates to adjust insulin injections very accurately in relation to the amount and type of food consumed, while only one T2DM participant on insulin pump (Gu Fang, age 29) counted carbohydrates. For patients not injecting insulin, carbohydrate counting for accuracy in food consumption was mostly irrelevant.

Overall, these demographic and disease results showed that the sample was diverse, consisting of diabetes patients from different subgroups. Due to the recruitment method most participants were part of a support group, and rather belonged to the active and motivated patients who had at least some diabetes education. However, five patients (Li Ting, Ei Tek, Rei Hong, Zhen Wei, Ming) were available who belonged to the group of patients at high-risk for health complications (in the following called "high-risk patients") because of lack of diabetes knowledge, insufficient self-management and unfavorable self-management attitudes, lack of motivation for self-management, and/or critical health conditions (e.g., high BG values). The diabetes patients who were considered high-risk in the sample were T2DM (Li Ting, Ei Tek, Rei Hong, Zhen Wei, Ming; see Table 7 in Appendix). In contrast to most participants who managed to keep their BG values stable in a medically uncritical range[13], dangerous BG shifts were reported in the high-risk patients. For example, Li Ting (age 49, T2DM) mentioned: "In the morning when I test my blood it's about, let's say ah, it's 15…. Then after that I inject insulin, right? After about two hours it goes… tremendously down to about 9…. Sometimes at night I have this uh, low hypo count. Always wake up in the [night]… then I feel all sweating, all this".

---

[13] Normal healthy BG: less than 5.6 mmol//l (less than 100 mg//dl); pre-diabetes: range between 5.6–6.9 mmol//l (100–124 mg//dl); diabetes: normal range between 7.0–7.9 mmol//l (126–142 mg//dl); diabetes: high from 8.0 mmol//l or higher (144 mg//dl), also see American Diabetes Association (2016).

Table 13. Interview Participants (Study 2)

No.	Name	Age	Gender	Diabetes type	Medication	Year (diag-nosis)
1	Sona	20	F	T1DM	Insulin injection	1999
2	Xin Qi	56	F	T2DM	Oral diabetes medication	2009
3	Bharat	66	M	T2DM	Insulin injection	1982
4	Li Ting	49	F	T2DM	Insulin injection + oral diabetes medication	2007
5	Gu Fang	29	F	T2DM	Insulin injection (pump) + oral diabetes medication	1996
6	Henna	60	F	T2DM	Insulin injection + oral diabetes medication	1992
7	Deng Li	68	F	T2DM	Oral diabetes medication	2012
8	Jie	64	M	T1DM	Insulin injection	1979
9	Kang	67	M	Pre-diabetes	No medication	2008
10	Ei Tek	60	M	T2DM	Insulin injection + oral diabetes medication	1985
11	Cheng	23	M	T1DM	Insulin injection	2007
12	Rei Hong	61	M	T2DM	Oral diabetes medication	2007
13	Xiu Wen	57	M	T1DM	Insulin injection	1984
14	Kaiyan	42	F	T1DM	Insulin injection	1980
15	Zhen Wei	47	F	T2DM (gesta-tional)	Oral diabetes medication	1998
16	Adit	22	M	T1DM	Insulin injection	2006
17	Ching Ching	64	F	T2DM	Oral diabetes medication	2006
18	Pang	19	M	T1DM	Insulin injection	2009
19	Shi Hui	35	F	T1DM	Insulin injection	1988
20	Ming	-	M	T2DM	Oral diabetes medication	2004
21	Navin	58	M	T1DM	Insulin injection (pump)	1978

Note. Names of participants were changed for reasons of anonymity; table adapted from Table 2 in Rossmann et al. (2019)

Table 14. Sample Description (Study 2)

Variable	n	% of N	M	SD	Min	Max
Age (in years)			48.35	17.46	19.00	68.00
Education						
BA graduate/college graduate	6	28.6				
Some college	7	33.3				
High school graduate	1	4.8				
Some high school	4	19.0				
Other education level	1	4.8				
Employment						
Full- time working	8	38.1				
Part-time working	3	14.3				
Homemaker	3	14.3				
Retired	3	14.3				
Student	3	14.3				
Family status						
Married	9	42.9				
Never married	8	38.1				
Separated/divorced	1	4.8				
Widowed	1	4.8				
Gender						
Men	11	52.4				
Women	10	47.6				
Nationality						
Singaporean	19	90.5				
Malaysian	1	4.8				
Unknown	1	4.8				
Diabetes Background						
Diabetes family history	12	57.1				
Diabetes type						
T2DM (incl. gestational)	11	52.4				
T1DM	9	42.9				
Pre-diabetes	1	4.8				
Diseases (other)	8	38.1				
Education on diabetes (received)	17	81.0				
Length of diabetes (in years)			19.89	12.07	4.00	38.00
Medication						
Insulin injection (syringe or pump)	14	66.7				
Oral diabetes medication	10	47.6				
(Self-) Management						
Check-up frequency (in months)			3.83	1.36	2.00	6.00
Diabetes app use	11	52.4				
Online health information seeking (HIS)	19	90.5				
Part of support group	15	71.4				
Part of diabetes program	2	9.5				

Variable	n	% of N	M	SD	Min	Max
Empowerment						
Psychological empowerment[a]			4.62	.54	3.33	5.00
Behavioral empowerment						
Decision-making style[b]			3.69	1.39	1.00	5.00
HCP-patient communication[c]			3.51	1.13	2.00	5.00

Notes. $N = 21$, results from background information questionnaire, additional interview data where necessary
[a] EMPOWER project scale (Mantwill et al., 2015), from 1 = strongly disagree to 5 = strongly agree
[b] Participatory Decision-Making Style (Heisler et al., 2002), from 1 = none of the time to 5 = all of the time
[c] Provider Communication (Heisler et al., 2002), from 1 = poor to 5 = excellent

13.2.2   Diabetes App Use in the Sample

As a preparation for the (non-) user typology (*RQ 2*), diabetes app use in the sample was examined, including reasons for the use or non-use, the types and names of diabetes apps used, the length of the app use, information sharing through the apps, or general interest in and knowledge about diabetes apps when not using them.

Generally, apart from two persons (Rei Hong and Ming), all participants said they looked for health information online: "You need to Google, and you need to find out yourself" (Xin Qi, age 56, T2DM). Previous app use for diabetes management differed among the participants, from no previous use, no interest in apps, and no knowledge about existing diabetes management apps, to infrequent and short-term app use, and to long-term app use (Table 15; Table 7 in Appendix). Some patients who had not used diabetes apps before, expressed no interest in diabetes apps (e.g., Ming, age unknown, T2DM), while some expressed interest but lacked knowledge of how to use the apps (e.g., Ei Tek, age 60, T2DM). Eleven participants (had) used diabetes-specific apps (Table 14), and 15 (had) used not necessarily diabetes-specific apps for their self-management (e.g., fitness trackers, see Table 9 in Appendix). Most participants were familiar with some apps for diabetes self-management, apart from patients who had no knowledge on app availability (e.g., Rei Hong and Zhen Wei).

Diabetes-specific apps used for self-management were limited to BG logbooks to record daily BG values and other health data (e.g., DAFNE online App, MySugr, Glooko, DiabetesM), and to food databases for receiving information on food ingredients such as carbohydrate levels, for example a food database app by the Singaporean Health Promotion Board. "They used to have these health promotion board app for Singaporeans,… Singapore food" (Adit, age 22, T1DM). Non-diabetes-specific apps used for diabetes self-management included medical information and appointment apps (e.g., Health Buddy by SingHealth, WebMD), BMI and health calculators, fitness apps (e.g., MyFitnessPal), heart rate monitor or step and sleep tracker apps (e.g., Jawbone), and Instant Messaging Apps (e.g., WhatsApp, see Table 9 in Appendix). Some participants reported using apps connected to external devices like BG meters, or step and sleep tracker wristbands (see Table 9 in Appendix). In rare cases the logbook app synchronized automatically with the BG meter or other devices (e.g., Henna, age 60, T2DM). Kaiyan (age 42, T1DM) mentioned that:

> I've been using a app called Glooko…; there's a log I can record my insulin, my… uhh… food, alright, even exercise; …I actually can also sync the steps into the log here…; So and then, I have a… I have a blood sugar meter that I carry with me all the time… So, at the end of the days, usually I'll sync it, sync the… blood sugar into it.

Some participants used diabetes apps connected to online clouds (Sona, Gu Fang, Henna, Cheng, Kaiyan) that automatically uploaded and stored information in the cloud, and in some cases allowed data access for several parties, e.g., the patient and the HCPs (e.g., DAFNE online app). Especially diabetes programs that included an app (DAFNE) used cloud systems to allow HCPs to access the recorded patient information. One DAFNE participant (Sona, age 20, T1DM) said that: "We also can use the app to record our blood sugar every day. Then uh, when we upload it online, it will be the nurses and the doctors and the dietician, they will be able to…yeah, they will be able to see [the data]".

If information sharing through a cloud was not possible, some diabetes patients reported information sharing by downloading the app data and sending it through email to their doctors, while some reported no information sharing with HCPs at all (see Table 9 in Appendix). Gu Fang (age 29, T2DM) reported:

> I will download the data in an Excel sheet. I will just like, edit it a bit, and then send like three months' worth of reading… over… through email…. They [HCPs] have a quick scroll through of my readings for the past three months, because it's color-coded, they can like… tell the trends.

Other patients pointed to difficulties in app data sharing. Xiu Wen (age 57, T1DM) said: "It's very difficult for them [doctors] to collect this information [app data], because there're so many patients, unless they have a project to track". If automatic data upload from external devices was not possible, participants reported using diabetes logbooks after testing BG values, and typing BG values and health data into the app manually (e.g., Cheng, age 23, T1DM).

The frequency of diabetes (logbook) app use particularly varied with the strictness, the frequency and the circumstances of BG testing and recording, with logbooks being used to monitor BG developments. Sona (age 20, T1DM) for example said: "I will forget [the BG recording in the app]… cause sometimes… I just check [the BG] like in a hurry ah". Detailed results on usage frequencies were not available from Study 2. Apart from logbook apps, food database apps informing about food content were mainly used before eating when food content was unknown (Table 9 in Appendix).

The majority of the participants reported using diabetes-specific apps or having used them for some period of time. A number of at least six participants had used a diabetes app for several months (Table 9 in Appendix). For example, Pang (age 19, T1DM) reported that he had tried two or three different apps for diabetes self-management, and that he had used one app for about one year when he was in secondary school. Table 15 summarizes characteristics of the previous app use for self-management as found in the sample.

After presenting sample description results and results on app use in the sample, the following chapter explains the representation of psychological (*RQ 2a*) and behavioral empowerment factors (*RQ 2b*), and of other factors influencing technology (non-) use (*RQ 2c*) and self-management (*RQ 2d*) in the interviews. These results were the foundation for comparing diabetes app (non-) user groups regarding these potential influencing factors. Table 16 delivers a summary of all factors collected from the interviews and based on the theory (theoretical empowerment approach in Chapter 7.1, factors from UTAUT in Table 2, technology rejection aspects in Chapter 5.5, and factors influencing self-management in Table 1).

Table 15. Diabetes App (Non-) Use Categories in the Sample (Study 2)

	Categories	Sub-Categories
Diabetes app use	Previous diabetes app usage (including length)	Never used diabetes apps before
		Short-term diabetes app use (few days to few weeks)
		Long-term diabetes app use (Several months minimum)
	Parallel usage of diabetes apps	One diabetes app
		Several diabetes apps – switching diabetes apps
	Parallel usage of online apps and channels for diabetes management	Diabetes non-specific mobile apps and channels only
		Diabetes apps and other apps/channels parallel
	(Reasons for diabetes app (non-) use)	Varying reasons
	Types of diabetes-specific apps used	Logbook/diary app
		Food database
	Types of diabetes non-specific apps used	Health information apps (e.g., Health-Buddy)
		Fitness apps and devices (e.g., step trackers)
		Instant messenger apps (e.g., WhatsApp)
	Sharing app information (e.g., with HCPs)	Sharing health data through clouds
		Sharing health data through email
		Sharing health data using printouts
		No health data sharing
App usage intention (non-use)	Interest in diabetes apps (in non-users)	No interest or interest in apps
	Knowledge of diabetes apps (in non-users)	No knowledge or knowledge of apps

13.2.3   Potential Antecedents of Diabetes App Use Represented in the Interviews

Empowerment

In relation to psychological empowerment (*RQ 2a*), text extract examples for the perceived relevance of self-management, the perceived competence for self-management, the perceived choice/self-determination in self-management, and the perceived impact on self-management outcomes were available (see extract examples in Table 6 in Appendix):

The *relevance* of diabetes self-management to avoid future health complications was emphasized by most participants (e.g., Sona, Henna, Deng Li, Jie, Kaiyan, Ching Ching, Shi Hui, Ming, and Navin), although some participants reported having other priorities, for example Rei Hong (age 61, T2DM) with his job being the most important, Pang (age 19, T1DM) primarily focusing on education, or Zhen Wei (age 47, T2DM) stressing the relevance of enjoyment.

With the sample including many motivated patients, rather high perceived *competence* for their own self-management was found (e.g., Ching Ching, age 64, T2DM, describing herself as the "model patient"), relatively high perceived *choice* in self-management/self-determination (e.g., Sona, age 20, T1DM), and both limited or high perceived *impact* on diabetes outcomes: While Deng Li (age 68, T2DM) perceived she could influence her BG values, Xiu Wen (age 57, T1DM) reported that he perceived it as very difficult to control BG outcomes (extract examples see Table 6 in Appendix, overview see Table 16).

As part of behavioral empowerment (*RQ 2b*), three types of decision-making styles appeared in the interviews (Table 16): The first group included independent patients taking health decisions mainly themselves with a minor role of doctors and HCPs (Sona, Xin Qi, Bharat, Deng Li, Jie, Kang, Xiu Wen, Zhen Wei, Ching Ching, Pang). This group mainly considered the doctor and other HCPs (nurses etc.) as advisors who delivered medical information as a foundation for their own patient decisions. The second group included patients who took diabetes-related decisions together with their medical supervisors (HCPs), and thus followed a shared decision-making approach with a mutual relationship between the diabetes patient and the HCPs (Gu Fang, Henna, Cheng, Kaiyan, Adit, Shi Hui, Navin). In this group, the doctor sometimes was considered something similar to a friend (e.g., Gu Fang and Henna). The third group included dependent patients following doctors' instructions who mainly did not make diabetes-related decisions themselves but relied on decisions taken by the HCPs (Li Ting, Ei Tek, Rei Hong, Ming). Here, the patients considered the doctors responsible for their treatment and were less active in decision-making themselves (e.g., Rei Hong, age 61, T2DM).

Results of HCP-patient communication revealed that there were large differences in the sample regarding this aspect, including the length of consultations, the offered support in consultations, as well as HCPs' willingness to share medical information in consultations, yet, many participants reported short consultations and limited time for advice from their HCPs: "The doctor is 5-10 minutes only" (Xin Qi, age 56, T2DM).

It could also be shown that the support from private social networks varied widely in patients. The relevance of the support from the family (e.g., Deng Li or Shi Hui) and friends (e.g., Xiu Wen, age 57, T1DM) was pointed out, as well as the support by other patients (support groups, e.g., Deng Li, age 68, T2DM). Deng Li (age 68, T2DM) mentioned that: "It's very important for the patient's family to accompany and to give the doctor… you know… explain to the doc everything". Yet, some participants reported managing their disease without family support (e.g., Ching Ching, age 64, T2DM) or even receiving negative support by their families: "They're involved in a negative aspect. They always say, 'Never mind la! Eat la, just eat'" (Kang, age 67, pre-diabetes).

Table 16 summarizes the categories on empowerment as a factor found in Study 2.

Factors Influencing Technology Adoption and Use from the UTAUT

Analysis of UTAUT factors (*RQ 2c*) as operationalized from theory (Table 2) showed that:

(1) The factors *perceived usefulness* of the diabetes app, and *extrinsic motivation* for its use could be supported by interview extract examples (the latter only insufficiently). Both represented the UTAUT factor *performance expectancy* being mentioned as

Table 16. Factor Collection Summary (Study 2)

	Factors from theory	Categories from interviews	Sub-categories from interviews
Psych. Em-powerment	Perceived relevance	Perceived self-management relevance	Low to high perceived relevance of self-management behaviors
	Perceived competence	Perceived competence for self-management	Low to high perceived competence for self-management
	Self-determination	Perceived choice in self-management	Low to high perceived choice in self-management/care
	Perceived impact	Perceived impact on self-management	Low to high perceived impact on diabetes outcomes by self-managing
Behav. Em-powerment	HCP decision-making	Style of health deci-sion-making	Independent patient with minor role of doctor (advisor)
			Dependent patient with major role of doctor (paternalistic)
			Shared decision-making
	HCP-patient communi-cation	Quality of HCP-patient communication	Little/insufficient time for feedback, HCP taking no time to explain care aspects in detail
			Sufficient time for feedback, HCP taking time to explain care aspects in detail
	Social support by private social net-works (also part of the UTAUT factor social influence)	Diabetes support group participation	Support group member
			Non support group member
		Support by family and friends, other patients	Support by family, friends, other patients in diabe-tes self-management
			No support by family, friends, other patients in diabetes self-management
Technology use – UTAUT	(Behavioral intention)	Interest in diabetes app usage, in combination with diabetes app knowledge	No interest in diabetes apps, no app knowledge
			No interest in diabetes apps, despite app knowledge
			Interest in diabetes apps, knowledge and use
			Interest in diabetes apps, but no use due to lacking app knowledge or other usage barriers
	Effort & performance expectancy (e.g., perceived useful-ness/potential, relative advantage, ease of use, effort, extrinsic moti-vation[a])	Perceived diabetes app usefulness/potential for self-management	Perceived as useful/potential for self-management
			Limited perceived usefulness/limited potential for self-management
		Reasons for starting diabetes app use (ex-trinsic motivation)	Incentives for diabetes app use, rewards for use
	Social influence	Reasons for starting diabetes app use	Recommendations by others
	Facilitating conditions	Reasons for starting diabetes app use	App as part of program
			Promotions/Advertising
	Voluntariness	Reasons for starting diabetes app use	Own interest/own initiation
	Experience	Online health info seeking[b]	Online health info seeking (preference for online information seeking)
			No online health info seeking (offline preference)

	Factors from theory	Categories from interviews	Sub-categories from interviews
Technology rejection/usage barriers (TPB, MPA)	Restriction evaluations	Reason for stopping diabetes app use/barriers to use	Financial aspects preventing app use (e.g., high app cost, insurance coverage) Technical aspects preventing app use (e.g., technical app failures) Temporal (time-related) aspects preventing app use (e.g., time-consuming app use) Cognitive aspects preventing app use (e.g., insufficient ability for app selection)
Diabetes self-management – personal factors	Demography (also part of the UTAUT)	Gender/age	Age group, men/women
	Individual adaptability, coping	Coping with diabetes expressed by self-management behaviors	Good diabetes self-management (regular BG testing, active patient, strict diet) Sufficient diabetes self-management (BG testing, at least partly active and following diet) Poor diabetes self-management (no BG testing, no exercise, no diet)
	Learning experience, knowledge, health literacy, (tech.) skills	(Perceived) diabetes knowledge	High perceived and actual knowledge (reading up a lot, attending talks, classes, asking HCPs) High perceived knowledge and low actual knowledge (misperceptions, no education classes attended, hardly reading up, etc.) Low perceived and actual knowledge (no education classes attended, hardly reading up, etc.)
	Personal/health beliefs, attitudes	Attitude towards self-management	Attitude description regarding self-management (e.g., fatalist, conservative)
		Interest in diabetes innovations	No interest in innovations, no information collection about innovations Medium interest, sometimes reading about specific innovations, or when becoming popular High interest, always up to date about innovations, interested in trying out new things
	Physical factors (e.g., interfering diseases etc.)	Diabetes type	T1DM T2DM (gestational diabetes/pre-diabetes)
		Diabetes medication	No insulin injection (pump/syringe)/no oral diabetes medication Insulin injection only (pump/syringe) Oral diabetes medication only Both insulin injection (pump/syringe) & oral diabetes medication
		Length of diabetes (since diagnosis)	Recently diagnosed (less than 5 years since diagnosis) Diagnosed some time ago (5-10 years since diagnosis) Diagnosed long ago (more than 10 but less than 20 years since diagnosis) Diagnosed very long ago (more than 20 years since diagnosis)
		Risk for diabetes complications	High-risk patient (high BG values or long-term complications showing, insufficient self-management, lacking motivation, lacking knowledge) No risk/normal risk (diabetes, but managing well, BG levels in medium range, sufficient to good motivation & knowledge)
		Health status	BMI, perceived health status, average BG values

	Factors from theory	Categories from interviews	Sub-categories from interviews
	Practical factors (e.g., socio-economic)	Self-management barriers	Self-management barriers described
	Psychological factors	General motivation for self-management	No motivation a) because of fear of receiving negative news about disease development → avoidance strategies hindering motivation for self-management b) due to lack in interest or indifference Sufficient to high motivation a) due to negative outcome expectations (e.g., danger of long-term complications) b) due to positive outcome expectations (e.g., benefits of self-management)
		Feelings, psychological problems	Depression, etc.
Diabetes self-management – provider/system factors	Access/care factors (e.g., availability of good quality health care[b])	Supervising HCP type	General practitioner (GP) Diabetes specialist/endocrinologist
		Perceived HCP quality	High quality doctor, content with supervision, recognizing the professional knowledge Low quality doctor, discontented with supervision, feeling that doctor doesn't know enough Indifference ("all doctors are the same")
		Diabetes program participation	Diabetes program attendee (like DAFNE program) No diabetes program attendee
	Communication (clinical relationships)	*See behavioral empowerment*	
	Education	Diabetes education	Diabetes education received No diabetes education received
	Social support (e.g., family and community support[b])	*See behavioral empowerment*	

Notes. Table based on theoretical Chapters 2 to 9; factors from empowerment approach as described in Chapter 7.1, factors from Unified Theory of Acceptance and Use of Technology (UTAUT) by Venkatesh et al. (2003), usage barriers based on restriction evaluations in Wirth et al. (2008), factors relevant for diabetes self-management based on Ahola and Groop (2013), K. M. Rodriguez (2013), and Wilkinson et al. (2014).
[a] Related factors see Table 2 on the UTAUT (root constructs) and Table 1 on self-management factors
[b] "The interaction of an individual – consumer, patient, caregiver or professional – with or through an electronic device or communication technology to access or transmit health information or to receive guidance and support on a health-related issue" (Robinson, Patrick, Eng, & Gustafson, 1998).

"root constructs" of performance expectancy in Venkatesh et al. (2003) (see Table 2, data extracts in Table 6 in Appendix). If an app was not perceived as useful it was unlikely that it was used, and it was mainly reported that the app had either not been used, or was no longer used. For example, Adit (age 22, T1DM) reported that he had stopped using diabetes apps after trying different apps and not finding them useful. Some diabetes patients perceived the self-management apps as very helpful, and reported that using an app had replaced the traditional BG recording into a book as one activity of self-management (logbooks, e.g., Kaiyan, age 42, T1DM). In contrast, others didn't find diabetes apps useful for self-management for several reasons including unattractive design, lack of features, or technical problems (e.g., Sona, age 20, T1DM). The general tendency regarding diabetes apps was positive, with reported perceived potential for improving diabetes self-management within the sample. However, the participants emphasized that they didn't perceive the apps as a solution to solving diabetes challenges, but rather as "just another tool" (Jie, age 64, T1DM).

Looking into extrinsic motivational reasons for app use, only two participants reported having received incentives for diabetes app use. Free special versions of an app (e.g., alpha version of MySugr, Gu Fang, age 29, T2DM) or app-related rewards (e.g., a voucher for counting daily steps, Deng Li, age 68, T2DM) delivered extrinsic motivation for an app adoption and maintained use.

(2) Regarding *effort expectancy*, the *ease* using the app (as a root construct and a fundamental aspect of *effort expectancy*, see Table 2) was mentioned by participants as an important precondition of using the app, for example "I want easy, simple thing" (Xin Qi, age 56, T2DM), while a high required effort for recording health data was reported to hinder continued use of the app, like the need to type all health data into the app (see usage barriers). Gu Fang (age 29, T2DM) said that: "It does take up a bit of time [to use diabetes logbooks] because you have to log in your entries". The interview extracts pointed to the conclusion that the ease of the diabetes app use was relevant for the app adoption or length of time an app was used.

(3) Considering the UTAUT factor of *social influences* on app use, the participants mentioned starting to use diabetes apps because of recommendations of an app by their HCPs, or by their own private social networks (family, peer patients, etc.). Sona (age 20, T1DM) for example explained that the HCPs were part of the DAFNE program and had recommended the DAFNE app to her, while Henna (age 60, T2DM) said that: "The supplier recommended this [app]". Only the three patients Sona (age 20, T1DM), Bharat (age 66, T2DM) and Henna (age 60, T2DM) confirmed that the

doctor had recommended an app for diabetes self-management before. All others did not receive app recommendations from their doctors: "I don't think they will, they will even recommend it to you. I don't think so. Because I think, I don't know what is the protocol of the hospital, but I feel they never introduce [apps] to us" (Li Ting, age 49, T2DM). Instead, several patients mentioned app recommendations by friends or other patients (e.g., Gu Fang and Cheng). Overall, as shown by the DAFNE member Sona (age 20, T1DM), app recommendations appeared to trigger and to facilitate the adoption of diabetes apps, especially when recommendations came from trusted sources (e.g., friends).

(4) Related to the latter, other *facilitating conditions* for app adoption or maintained diabetes app use could be found, for example the inclusion of apps in specific diabetes programs and therefore a facilitated access to the app for the program participants (e.g., DAFNE, Sona and Shi Hui), or promotions of an app that made the app more visible to the patients. Kaiyan (age 42, T1DM) for example mentioned promotions of the BG test stripes vendor.

(5) In relation to the UTAUT factor *voluntariness* of the app use, an obligatory use of apps was not preferred by most participants, e.g., the idea of the prescription of an app by the doctor similar to the prescription of medicine. Some participants preferred to make their own decisions and app use initiation (Sona, Gu Fang, Ching Ching, Pang, Navin), while some thought a prescription of apps would be helpful to make the diabetes patients use it (Xin Qi, Deng Li, Ei Tek, Zhen Wei, Ming). Other patients reported that the success of an app prescription depended on the target group and specific circumstances the patients were in (Bharat, Henna, Jie, Xiu Wen, Kaiyan, Adit; see extract examples in Table 6 in Appendix). Thus, an obligatory use of diabetes apps was found not necessarily to promote an adoption and use of diabetes apps. The participants rather expressed that they wanted to have a choice which app to choose or if to use diabetes apps for self-management at all.

(6) In relation to the UTAUT factor *experience*, information on previous online health information seeking and the usage of online media for diabetes management was available from the interviews (Table 9 in Appendix). Information on diabetes app usage experience already was introduced in Chapter 13.2.2 on diabetes app use in the study sample. Overall, previous online usage experience was found likely to facilitate diabetes app adoption and use. For example, patients not using online media at all, like Ming (age unknown, T2DM) who had never searched for health information online, were also found either to show no interest in diabetes apps, or lacked the technological knowledge about how to use apps. In contrast, tech-savvy participants using online media for seeking health information and for their diabetes management were found to use diabetes-specific or other apps for their self-management in addition. Cheng (age 23, T1DM) reported using a diabetes logbook, MyFitnessPal, and WhatsApp for his diabetes management, and searching for health information online.

(7) An example that pointed towards the potential influences of the demographic UTAUT factors *age* and *gender* on diabetes app use was sought (Table 16). Older diabetes participants in the sample were either not interested in using diabetes apps or were unable to cope with the technology. Xiu Wen (age 57, T1DM) emphasized: "The ladies out there who are in their fifties, sixties,… seventies, they will not Bluetooth and all these…; with the seventies, you don't ask them to do this keying in [data in logbook app] (laughter). Nobody is going to do that. But… if it's the young, young environment,… people will be interested". His comment suggested the relevance of gender as well, with men potentially being more tech-savvy than women. However, a closer analysis of these aspects is needed.

(8) The development of the UTAUT considered *attitude* to using technology, but excluded this aspect from the final model, with attitude not found to have any direct influence on behavioral intention, similar to anxiety (Venkatesh et al., 2003). In the interviews, some diabetes patients were generally not interested in using apps and showed rather skeptical attitudes towards diabetes app adoption (e.g., Xin Qi, Deng Li, Jie), while others were generally interested but lacked knowledge about app availabil-

ity (e.g., Zhen Wei, age 47, T2DM), or knowledge how to use apps: "Yes, yes. But I can't. I don't know how to operate" (Ei Tek, age 60, T2DM). Anxiety was expressed regarding diabetes outcomes: "I'm just too afraid to go for an operation… I'm just too afraid, yeah; yeah, because sometimes we feel that, we are afraid of, you know, to know the actual thing that's happening to us" (Zhen Wei, age 47, T2DM).

Factors Inhibiting Technology Usage

The reported diabetes app use barriers mainly fell within the four theoretical restriction evaluation categories used in the MPA (Wirth et al., 2008): financial, temporal, cognitive, and technical (Table 16). Respondents pointed out technological failures of apps with apps crashing and therefore a lack of reliability (e.g., Cheng, age 23, T1DM), or technological incompatibility with BG meters: "I think the importer wasn't compatible with my meter at the moment" (Gu Fang, age 29, T2DM). Another technological limitation of apps were interfaces being perceived as too simple, with sometimes unattractive interfaces. Sona (age 20, T1DM) explained that the DAFNE app "where we key in the the background… is not very nice ah, not very uh… attractive or what, so sometimes… I also think it's uh, that's an issue ah".

Regarding financial barriers, some participants expressed unwillingness to pay for diabetes apps: "It boils down to cost" (Shi Hui, age 35, T1DM). The time consuming use of app logbooks when recording health data manually was reported as a temporal barrier: "They ask you to input your, your… food, when you eat… but it takes a lot of efforts to to do that" (Xiu Wen, age 57, T1DM).

The lack in knowledge about app availability was mentioned as one of several cognitive barriers: "My major problem is… there're so many applications out there, you do not know which one to take" (Xiu Wen, age 57, T1DM). Several participants expressed that certain patient groups might not be able to use diabetes apps, like older people lacking technological or cognitive skill, mentioned for example by Deng Li (age 68, T2DM). Xiu Wen (age 57, T1DM) referred to age group limitations: "If you're targeting uhh… youngsters, then, it, it may work…. But if you're targeting those people who are in seventies [laughter], it'll be a, a challenge". The results showed that the interview participants perceived the potential of diabetes apps for older people as being less high than for young adults, and less high for the uneducated than for the educated. Zhen Wei (age 47, T2DM) said that diabetes apps were probably useful for patients who can read and understand app content because the phone as a tool was always with them. Moreover, Ching Ching (age 64, T2DM) believed that diabetes apps were useful only if there was enough self-discipline: "It depends on first your self-discipline to follow what is instructed to do". Thus, motivation was a crucial aspect appearing in the interviews. The previous app use in the sample participants mainly confirmed these reported perceptions.

In addition to the four categories, there was a data privacy concern that hindered app adoption or continued use for diabetes management (mentioned by Kang and Xiu Wen). The trust in private data protection was reported to be a major concern. Xiu Wen (age 57, T1DM) said: "This is medical information, so if you put medical information on the cloud, then this becomes a data privacy issue".

All mentioned diabetes app adoption und usage barriers are listed in Table 7 in the Appendix.

Factors Influencing Diabetes Self-Management

Chapter 2.3 introduced research on factors influencing diabetes self-management. Some of these factors were expected to be relevant for diabetes app use as part of the overall diabetes self-management (*RQ 2d*). Personal factors influencing diabetes self-management were distinguished from provider or health system factors as outlined by Ahola and Groop (2013), K. M. Rodriguez (2013), and Wilkinson et al. (2014) in Table 1. Table 16 displays how these factors were represented in the interviews.

(1) Apart from the sociodemographic background, personal factors included (2) the ability to manage and cope with diabetes which was displayed by the sum of previous self-management activities. Generally, the sample managed their condition rather well with some exceptions of high-risk patients (Ei Tek, Li Ting, Ming, Rei Hong, Zhen Wei).

(3) Perceived knowledge about diabetes was assessed in each interview. Some patients revealed high perceived diabetes knowledge, reporting a high level of "expert" knowledge about diabetes. Navin (age 58, T1DM) for example said: "At the conference I learnt a lot of things about the importance of blood glucose levels.... I attended a lot of scientific lectures...; I was hungry... I wanted to learn". Others reported insufficient perceived knowledge ("Don't know what ah, those tests, right?", Ei Tek, age 60, T2DM) or showed misperceptions about their diabetes knowledge, believing that they had good knowledge while reporting wrong diabetes facts or gaps in knowledge. Ming (age unknown, T2DM) for example reported: "Every time they got class, I come and listen... know... lot of knowledge; ... I study not very hard...; ...definitely eat a lot of sugar so at last I got type 2 already" (believed that he had a lot of knowledge but at the same time reported that he didn't read and understand facts, believed he had diabetes because he had eaten a lot of sugar in the past, too simplified). Similarly, Zhen Wei (age 47, T2DM) said: "We see, we know what is it [diabetes]...; to cut down [food], yeah. And more veggie, no coffee, yeah. That is ridiculous, right?"

(4) Personal and health beliefs could be evaluated when looking at diabetes patients' general and diabetes-related attitudes. Diabetes-related attitudes were for example found in interest towards diabetes innovation (e.g., sensor patches), while general attitudes towards life could be found in general optimism or pessimism expressed in the context of diabetes self-management. Pessimistic attitudes were especially found in diabetes patients not managing and coping well (Ming, Zhen Wei), while optimistic attitudes were found in motivated patients managing without problems (e.g., Pang, Shi Hui, Kaiyan, Table 10 in Appendix). Zhen Wei (age 47, T2DM) for example expressed pessimistic attitudes when saying: "If you have it from your mom, your grandma, who have this diabetes from the gene, ...it can never go off, it will stay there forever. So I feel like, it's no point". Xiu Wen (age 57, T1DM) emphasized the importance of optimism for diabetes management, saying that "the key is that they're (friends and family), they're not uhh... really that negative on this [diabetes]". Simi-

larly Kaiyan (age 42, T1DM) advised: "When you have a problem, you don't just keep it to yourself, always talk to friends. And, talk to people who are positive…".

(5) Physical factors, including diabetes background on the type of diabetes, medication, length of disease since diagnosis, risk of complications, and health status, were reported by the diabetes participants in both the interviews and the background information questionnaire, and results can be found in Chapter 13.2.1 on the sample description.

(6) Socioeconomic factors were assessed as part of the personal practical factors because they were found to play a major role for diabetes self-management. Financial constraints were reported by the majority of the participants. In many cases, consultation or medication costs had to be covered by patients themselves, as Henna (age 60, T2DM) explained: "Not in Singapore. The insurance do not cover all these… In fact, I think it's considered um… a chronic disease. So there is no accommodation… if it's an existing condition, the insurance don't want to cover you for hospital or… or medical" (Henna, age 60, T2DM). Economic pressure mentioned by several participants led to busy lifestyles and job-related priorities affecting the overall diabetes self-management: "Race kind of… economy" (Rei Hong, age 61, T2DM).

(7) Psychological factors included motivation for diabetes self-management. Motivation for self-management was found to split in positive motivation from success in self-management (Xiu Wen, age 57, T1DM), and negative motivation from fear of diabetes complications or negative long-term consequences (Ming, Deng Li, Ei Tek, Adit, Shi Hui). Fear of complications was frequently reported as a motivating factor by many participants (Tables 7 and 10 in Appendix, Table 16). However, in some participants fear of diabetes complications was also found to hinder motivation for self-management when resulting in avoidance strategies. For example, Zhen Wei (age 47, T2DM) who mentioned: "Sometimes we feel that, we are afraid of, you know, to know the actual thing that's happening to us".

As a second psychological factor, depression was mentioned as an important factor influencing self-management. The inconveniences that came with insulin injections, for example problems related to insulin injections in public were reported by individuals who injected insulin (e.g., Adit, age 22, T1DM), frequently leading to depressive feelings due to the rigidity of the required adherence. Moreover, depressive periods were reported after the fist disease diagnosis with a lack of knowledge about how to manage diabetes (e.g., Xiu Wen, Kaiyan, Adit), as well as for times when self-management became difficult due to difficult life circumstances such as stress in the job, other diseases, or during school graduation (e.g., Shi Hui, Adit). Educational diabetes classes and support were reported to be helpful in overcoming depressive periods (e.g., Adit, age 22, T1DM). However, overall the participants reported that too little attention was given to psychological support in addition to medical support in diabetes care. Navin (age 58, T1DM) mentioned that: "When I look back I have realized the importance of psychological support… it should be something that a doctor [provides]… help you see a dietician, help you to arrange to see a a psychotherapist for that". Overall, the relevance of psychological aspects of self-management as well as the lack of psychological support in diabetes care were pointed out by study participants (e.g., Navin, age 58, T1DM).

(8) Examining provider or health system factors, the HCP types used for diabetes care and supervision were found to be a relevant background factor for diabetes self-management (Table 16), with reported differences between diabetes specialists (endocrinologists) and general practitioners (GPs) regarding supervision quality. The quality of GPs consulted for diabetes care was experienced as insufficient by the interviewees (e.g., mentioned by Xin Qi, Bharat, Jie, Kang, Zhen Wei), while patients previously consulting endocrinologists or diabetes specialists reported high perceived quality of care (mentioned by Gu Fang, Henna, Ei Tek, Cheng, Shi Hui, Navin). While the specialists were reported to offer intense supervision supported by specialized knowledge, the GPs were accused of lacking knowledge about diabetes, and a lack in support (e.g., Zhen Wei, age 47, T2DM; Table 16) or even negative behaviors towards the patient (e.g., threatening the patient, Li Ting, age 49, T2DM). Despite the lack of

supervision by GPs, patients reported that they consulted GPs because they were cheaper (e.g., Deng Li, age 68, T2DM). This was connected to economic pressure as described previously. For example, Deng Li (age 68, T2DM) reported that she made sure that she would always see the same GP she chose at a polyclinic, with the advantage that polyclinics were cheap and had a database for medical results that could be accessed by all polyclinics.

The relevance of nurses (in Singapore called DNEs: diabetes nurse educators, see Bharat, age 66, T2DM), dieticians and other HCPs stayed unclear from the interview statements. Some patients consulted them in addition to the doctors, some didn't have nurses or dieticians in their care at all, and some received more support from them than from the doctors. Adit (age 22, T1DM) reported that he could call the nurse educators on a 24-7 hotline, where they would always be available, if necessary.

(9) The interviews showed that participants of specialized diabetes programs displayed detailed and specialized knowledge of diabetes self-management, based on intense training, a high level of support, and frequent HCP-patient communication. (e.g., Sona and Shi Hui were part of the DAFNE program, dose adjusting for normal eating, SingHealth, 2017). "Going through DAFNE program is not easy... you have to be disciplined... because the course is actually um a full five day course" (Shi Hui, age 35, T1DM).

(10) Diabetes education was found to be a common background for diabetes self-management, and was analyzed in relation to perceived diabetes knowledge. Most patients in the sample had received diabetes education as part of their diabetes care. However, this might also relate to sample selection, with most participants being part of support groups.

Table 16 summarizes all factors as explained in this chapter, while specific extract examples can be found in Table 6 in the Appendix.

13.2.4 Diabetes App (Non-) User Group Differences – Typology

Four broader diabetes app user and non-user types evolved from the interviews when grouping (non-) users together based on diabetes app usage and non-usage characteristics in the sample, including the previous app use or non-use, reasons for the use or non-use, the length of the use, the types of apps used, app information sharing with HCPs, knowledge about apps, and interest in apps (see Table 15). These characteristics included both usage and non-usage aspects, as well as behavioral intention aspects in non-users (interest in apps and app knowledge). The resulting (non-) user types are listed in Table 17. The non-users of diabetes apps split into non-users without interest in diabetes apps, and non-users generally interested in diabetes apps but facing barriers. The diabetes app users split into short-term users who were either dissatisfied diabetes app adopters, or experienced app switchers using apps parallel, and long-term users who used one main app over a minimum period of several months (Table 17). The typology confirmed that a one-sided look at users ignoring non-users could not be justified, and that inhibiting factors or usage barriers towards diabetes app use were found important to be considered. Table 7 in the Appendix delivers further details about the (non-) usage characteristics the typology was based on.

Table 17. Diabetes App (Non-) User Typology (Study 2)

	Non-User of Diabetes Apps		Diabetes App User		
	The diabetes app non-user without interest in diabetes apps	The interested non-user of diabetes apps	The dissatisfied adopter of diabetes apps	The experienced diabetes app switcher	The consistent long-term diabetes app user
Explanation	Does not use diabetes apps and is not interested, partly app knowledge, partly uses and prefers other non-diabetes-specific (mobile) channels (health information apps, WhatsApp for information exchange)	Does not use diabetes apps but is generally interested, no app knowledge, rarely uses other health apps	Adopts and tries diabetes apps (logbooks, food databases) short-term, but does not continue use due to perceived app insufficiency, preference for other online/offline channels (other apps, partly using clouds, partly turning back to pen and paper), info sharing in various ways	Adopts and uses various types of diabetes apps parallel (various devices and apps for self-management), and frequently switches apps, "playing around" with apps, info sharing in various ways (no clouds)	Adopts and uses one major diabetes app (logbook) over a longer period of time (several months to years), sticking to one app in combination with external devices and clouds, automatic synchronization of data, info sharing though clouds

Notes. Based on Study 2 interviews; based on the following (non-) usage characteristics: previous (non-) use, reasons for (non-) use; users: length of app use, app types used, app information sharing; non-users: app knowledge, app interest

The types of (non-) users were compared for psychological empowerment (*RQ 2a*), behavioral empowerment (*RQ 2b*), described factors influencing technology use and non-use (*RQ 2c*), and described factors influencing self-management (*RQ 2d*) as listed in Table 16. This allowed the researcher to discuss the potential relevance of the factors as antecedents of diabetes app use, and delivered a first exploratory step towards examining empowerment as an antecedent of diabetes app use in addition to other antecedents.

Overview on Types of Diabetes App (Non-) Users Compared for Influencing Factors

Non-Users of Diabetes Apps for Self-Management Without Interest in Diabetes Apps
The first group included older diabetes app non-users without interest in diabetes apps (Deng Li, Xin Qi, Kang, Jie, partly Ching Ching). The group contained diabetes patients above 60 years of age suffering from all types of diabetes, and sometimes other interfering diseases (e.g., cancer, Ching Ching, age 64, T2DM). They were mostly active, sometimes with busy lifestyles, and managed their diabetes well (no risk group). Some followed a very strict self-management regimen with perfectionist tendencies with very strict diet and regular exercise (e.g., Kang, age 67, pre-diabetes; Ching Ching, age 64, T2DM). The strictness was partly also perceived as a barrier towards quality of life, as well as related emotions and psychological aspects.
They displayed some knowledge about diabetes apps for self-management, but showed no interest in using the apps. They perceived the usefulness of diabetes apps as limited or were skeptical towards diabetes app use. This was related to partly conservative self-management attitudes. They expressed no need for diabetes apps, or barriers towards app use with the apps not being suitable for older people (e.g., eyesight), being too commercial, or not compatible with phones using older operating systems. Moreover, the apps were perceived as difficult to use (effort, time consuming), or as difficult to select. Moreover, concern about privacy and cost of the app use were expressed. Despite rejecting the use of diabetes apps, they looked for health information online, used email, and used other health information apps (WebMD, HealthBuddy), or WhatsApp for support group chats.

Looking at psychological empowerment, the group reported high perceived relevance of their diabetes management. They reported a feeling of competence, going along with reported experience in self-management, and good diabetes knowledge due to frequent information collection about diabetes. This also was connected to a feeling of independence from HCPs and feelings of self-determination, as well as reported perceived control over BG values (perceived impact, see Table 7 in Appendix). Overall, the group showed high psychological empowerment scale scores.

As for behavioral empowerment and self-management provider factors, the group mainly used GPs for consultation and reported that they selected their doctors themselves or chose doctors at the polyclinics due to patient databases that shared patient data across polyclinics (beneficial for emergencies, Deng Li, age 68, T2DM). With cost being reported as a barrier towards self-management, the conscious selection of GPs (being cheaper than specialists) could be explained with financial constraints. If there was a lack in HCP supervision it was compensated with independent self-management in this group (see Table 7 in Appendix). Most diabetes patients in this group mentioned that they mainly managed their condition alone, with limited support from social networks. However, they participated in support groups, sometimes as a leading figure for group activities (e.g., Jie, age 64, T1DM administrator of WhatsApp support group chat).

Interested Non-Users of Diabetes Apps for Self-Management

The second group of diabetes app non-users included patients who were generally interested in diabetes apps due to their critical condition or previous diabetes complications, but lacked knowledge about diabetes apps for self-management (Ei Tek, Li Ting, Ming, Zhen Wei, partly Rei Hong). The group mainly included middle aged to higher aged T2DM patients. Despite the length of their condition (mostly diagnosed 10 or more years ago) they displayed insufficient self-management, and dangerous health behaviors. The group was found to be at high risk for diabetes complications from lack of motivation for self-management, avoidance strategies (denial of health condition, e.g., Li Ting, age 49, T2DM), as well as pessimistic and sometimes fatalist attitudes (Rei Hong, age 61, T2DM).

They had not used diabetes apps before due to perceived high barriers (e.g., choosing an app, language barriers, technological barriers) or lack of knowledge about diabetes app options. They rarely used other mobile channels for their diabetes management (WhatsApp, HealthBuddy). Some never or rarely looked for health information online, or preferred face-to-face consultation. In a few cases they used online channels instead of consulting the doctor (misperceptions about own knowledge). Due to their serious conditions, they were generally interested in diabetes apps, and perceived the apps as useful after introduction to the MySugr App Series: "Maybe next time I can think… my blood sugar getting higher maybe I need this [app]" (Ming, age unknown, T2DM). They only partly acknowledged the relevance of diabetes self-management when analyzing psychological empowerment. They displayed limited perceived competence in self-management, going along with a lack of perceived diabetes knowledge or misperceptions about the own knowledge. Due to high perceived self-management barriers, the perceived impact on self-management outcomes was limited. Barriers to self-management mainly included lack of motivation, depression and phobias, denial, work stress, and financial constraints. Overall psychological empowerment scores were lower than in all other groups (see Table 7 in Appendix).

Regarding behavioral empowerment and provider factors, they mainly felt dependent on their HCPs (GPs).,with whom they were dissatisfied due to lack of professional competence and support. Some felt partly independent from their HCPs, connected to dangerous health decisions due to misperceptions about their own diabetes knowledge. Despite the perceived insufficient HCP support, this group did not actively seek much support from diabetes support groups; nor did they receive or seek much support from their private social networks. Behavioral empowerment scores were in the low to medium range (see Table 7 in Appendix).

Short-term Diabetes App Users and App Switchers
The third type of users included patients using diabetes apps short-term, trying various diabetes apps, using apps parallel, or switching apps. These short-term diabetes app users presented detailed knowledge about diabetes apps due to the trial of several apps. Moreover, they frequently searched for health information online, showed interest in

diabetes innovations (e.g., sensor patches), and managed their health conditions well (no risk group). The group showed very good and specialized diabetes self-management knowledge related to intense diabetes training, or to frequent reading about diabetes. Concerning psychological empowerment, they reported a feeling of competence, independence and perceived impact on self-management outcomes, with resulting psychological empowerment scores ranging high (see Table 7 in Appendix).

Apart from these characteristics, two subgroups appeared that mainly differed in age. One subgroup included young T1DM patients in their early 20s or younger, who were diagnosed with diabetes early in life, and were dissatisfied adopters of diabetes apps (Adit, Sona, Cheng, Pang). Their innovative attitudes were visible in attitudes about diabetes apps for self-management. They searched for apps themselves or followed friends' recommendations, or participated in diabetes programs that included apps. The adoption and trial of several diabetes apps, including diabetes logbooks and food databases, left them dissatisfied with the state of the apps. Thus, after the app trial they decided that diabetes apps were of limited usefulness, and stopped the app to turn to other mobile online channels (fitness apps, WhatsApp), or to turn back to pen and paper for BG recording (e.g., Pang, age 19, T1DM). They criticized the unattractive design of the apps, the lack of user-friendliness, cost, compatibilities with other devices, lack of reliability, technological failure, and missing features.

In relation to behavioral empowerment and provider factors, this subgroup reported good supervision by diabetes specialists and additional other HCPs (nurses), and reported being satisfied with the HCP supervision quality. They made medical decisions together with their HCPs (shared decision-making), or made decisions independently and carefully, listening to medical advice before making decisions. They communicated with their HCPs both online and offline (e.g., WhatsApp with doctor, email, or cloud, or nurse hotlines). Due to their youth, they additionally had received intense support from parents, other family members and diabetes support groups. Some of them volunteered in support groups to educate other young patients (e.g., Adit, age 22, T1DM). The intense supervision went along with high behavioral empowerment scores in this group (see Table 7 in Appendix). Stress from school or military service was mentioned as a barrier to self-management, as well as psychological pressure to cope with diabetes (e.g., injecting in public as a problem) and normal adolescent life, leading to frustration. Furthermore, they differed from other groups in putting much focus on finding a balance between strict diabetes self-management and a normal life as a young person. This led to experimenting with what worked best for them in their self-management (trial and error).

The second short-term diabetes app user subgroup included experienced diabetes app switchers who used several diabetes apps in parallel and in contrast to the previous group reported perceived app usefulness. This group especially included tech-savvy and innovation interested middle to higher aged patients with T1DM or T2DM (Navin, Bharat, Xiu Wen). They were very experienced in their self-management (diagnosed long ago), and managed their condition well. Due to their high interest in innovation, the tech-savvy attitudes, and the perceived need to be always on top of diabetes self-management, they used many diabetes apps, other apps (e.g., step trackers), and connected devices in parallel. The group mainly called it "playing around" with diabetes apps, and mainly expressed perceived usefulness of diabetes apps. They also used support group chats, and online communication with their HCPs (email). However, they were concerned about data privacy aspects when using clouds, and thus rather avoided cloud-based systems, using printouts to share the app results with HCPs instead (e.g., showing the app logbook results to HCPs). Thus, their attitude was more responsible and traditional than in the younger subgroup. Other barriers to maintained app use were the constant search for the best apps, as well as effort and time for data recording, and cost of unsubsidized diabetes apps.

Regarding behavioral empowerment and provider factors, in contrast to the younger short-term diabetes app users they reported very strong independence from HCPs, with some HCPs (GPs) reported to know less about diabetes than the patients themselves. This was reflected in dissatisfaction with medical supervision in some participants, and partly low behavioral empowerment scores (see Table 7 in Appendix). Support from families and especially spouses was mentioned, as well as participation in support groups (sometimes leading positions).

Long-term Diabetes App Users

The fourth group included patients using one main diabetes app over a period of several months to several years (Gu Fang, Henna, Kaiyan, Shi Hui). In the sample, this user type included experienced T1DM or T2DM patients of all age groups, who were mostly part of a specific diabetes or an app pilot program (e.g., DAFNE). This group also managed diabetes actively and well (no risk group). Self-management attitudes found were responsibility, self-determination, consistency in self-management, and optimism. Nevertheless, barriers to self-management were similar to other diabetes groups, mainly including work-related stress and busy lifestyles, limited insurance coverage, or psychological problems (denial, depression, or social pressure). Moreover, this group reported competitiveness among patients as an additional barrier, as well as problems following strict routines in diabetes programs (e.g., regulated food intake).

Attitudes towards mobile diabetes technology were positive, with reported perceived usefulness of apps, and interest in technological diabetes innovation. The apps mainly were part of the program the patients participated in, including BG logbook apps, and were used over a minimum period of several months. They were used in combination with other external devices (BG meter, step trackers, etc.), connected to cloud systems the HCPs had access to, in addition to online health information seeking. Automatic data synchronization between devices and online platforms was used as a foundation for sharing data with HCPs. Additionally, texting and email were used to communicate diabetes-related topics with HCPs. Barriers to the use of diabetes apps were seen in design aspects, compatibility and other technological problems (app reliability), lacking app tailoring, cost, and partly effort required to use the app.

For psychological empowerment, intense program training related to perceived specialized diabetes knowledge, and related to a feeling of competence for self-management. The group showed high motivation for self-management, and perceived the relevance of self-management as very high. A feeling of good control, independence, and perceived impact of diabetes outcomes was reported, with high psychological empowerment score results shown (see Table 7 in Appendix).

Regarding behavioral empowerment and provider factors, due to the program participation these patients received intense supervision by diabetes specialists together with additional HCPs (nurses). Close relationships with the HCPs resulted from program participation. Health-related decisions were made in a shared way together with HCPs. High behavioral empowerment scores (see Table 7 in Appendix) reflected good relationships with HCPs and satisfaction with the HCPs' supervision. Additional support partly came from friends and families, support groups, or other program members. Long-term app users mainly took leading positions in support group or program activities. Table 18 summarizes the main relevant factors the diabetes app (non-) user groups were compared for, while Table 7 in the Appendix delivers further details about the comparisons.

Comparing Types of Diabetes App (Non-) Users for Empowerment – Hypotheses
To understand the role of psychological and behavioral empowerment for diabetes app use, similarities and differences in types of diabetes app users and non-users were analyzed in more detail to draw a first conclusion (*RQ 2a* and *RQ 2b*, Table 4). Additionally, hypotheses to be tested in study 3 were developed from Study 2 results.

(1) Psychological empowerment: All types of diabetes app users showed high psychological empowerment scores (Table 7 in Appendix), and reported perceived relevance of diabetes self-management, perceived competence, a feeling of independence and self-determination, and perceived impact on diabetes outcomes accordingly (e.g., the possibility of influencing BG values with diet and exercise). In contrast, the interested non-user group displayed lower psychological empowerment scores (Table 7 in Appendix), reported limited perceived relevance, limited perceived competence for both self-management and for diabetes app adoption (selecting apps) and use (understanding, technological skill, knowledge, etc.), a feeling of dependence on HCPs, and limited perceived impact on diabetes outcomes. This group contained patients at high risk of complications. Concerning psychological empowerment, the interested non-user group at high risk of complications differed from all diabetes app user groups. Thus, more generalized the first derived hypothesis from Study 2 results said that *diabetes*

app users showed higher psychological empowerment than non-users of diabetes apps (*H 1*, Table 19).

Table 18. Types of App (Non-) Users Compared for Factors Potentially Influencing App Use (Study 2)

		Non-User of Diabetes Apps		Diabetes App User		
		The diabetes app non-user without interest in diabetes apps	The interested non-user of diabetes apps	The dissatisfied adopter of diabetes apps	The experienced diabetes app switcher	The consistent long-term diabetes app user
Empowerment	Psych and behav. empowerment	High perceived psych. empowerment (for all four indicators); behav.: independent decision-making	Relevance of self-management partly seen, limited perceived competence & impact; behav.: dependent, or independent with dangerous health behaviors	High perceived psych. empowerment (for all four indicators); behav.: independent but listening to advice, or shared decision-making	High perceived psych. empowerment (for all four indicators); behav.: independent, HCPs just for advice	High perceived psych. empowerment (for all four indicators); behav.: shared decision-making with close relationships
Technology (non-) use – UTAUT factors	Perceived usefulness & facilitating/inhibitin g conditions	Limited perceived usefulness, perceived high use barriers (no interest or skeptical despite app knowledge)	Perceived as useful, perceived high use barriers (interested but lacking diabetes app knowledge)	Limited perceived usefulness, dissatisfied with the current state of diabetes apps	Perceived usefulness (but improvement suggested)	Perceived usefulness, part of diabetes program
Self-management – personal factors	Age	Higher age	Middle aged to higher age	Young	Middle aged to higher age	All age groups
	Self-management and risk	No risk group, experienced with good perceived diabetes knowledge, mainly good self-management	Diabetes risk group, perceived lacking diabetes knowledge or misperceptions about knowledge, unmotivated, avoidance strategies, insufficient self-management, dangerous health behaviors	No risk group, good perceived diabetes knowledge (educated at young age), good self-management	No risk group, very good perceived diabetes knowledge, very good self-management, experienced, strict regimen	No risk group, specialized perceived diabetes knowledge, intense diabetes education, good self-management, strict carb counting, active
	Attitudes	Conservative, perfectionist, self-determined	Insecure, partly fatalist, pessimistic	Innovative, partly back to the roots	Innovative and always on top , tech-savvy, responsible, unconventional	Consistent, responsible, determined, optimistic
Self-management – provider factors	HCP types, support	Mainly GPs (partly dissatisfied), support groups	Mainly GPs (dissatisfied), partly no support group	Diabetes specialists (satisfied), support groups	GPs or diabetes specialists (satisfied or dissatisfied, depending on HCP type), support groups	Diabetes specialists (satisfied), doctors as "friends", support groups

Notes. Study 2 interview results, abbreviations: BG = blood glucose, HCP = healthcare professional, GP = general practitioner

Looking at each psychological empowerment indicator, there was a difference between high risk non-users of diabetes apps and other user and non-user groups regarding the perceived relevance of diabetes self-management. Only interested non-users at high risk of complications partly reported limited perceived relevance of self-management. For example, Zhen Wei (age 47, T2DM) did not take the condition seriously until complications started to appear. She said that the doctor "warns me to eat properly, to eat two… two spoons of rice, but I can't do that…. to cut down, yeah. And more veggie, no coffee, yeah. That is ridiculous, right? Yeah, we don't care". Other non-users of diabetes apps mainly reported high perceived relevance, but partly said they had other priorities that were more important than their diabetes condition. Rei Hong (age 61, T2DM) prioritized his job, being self-employed, and said that diabetes is "very important, but sometimes we… tend to forget", while Ching Ching (age 64, T2DM) had to prioritize breast cancer for a certain period of time. The diabetes app users reported high relevance, and especially T1DM app users said that self-management was essential for their daily lives, to avoid hyper- or hypoglycemia incidences (e.g., Cheng, Xiu Wen). Kaiyan (age 42, T1DM) called diabetes her "friend" she had to take care of, and said: "I realized that I need to put my diabetes as number one". She considered: "Diabetic is a condition that, if you don't take care, …this friend will go and look for other friends in your body right… eyes, the legs…". Overall it was hypothesized *that diabetes app users showed higher perceived relevance of self-management than non-users of diabetes apps* (*H1 a*, Table 19).

In contrast to all other groups showing high perceived competence for self-management, the interested non-users reporting low perceived competence (e.g., Li Ting, age 49, T2DM), were insecure in their self-management and perceived they lacked diabetes knowledge (Li Ting, Ei Tek, Rei Hong, and Zhen Wei), showed less self-management initiative, did not know how to use diabetes apps, or did not feel competent to use apps for self-management. Perceived competence at least partly went along with perceived diabetes knowledge (resulting from diabetes education), and perceived self-management experience. In patients with a long history of the condition, the perceived competence was shown as high. For example, Jie (age 64, T1DM, diagnosed 1979) mentioned: "I mean… being a diabetic for so long, I think… primarily, I know everything already... So if I were to tell the doctor something – and I'm from the Diabetic Society, I'm so many years having this history – this and that... they always believe me". Generally in all (non-) user groups, perceived competence seemed to relate to general self-management behaviors – the patients managing well reported that they felt competent, while patients with insufficient self-management and at high risk of complications (Li Ting, Ei Tek, Rei Hong, and Zhen Wei) mostly didn't express the feeling of competence. Perceived insecurity was reported by all users and non-users on how to deal with the disease at the beginning of diagnosis, changing to a feeling of greater competence after gaining experience with the disease, and after having participated in educational diabetes classes (e.g., Adit and Pang). Furthermore, the interview results showed that perceived competence for self-management could be problematic when misperceptions about competence occurred. In summary, to test for general differences it was hypothesized *that diabetes app users showed higher perceived competence for self-management than non-users of diabetes apps (H1 b*, Table 19).

Some users and non-users expressed a very strong feeling of independence and self-determination (e.g., Deng Li, Ching Ching, Tan). For example, Ching Ching (age 64, T2DM) reported that: "The day I reach 5.9 [BG value] I will be satisfied...; I love challenges.. and I looove to see improvements.... I want to see a better result and I am still like trying any way I can to get a 5.9". The interviews supported the view that self-determination might increase the likelihood of initiating diabetes app use on one's own, actively searching for apps, and switching apps to find the best apps. This is because self-determined participants like Ching Ching reported looking for strategies to improve self-management. However, this was also related to other factors, like general interest in diabetes apps. The group of older non-users for example showed no interest in diabetes apps despite high perceived independence/self-determination in their self-management. To test for general differences, it was hypothesized *that diabetes app users showed higher perceived independence in self-management than non-users of diabetes apps (H1 c*, Table 19).

Most users and non-users said they felt that they knew how to influence their BG values using self-management activities (exercise, diet), and thus perceived they had impact on their diabetes outcomes (see Table 7 in Appendix, and extract examples in Table 6 in Appendix). For example, Deng Li (age 68, T2DM) said: "I realized how to bring it [BG] down". In app users, perceived impact regarding diabetes app use was visible when the development of health data like BG values could be tracked with a diabetes app and changes in BG became visible in graphic form. This made results of the user's self-management and the app use visible to app users (e.g., Pang, age 19, T1DM; see extract examples, Table 6 in Appendix) and increased perceived utility of the app. However, several diabetes app users injecting insulin said it was very difficult to influence BG outcomes because their BG values fluctuated with the amount of insulin injected and the physical activities executed (e.g., Sona and Xiu Wen). Xiu Wen (age 57, T1DM) said: "It's, it's very difficult to control [the BG]. Because uhh... it, it depends on what you take [eat], and you... you really cannot tell... the amount of sugar that's in there". In contrast to other groups, the group of interested non-users reported no perceived impact of their activities on diabetes outcomes. Li Ting (age 49, T2DM) expressed the feeling of helplessness when it came to bringing BG values down. It was hypothesized *that diabetes app users showed higher perceived impact on self-management outcomes than non-users of diabetes apps (H1 d, Table 19)*.

The additional psychological empowerment scores from the EMPOWER project scale (Mantwill et al., 2015) in the background information questionnaire confirmed the interview results on psychological empowerment (Table 14, Table 7 in Appendix). Participants who communicated a feeling of self-management relevance, and feelings of competence, independence and impact also were found to show high scores on the psychological empowerment scale (scores above 4.0 on the 5-point scale).

Psychological empowerment scores of non-users without interest in diabetes apps were as high as those of app users (Table 7 in Appendix), and the results regarding all four psychological empowerment indicators resembled the results of diabetes app users. Thus, apart from hypothesizing general differences between diabetes app users and non-users regarding psychological empowerment (*H 1 a-d*), reasons for the non-use of diabetes apps had to be analyzed more closely to find potential explanations as to why some non-users differed from users in psychological empowerment, and some didn't. Other factors had to be considered in addition to psychological empowerment to get a detailed picture.

(2) Behavioral empowerment: The interested non-users at risk of complications mostly reported a feeling of dependence on their HCPs. For example, Rei Hong (age 61, T2DM) said that: "I got to depend the... the... what you call that... the doctor to look after me". Support from both HCPs and social networks was mostly perceived as limited in the interested non-users, and partly there was no support group participation. As an exception in this group, Zhen Wei (age 47, T2DM) partly reported independence that was found to relate to dangerous health behaviors (Tables 8 and 10 in Appendix).

The group of older non-users who were not interested in diabetes apps reported very short consultations with HCPs, and limited support by HCPs. Moreover they said they managed their disease mostly alone, with limited support from their social networks. Deng Li (age 68, T2DM) mentioned that: "Nobody actually uh, advise me how to manage it... he [doctor] just gave me the medication". Thus, both non-users groups reported lower behavioral empowerment than most users, and the second resulting hypothesis stated *that diabetes app users showed higher behavioral empowerment than non-users of diabetes apps* (*H 2*, Table 19).

In contrast to diabetes app non-users, both the young dissatisfied adopters of diabetes apps and the long-term app users displayed high behavioral empowerment scores (Table 7 in Appendix), reported shared decision-making or independence from HCPs but taking their advice into consideration, and satisfaction with HCP supervision. For example, Shi Hui (age 35, T1DM, long-term diabetes app user) said: "My dieticians, my nurses are all very nice because of the DAFNE program and it becomes like we are very... we are more like family yeah... ; and they are very supportive". From the results the hypothesis was formulated that shared decision-making only appeared in diabetes app users, while paternalistic decision-making only appeared among diabetes app non-users; or *that diabetes app users reported more shared decision-making than app non-users* (*H 2a*, Table 19).

Similarly, results on HCP-patient communication additionally implied *better and more participatory HCP-patient communication in diabetes app users than in non-users* (*H 2b*, Table 19). Xiu Wen (age 57, T1DM, app user) reported that: "They [doctors] spend time, really spend time to discuss". However, the experienced diabetes app switchers slightly differed from the rest of the app users with some patients presenting low scores for HCP-patient communication, and some dissatisfaction with HCP supervision. For example, Bharat (age 66, T2DM) said: "Doctor is uh… not in the picture… doctor only give you medicine. Uh, he'll ask you how much you want. Next…". Thus other factors additionally were likely influencing the potential relationship between HCP-patient communication and diabetes app use (see Chapter 13.2.4.2).

In relation to support from private social networks, the overall tendency showed that *non-users of diabetes apps reported less behavioral empowerment by their social private networks (family and friends) than diabetes app users* who mostly showed high support by them (*H 2c*, Table 19). The support by other patients (e.g., through support groups) seemed to matter for all diabetes app users, and for some non-users. Only the group of interested non-users of diabetes apps at risk of complications included patients not using any support group or contact with other patients for support in self-management (Li Ting and Zhen Wei). The rest of the participants attended support group meet-ups and used chats to communicate with other patients (e.g., Diabetes Singapore WhatsApp chat group, lead by Jie, age 64, T1DM)[14]. According to the participants' reports, the main contact persons within diabetes support groups were other patients rather than organizations' staff. Some patients engaged actively in support groups' administrative organization (e.g., Bharat, Jie, Gu Fang, Adit). The relevance of support from other patients and support groups was reported to be high for empowering support in daily self-management. Throughout the interviews, the results revealed that diabetes support groups possibly could even deliver more empowering support than HCPs. Pang (age 19, T1DM) said that he had learned to cope better from other patients suffering from the same condition. Deng Li (age 68, T2DM) summa-

---

[14] It has to be noted that the majority of the sample was part of a diabetes support group (Diabetes Singapore and TOUCH support groups in Singapore) due to the sampling recruitment method.

rized that: "It was from the group that I learnt a lot. I wish I had joined them earlier". The patients mentioned financial, motivational, emotional, and educational support by these groups and their other diabetes members. Financial support programs, walking events, educational classes for newly diagnosed and other means of support played a relevant role in their self-management. In addition, online and offline support groups were found to be a potential channel for exchanging information on diabetes app usage (e.g., in Diabetes Singapore WhatsApp chat). However, despite the empowering support, a competitive aspect was also mentioned by the patients. Support group members reported that they sometimes held back private diabetes-related information (e.g., the state of BG values) due to perceived competition between members regarding success in BG control (mentioned by Henna, age 60, T2DM). This hindered the effectiveness of support group interaction and information exchange.

Examining additional behavioral empowerment scale results from the background information questionnaire, non-user groups mostly displayed lower scores for participatory decision-making (PDMstyle) and for HCP-patient communication (PCOM) than users, with exception of Ei Tek who showed a higher PCOM score (see Table 8 in Appendix). Generally, the behavioral empowerment scale results delivered additional reasoning for the formulation of the hypothesis *H 2* (Table 19).

(3) The relation between psychological and behavioral empowerment: Following the theoretical argumentation on relationships between psychological and behavioral empowerment in Chapter 7.1.2, the interviews delivered results showing a potential influence of behavioral empowerment on psychological empowerment. High behavioral empowerment in diabetes app users (with exceptions) went along with high psychological empowerment (e.g., Sona, Henna, Cheng, Kaiyan, Adit, Pang, Gu Fang, Shi Hui). Thus, it was hypothesized *that psychological empowerment positively related to behavioral empowerment in diabetes app users* (*H 3*, Table 19).

For diabetes app non-users, hypotheses regarding a relationship between psychological and behavioral empowerment had to be formulated taking differences in non-users into account. *Paternalistic decision-making (found in interested non-users) was expected to result in lower psychological empowerment than shared decision-making in all app user and non-user groups* (*H 4*, Table 19). Patients dependent on doctors' instructions tended to be patients not managing diabetes well, with high risk of complications, and reporting lower psychological empowerment than other patients, for example Li Ting (age 49, T2DM), or Zhen Wei (age 47, T2DM). Specifically looking at the group of interested non-users it could be hypothesized *that psychological empowerment positively related to behavioral empowerment in diabetes app non-users at risk of complications* (*H 5*, Table 19). In contrast, the group of older non-users without interest in diabetes apps differed from these tendencies, with reported high psychological empowerment despite low behavioral empowerment results (e.g., Ching Ching, Jie, Kang). This led to the hypothesis that *psychological empowerment negatively related to behavioral empowerment in older non-users of diabetes apps over 60 years of age* (*H 6*, Table 19). Similarly, the group of experienced diabetes app switchers partly displayed high psychological empowerment despite lacking HCP-patient communication (e.g., Navin, age 58, T1DM).

The decision-making style appeared as a potential explanation for the mentioned differences in otherwise relatively homogeneous tendencies in user and non-user groups regarding a relation between psychological and behavioral empowerment: The diabetes app non-users without interest, and the app switchers – displaying high psychological empowerment despite lower behavioral empowerment (see Table 7 in Appendix) – reported to take health decisions very independently with medical supervisors taking a minor role. For example, independently managing Xiu Wen (age 57, T1DM, app switcher) said: "[seeing the doctor] that's for the [insulin] supply, that's all". The sample characteristics in these independent groups pointed towards the conclusion that strong independence in health decision-making in combination with diabetes expertise, experience, and own information collection could lead to high psychological empowerment despite lacking HCP support. Xiu Wen for example reported high psychological empowerment including the feeling of good competence for self-care, while managing diabetes himself, using GPs only for getting medication, attending talks on diabetes, using different apps and searching for information himself, reading up a lot about diabetes, and having been very self-disciplined for some time ("very rigid"). He said: "It's all control by myself," and that he managed everything around his diabetes himself, despite difficult periods at times (e.g., depression). Active self-management and importance of support from other diabetes patients was reported by most patients managing their condition independent from HCPs: "It was from the [support] group that I learnt a lot. I wish I had joined them earlier" (Deng Li, age 68, T2DM, very independent). Thus, for independent patients behavioral empowerment by other patients might be more dominant than empowerment by HCPs. Further research is necessary on this aspect.

For the app non-users without interest in diabetes apps the emphasis on independent decision-making also might help to explain why this group didn't want to adopt and use diabetes apps despite knowledge of the availability of diabetes apps (Table 7 in Appendix). In this group it was mostly a conscious decision to refrain from using diabetes apps because of perceived limited usefulness or lacking lack of interest. They expressed no need for diabetes apps, seeing them as unsuitable for older people, and requiring significant effort to use (Table 7 in Appendix). Their independence led to informed choice against diabetes apps, Xin Qi (age 56, T2DM, non-user of apps) for example mentioned that: "I think more or less, some [apps] they are not that good la… I don't think they are that useful… more or less they are quite similar, in fact". In contrast, the group of interested app non-users at risk of complications did not take such a conscious informed decision but rather generally lacked knowledge about diabetes apps and diabetes app usage ("I didn't know", Zhen Wei, age 47, T2DM).

Apart from independent decision-making, the medical specialty of the supervising HCP appeared as a second crucial factor that could help explain relationships between psychological and behavioral empowerment in relation to diabetes app use in greater detail. The HCP type/specialty is a *provider or care access factor* that was described as influencing self-management in Table 16 (based on theory in Table 2). The following chapter focuses on factors generally influencing self-management to explain diabetes app (non-) user differences (*RQ 2d,* Table 4) in addition to empowerment, starting with the type/medical specialty of the supervising HCP.

Comparing Types of Diabetes App (Non-) Users for Technology Adoption and Self-Management Factors – Hypotheses

(1) Self-management factors:

Firstly, the *type/medical specialty of the doctor* providing diabetes care was a potential reason for lower behavioral empowerment in some app switchers and in the uninterested non-users compared with other groups with high psychological empowerment. These groups consulting GPs reported dissatisfaction with GP supervision, believing that GPs lacked knowledge of diabetes management, and provided insufficient support for diabetes self-management:

> They [GPs] are all, not to say they are no good doctors but they are not specialized in this field… being a long-term diabetic so to speak ah, I'm well aware what the doctors say and I know whether the doctor is telling me something which is different from what they are practicing. (Jie, age 64, T1DM)
>
> I told him [GP] that my eye is blur, my right eye. I can't…, you know… why is it so irritating? I can't see clear. They said… he… he just like – I don't know what kind of doctor is he – so, he said: 'No, nothing, you just have to cut down on your food, and take care of your diabetes'… every month he [GP] keeps telling the same… show me the same pictures of the rice and noodle, you know, the same old things. (Zhen Wei, age 47, T2DM)

Li Ting (age 49, T2DM) even reported negative behaviors of GPs threatening her instead of supporting her: "They [doctors] just want to see improvement, but sometimes they get angry". Most patients consulting GPs reported short consultations due to the large patient numbers. Some patients reported that they hardly spent any time with their GPs, and that the doctors were not helpful in their diabetes management (Xin Qi, Li Ting, Kang, Rei Hong, Zhen Wei). Jie (age 64, T1DM) said that GPs at polyclinics "have to see hundreds of people, maybe, I'm not sure how many, but they're always rushing".

On the contrary, the groups consulting diabetes specialists (diabetes app users apart from some independent app switchers) reported intense and satisfying supervision in their self-management. Especially patients with a close relationship with their specialist reported good supervision quality. Some diabetes app users reported significant communication with their doctors, including instant feedback via email, chats, or telephone (email with HCPs, Xin Qi and Navin; WhatsApp chats with doctor, Cheng; texting with HCPs, Shi Hui).

To summarize, from the analysis shared decision-making with diabetes specialists appeared to result in the best perceived doctor-patient communication, and highest satisfaction with consultation, potentially relating to high psychological empowerment. Adit (age 22, T1DM) for example reported that he had known his doctor for a long time and made decisions together with his HCPs, frequently exchanging information with HCPs (could call nurses any time on nurse hotline). He was satisfied with his supervision. At the same time he showed high psychological empowerment in the interview analysis. Shared decision-making with diabetes specialists further could relate to maintained diabetes app use over time in some patients (e.g., Shi Hui, age 35, T1DM, long-term DAFNE app user, good relationship with DAFNE HCPs). Paternalistic decision-making styles by GPs with dependent patients potentially related to lack of supervision, dissatisfaction, lack of diabetes knowledge, low motivation for self-management, and lower psychological empowerment in the sample (e.g., Li Ting, age 49, T2DM, supervised by GPs, dependent on HCPs, insecure, lacking knowledge, non-user of apps). The respective group did not adopt or use any diabetes apps, despite perceived severity of the health condition, and the urgency for self-management improvement (see e.g., Li Ting, age 49, T2DM). To summarize, the hypotheses were elaborated that *the type/medical specialty of the supervising HCP related to the decision-making styles and to the quality of HCP-patient communication in both user and non-user groups* (*H 7*, Table 19), and *that diabetes app users rather consulted diabetes specialists while non-users consulted general practitioners* (*H 8*, Table 19).

As described before and as an exception, there were some patients consulting GPs, but showing strong independence from their doctors, which potentially led to good diabetes self-management and high psychological empowerment despite lacking HCP supervision by GPs. Due to strong independence, and based on informed decisions, there was either interest in diabetes apps, leading to trial of various apps and to the search for the best apps (app switchers, e.g., Xiu Wen, age 57, T1DM), or to diabetes app rejection (non-users without interest, e.g., Kang, age 67, pre-diabetes, compare *H 6*).

Secondly, another aspect that appeared to be potentially influence (maintained) diabetes app use was found in *participation in diabetes programs* as a facilitating condition (e.g., DAFNE, Shi Hui, app pilot program, Henna). Especially the inclusion of diabetes apps in specialized diabetes programs (e.g., DAFNE) could deliver motivation for the app use, could increase the perceived relevance of the app with regular HCP feedback on app data, and could create increased involvement for the app use (Shi Hui, age 35, T1DM). It was therefore hypothesized *that the participation in diabetes programs related to longer diabetes app use* (*H 9*, Table 19).

Thirdly, it could be shown *that lack of diabetes knowledge was likely related to dependence in decision-making, and to the non-use of diabetes apps* (*H 10*, Table 19), with the use of diabetes apps requiring a sufficient amount of diabetes knowledge and diabetes education. For example, Li Ting (age 49, T2DM, diagnosed 2007) expressed that she felt she lacked diabetes knowledge and that she felt insecure in her management. Additionally, she never attended courses about diabetes management, was not part of any diabetes support group, did not receive supporting input from her HCPs, and did not know about diabetes apps available for self-management. On the other hand, Navin summarized that (age 58, T1DM) if the required diabetes knowledge was there, using apps that showed a trend of BG reading results could lead to self-reflection, which could empower the patient to improve and to make better health decisions. In the sample, all diabetes app users showed good or very good knowledge about diabetes, sometimes in combination with long experience in diabetes self-management. As part of the diabetes app users, Navin (age 58, T1DM, diagnosed 1978) for example said that he felt very experienced and knowledgeable about diabetes management, and reported that he read a lot about diabetes, attended conferences about diabetes topics, and showed that he had detailed diabetes knowledge. However, the group of non-users without interest showed that diabetes knowledge did not necessarily lead to diabetes app use, e.g., when there was no interest in diabetes apps despite diabetes knowledge and knowledge about diabetes apps. Thus, other preconditions had to be fulfilled for diabetes app use to be carried out in addition to available diabetes knowledge.

Fourthly, similarly to diabetes knowledge, *lacking technological skill and experience, e.g., shown by lacking app use experience or lacking online health information seeking, was hypothesized to relate to the non-use of diabetes apps* (*H 11*, Table 19). On the one hand, the interested diabetes app non-users reported general barriers like reading and understanding problems (including technology), and lacking technological knowledge. Older diabetes app non-users without interest in diabetes apps partly reported barriers to diabetes apps specifically for older target groups (use of outdated technology, reading difficulties on technological devices, etc., e.g., Kang, age 67, prediabetes). On the other hand, diabetes app user groups reported frequent health information seeking, interest in technological innovation, and being tech-savvy (e.g., Xiu Wen, age 57, T1DM). Most participants searching for online health information (HIS) reported having tried to use apps, while those never using online media for self-management also reported no previous diabetes app use (Rei Hong and Ming, see Table 9 in Appendix).

Fifthly, when trying to understand why interested non-users of diabetes apps generally reported interest in using diabetes apps in contrast to the older non-users who were not interested, the researcher found that the *severity of the health condition* potentially explained this interest and perceived app potential. The high-risk group expressed general interest in diabetes apps despite lacking knowledge about app options, and perceived the app potential as high after introduction to app options in Study 2. The interviews showed that occurring diabetes complications drew the attention of otherwise unmotivated patients to the seriousness of the health condition. For example, Zhen Wei (age 47, T2DM) started to recognize the relevance of diabetes management when one of her eyes started to get blurred. Thus, she was forced to overcome her general avoidance strategies when complications started to occur because she could not deny her condition any longer. When she realized the seriousness of the condition and the possibility of general diabetes self-management, the first introduction of diabetes apps sparked her interest in apps as potentially easy to use self-management tools. Thus, the severity of the condition at least partly could helped explain increased interest in additional tools for self-management. The hypothesis was elaborated *that a higher perceived severity of the health condition related to a higher perceived potential of diabetes apps for self-management* (*H 12*, Table 19). Moreover, it was hypothesized *that diabetes app users and non-users differed in health status and demographics* (*H 15*).

Sixthly, this was also influenced by *general attitudes* towards life. For example, patients showing fatalist or self-destructive attitudes were found to manage their disease insufficiently, e.g., "What can you do? You can't do anything" (Rei Hong, age 61, T2DM). Moreover, they either did not know about diabetes apps, or showed no interest in diabetes apps (e.g., Rei Hong, age 61, T2DM showed limited interest in apps). *General negative attitudes towards life (e.g., pessimism) were therefore hypothesized to relate to the non-use of diabetes apps, while general positive attitudes (e.g., optimism) were hypothesized to relate to the diabetes app use* (*H 13*, Table 19).

Other psychological, physical and practical diabetes self-management factors potentially explaining differences in diabetes app use could not sufficiently be supported by interview extracts. The results did not allow an interpretation of user and non-user differences regarding these factors. This included psychological aspects like the motivation for self-management, feelings, and psychological problems (e.g., depression), physical factors including the type of diabetes, the diabetes medication used, the length of the disease, and practical factors like socioeconomic influences. For example, it was unclear if user and non-user groups differed in types of diabetes. T2DM participants fell under the category of non-users of diabetes apps to a larger extent than T1DM, while the majority of T1DM participants were part of the diabetes app user group. However, there were T2DM users (Bharat, Gu Fang, Henna, Deng Li) and T1DM non-users (Jie). Similarly, it was unclear if user and non-user groups differed in the type of medication used (insulin injections or oral medication). The results only showed that some apps might be considered more relevant to patients injecting insulin than the ones using oral medication or using no medication. For example, food data-bases giving information on food ingredients were reported as relevant only by pa-tients injecting insulin (Adit, Pang, Shi Hui), to adjust insulin dosages to the amount of carbohydrates consumed.

(2) Technology Adoption Factors (UTAUT Factors and Technology Usage Barriers):

Firstly, as part of demographic factors (*H 15*) *age* is relevant in the UTAUT and was possibly a factor relevant for diabetes app adoption and usage, leading to diverse atti-tudes towards diabetes app adoption and use in different age groups. The user and non-user typology showed that the young diabetes adopters (e.g., Adit, age 22, T1DM, being dissatisfied with apps) differed in their attitudes about diabetes apps from the older diabetes, app switchers or long-term users (more satisfied with apps, e.g., Shi Hui, age 35, T1DM), while the older non-users of diabetes apps fully rejected diabetes app usage (e.g., Jie, age 64, T1DM).

Secondly, as shown by demographic factors, some self-management, UTAUT and empowerment factors overlapped. For example, the inclusion of diabetes apps in dia-betes programs (*H 9*) like DAFNE could be considered part of the UTAUT factor *fa-cilitating condition* for diabetes app adoption and use, as well as an *access or care factor* when looking at diabetes program participation (Table 16). Similarly, techno-logical experience (*H 11*) was reported as a self-management factor when looking at *diabetes skills and knowledge*, but is also an aspect of the UTAUT factor *experience*. Thus, the UTAUT factors *facilitating condition* and *experience* were already men-tioned when talking about self-management factors in the previous paragraphs.

Thirdly, other UTAUT factors were likely results of self-management factors. For example, the *perceived usefulness and potential* of diabetes apps for example was found to be likely related to the perceived seriousness of the health condition (*H 12*). In both users and non-users there were groups perceiving diabetes apps as useful (in-terested non-users, diabetes app switchers, long-term diabetes app users), and groups evaluating the diabetes app usefulness as limited (non-users without interest, dissatis-fied app adopters). For example, Kaiyan (age 42, T1DM) said that: "Before this I to-tally don't have any app, so usually umm… I will record it in the book but that's a little cumbersome, and I normally don't follow through. So I find this thing [app] uhh… it's very helpful". In contrast, Sona (age 20, T1DM) said:

> I don't think it's really helpful [logbook app]. Sometimes um uh because we have to manually record, right? Then sometimes… if we are lazy, we don't really record. So like uh, initially, okay I think it's okay to record… After like halfway through ah… I'm too lazy to record, so I just leave it.

The perceived app usefulness or the perceived app potential were likely related to actual diabetes app adoption and (maintained) usage in diabetes app users, and thus it was hypothesized *that diabetes users reported higher perceived app potential for self-management than non-users* (*H 14*, Table 19).

Fourthly, there were insufficient extract examples about the factors *extrinsic motivation* for diabetes app use (incentives for the app use hardly reported in the sample) and the *voluntariness* of the app use (obligatory diabetes apps use as part of a program not reported by any patient), and no conclusions about (non-) user differences could be drawn. *Social influence* as part of the UTAUT overlapped with behavioral empowerment indicators (*H 2*).

Fifthly, *restriction evaluations* were mostly covered by self-management and technology adoption factors as non-fulfilled preconditions (reverse, negatively influencing factors). For example, financial barriers hindering diabetes app use could be categorized as part of financial restrictions, or as the mentioned socioeconomic factors influencing self-management (practical self-management factors). Technological experience was mentioned as a self-management factor likely to enhance app use (e.g., Xiu Wen, age 57, T1DM reported good knowledge about apps due to his IT related job), and as a usage barrier if there was a lack of technological experience: "I didn't know [about diabetes apps]" (Zhen Wei, age 47, T2DM).

To summarize, hypotheses on the relationships between empowerment as an antecedent factor, other self-management and technology adoption factors, and the diabetes app use were derived from the Study 2 interview results as summarized in Table 19.

(3) Other Relevant Factors:

Apart from the factors derived from theory, *health system characteristics* appeared relevant for diabetes app use on a more general level. For example, most doctors did not push their patients towards using additional technological tools for self-management. Doctors related to the DAFNE program (dose adjusting for normal eating) supported an app use because the DAFNE program included a diabetes logbook app for BG recording (Sona and Shi Hui). One reason for the lack of promoting online mobile tools for diabetes self-management was found in specific health system characteristics in Singapore, with a top-down structure in health policies and healthcare.

> So they [doctors] have to be careful [when recommending apps]: ... If let's say for example, doctor say 'Oh. Try this app.' Then if something goes wrong, they will publish [it] in the newspaper, they'll write [it] into the forum, or they put [it] on Facebook and say, 'Oh, this doctor ah. Tells me to use this ah and went wrong.' So the doctors are... they will never push it unless if it's through the government. Okay la, for example, one of the channel is the Health Promotion Board, Health Buddy. Okay. And then they say, 'Oh, you want information? Go to the Health Buddy and they will have information for you.' So the government will bear the brunt of the... any feedback after this, you see... The government says 'We support this app.' You know? They have to ascertain information is good and all that, you know. 'It's not 100%, you know... but, these are the apps we do support'. (Kang, age 67, pre-diabetes)

The example shows that the Singaporean government was reported to be rather hesitant with new technology introduction for diabetes management. Cheng (age 23, T1DM) said that: "New technology when it's tested overseas [needs] like, a period up to ten years, and that's like, nothing has gone wrong within this ten years, then they start importing the device in". As reported by the study participants, before introducing new technology to patients, HCPs waited for an official approval by the government (also concerning apps).

Additionally, influences on technology-supported self-management could for example be found in a lack of insurance coverage for chronic diseases, financial aid for patients

Table 19. Summary on Hypotheses Deriving from Study 2 Results

Theory	Factor	No.	Hypotheses
Psych. emp.		1	Diabetes app users show higher psychological empowerment than non-users of diabetes apps:
	Relevance, competence, self-determination, impact		a) Diabetes app users show higher perceived relevance of self-management, b) higher perceived competence for self-management, c) higher perceived independence in self-management, and d) higher perceived impact on self-management outcomes than non-users of diabetes apps.
Behav. emp.		2	Diabetes app users show higher behavioral empowerment than non-users of diabetes apps:
	HCP decision-making, HCP-patient communication, support by social networks		a) Diabetes app users report more shared HCP decision-making, b) better and more participatory HCP-patient communication, and c) more support from private social networks than non-users of diabetes apps.
Psych. & behav. emp.		3	Psychological empowerment positively relates to behavioral empowerment in diabetes app users.
		4	Shared decision-making results in higher psychological empowerment than paternalistic decision-making in both diabetes app users and non-users.
		5	Psychological empowerment positively relates to behavioral empowerment in diabetes app non-users at risk for complications.
		6	Psychological empowerment negatively relates to behavioral empowerment in older diabetes app non-users above 60 years of age.
UTAUT & self-management	Facilitating conditions/ social influence/ provider factors	7	The type/medical specialty of the supervising HCP relates to decision-making styles and to quality of HCP-patient communication in both user and non-user groups.
		8	Diabetes app users consult diabetes specialists while non-users consult general practitioners.
		9	Participation in diabetes programs relates to longer diabetes app use.
	Experience/ knowledge/skill	10	Lacking diabetes knowledge relates to dependence in decision-making, and to the non-use of diabetes apps.
		11	Lacking technological skill and experience relates to the non-use of diabetes apps.
	Health condition	12	The higher the perceived severity of the health condition the higher the perceived potential of diabetes apps for self-management.
	Attitudes	13	General negative attitudes towards life relate to the non-use of diabetes apps, while general positive attitudes relate to the use of diabetes apps.
	Performance & effort expectancy	14	Diabetes users report higher perceived app potential for self-management than non-users.
	Demography	15	Diabetes app users and non-users differ in demographics and health status.

by diabetes organizations, the structure of healthcare facilities (e.g., general practitioners at polyclinics versus diabetes specialists at diabetes centers), high economic pressure (housing prices, prices for medication), pressure to succeed in a working career (attitude towards work), and general culturally influenced attitudes (e.g., on diabetes research). Lack of insurance coverage, high economic pressure, and lack of financial aid could for example influence willingness to pay for diabetes apps (mentioned by Henna, Rei Hong, Xiu Wen).

The interviews further confirmed that the technological characteristics of the apps could likely influence the decision to adopt or to reject an app, or the decision to maintain or to stop using an app. This was in line with usage and app feature preferences. For example, amongst the users, young adopters were dissatisfied with diabetes apps, criticizing diabetes app designs and interfaces, app reliability, costs of app usage, and further problems inherent in the apps. These results at least partly confirmed Study 1 results on diabetes apps that found insufficient app quality and low potential for empowered self-management. However, differences between user and non-user groups regarding preferred app characteristics could not be interpreted from Study 2 results, and thus the relevance of app characteristics for diabetes app use in different (non-) user groups was not clear. Further research is necessary examining the influence of app characteristics on diabetes app usage in various (non-) user groups.

13.3 Discussion

Diabetes App Use as Part of Self-Management

Study 2 results delivered an insight into diabetes app (non-) use in the Singaporean sample. As suggested theoretically in Chapter 4.1, the interview results showed that diabetes app use had to be considered as only one self-management behavior in addition to other self-management behaviors like BG measurement and recording, diet, exercise, foot care, checkup adherence, online health information seeking, and other behaviors. Diabetes apps were considered tools that could support and potentially improve the overall self-management by e.g., structuring BG measurements and insulin injections (logbooks), delivering educational information (educational videos), improving an adjustment between diet and insulin intake (databases for carbohydrates), or making self-management more fun (interactive gamification of self-care). Yet, perceived usefulness of diabetes apps for self-management and app preferences varied largely in patient groups, and led to varying usage patterns as described by the (non-) user typology.

Empowerment and Diabetes App (Non-) Use

With empowerment being an antecedent of self-management behaviors (Funnell & Anderson, 2003; Tol et al., 2015), the theoretically derived hypothesis *H II* (Table 4) had been elaborated that empowerment was an antecedent of diabetes app use in the same way as it is for other self-management behaviors, and that it complemented other antecedent factors (*H III*, Table 4). The Study 2 results on differences in (non-) user groups leaned towards a first confirmation of the relevance of (both psychological and behavioral) empowerment as an antecedent of diabetes app use in addition to other antecedent factors. The interviews and data from the background information questionnaire delivered support for the relevance of the psychological empowerment indicators perceived relevance, perceived competence, and perceived impact and the behavioral empowerment indicators HCP decision-making, HCP-patient communication and support by private social patient networks for the adoption and (maintained) use of diabetes apps for self-management. Furthermore, with the additional psychological (and behavioral) empowerment scale results in the background information questionnaire confirming interview results, consistency across the data could be found. Thus, the interviews confirmed the validity of the scales in addition to available reliability and validity test results.

Comparing study results with previous research, the types of doctor-patient relationships found in the interviews were almost identical to the four models of doctor-patient relationship by Emanuel and Emanuel (1992) described in Chapter 7.1.2. Three types of relationships similar to the theoretical model evolved from the interviews, including patients managing diabetes independently from their HCPs (informative), patients depending on their HCPs (paternalistic), and patients following shared decision-making with their HCPs (deliberative). Shared decision-making appeared to be relevant for diabetes app adoption and maintained app use over time, and appeared to be likely the most successful approach for supporting both self-management and diabetes app use in the interviews.

With participants emphasizing the relevance of support from private social networks (family, friends, other patients, support groups), the relevance of social support by private networks could be confirmed. Moreover, Study 2 results delivered at least some support for the theoretical argumentation in Chapter 7.1.2 that support by private patient networks should be considered part of behavioral empowerment in addition to support by HCPs.

Other Relevant Factors for Diabetes App Use

From Study 2 central factors for diabetes app use besides empowerment appeared to be the type of supervising doctor (in combination with the decision-making style as part of behavioral empowerment), the participation in diabetes programs (including an app), diabetes knowledge, previous technological experience, the severity of the health condition (e.g., high BG values or symptoms of diabetes complications showing), general attitudes towards life (optimism and pessimism), age, and the perceived usefulness of diabetes apps. These factors were indicated differences in the overall self-management, and/or differences in diabetes app user and non-user groups.

Regarding results on the relevance of diabetes knowledge for self-management (lack of diabetes knowledge going along with lower psychological empowerment and dangerous health behaviors) the Study 2 results were consistent with previous research stating that "health literacy without patient empowerment comes down to wasting health resources, while empowerment without health literacy can lead to dangerous or suboptimal health behaviour" (Eyuboglu & Schulz, 2016, p. 1).

Furthermore, Study 2 confirmed previous research which found that vulnerable diabetes target groups were unprepared for digital disease management tools (Mathiesen et al., 2017). The group of interested diabetes app users with high risk of complications and lacking diabetes knowledge fitted into definitions of vulnerable target groups, including poor diabetes management, low (diabetes) education levels and low health literacy, lifestyle risk factors, and the presence of comorbidities (Mathiesen et al.,

2017). The text extracts on this non-user group also confirmed reported psychological avoidance mechanisms (e.g., Zhen Wei, age 47, T2DM), non-usage of digital self-management tools, as well as preferences for human interaction instead of digital contact (e.g., Rei Hong, age 61, T2DM) (Mathiesen et al., 2017).

Apart from the factors potentially influencing diabetes app use derived from theory, it had to be discussed whether more general health system and society characteristics not appearing in the theory needed to be considered when evaluating antecedents of health app use. Study 2 interviews pointed to a dependence of adoption and successful diabetes app use from general Singaporean health system characteristics. HCPs were reported to be hesitant to recommend diabetes apps for self-management, and an official approval of apps in the diabetes context is needed for the HCPs to gain confidence to include apps in diabetes care. Other studies found similar results to these findings (L. Boyle, Grainger, Hall, & Krebs, 2017). General health system characteristics are expected to play a role in the adoption and use of diabetes apps, not only when comparing study results across different health systems (i.e., across countries), but within one health system as well. These results confirmed theoretical argumentation by Menon (2002) who suggests individual psychological health empowerment taking place in the context of health policy and the health system (Chapter 7.1.1). In future research, comparative studies on the use of diabetes apps for self-management should be conducted to provide an insight into differences between systems, and an understanding how society and the health system relate to the role of mobile smart tools for diabetes self-management. Diabetes self-management in Singapore might differ significantly from other societies due to the differences in health system structures. Comparative approaches would also help to define the relevance of diabetes app usage barriers, like financial barriers. The financial aspect occurred in almost all self-management related themes in the interviews, and was found to be a major barrier towards good self-care.

13.4 Study Limitations

Some Study 2 limitations had to be addressed. Firstly, a (non-) user typology is useful for both research and for practice. Based on an app user and non-user typology, guidelines on how to tailor diabetes apps for specific diabetes (non-) user groups can be developed. However, the developed (non-) user typology showed some methodological limitations. With every patient managing the disease individually, the user typology offered only broad user and non-user types with dynamic borders, and mixed forms (some patients might fall under several user groups/types). Criticism of over-generalization using broad types of diabetes app (non-) users might be expressed here. However, the typology as a generalized categorization was useful to help understand diabetes app (non-) user groups, usage differences, app use in general, and the relevance of empowerment as an anteceding factor.

Secondly, diabetes apps for self-management were focused on. However, the text extracts showed that frequently it was not diabetes specific apps that were used as part of self-management, but other tools on mobile devices, like WhatsApp group chats in diabetes support groups (e.g., Diabetes Singapore chat on WhatsApp, e.g., Ei Tek, age 60, T2DM). For example, Ei Tek (age 60, T2DM) reported participation in diabetes support group chats using WhatsApp to exchange diabetes-related information between support group members. Follow-up studies should examine the use of mobile smart devices for diabetes self-management more broadly, and include all mobile tools that are used as part of the self-management process. Alanzi, Bah, Jaber, Al-shammari, and Alzahrani (2016) looked into the usage of WhatsApp for diabetes self-management. They found significant improvement in patients' knowledge and self-efficacy when using WhatsApp for diabetes management compared with a control group. More research looking into various mobile tools as part of diabetes self-management is necessary to extend the scope from diabetes apps for self-management to other channels on mobile smart devices.

Thirdly, Study 2 mainly focused on the doctor-patient relationship and communication, with the relevance of diabetes nurses and dieticians being possibly underexposed in the interviews. It could be shown that every diagnosed patient in the sample regularly consulted a doctor, while only a few patients consulted diabetes nurse educators (DNEs), dieticians, podiatrists, or other HCPs. Only participants of some diabetes care programs, like the DAFNE program (dose adjusting for normal eating, SingHealth, 2017), reported consulting nurses and dieticians at regular checkups with the doctor (e.g., Sona, age 20, T1DM). A few participants reported frequent contact with nurses and nurse educators (chat with nurses, Sona; app communication with nurse educators, Bharat; nurse hotline, Adit;). Overall, the extent to which other HCPs apart from doctors were part of behavioral empowerment could not fully be clarified from the interviews. Further research should put a stronger focus on other HCPs involved in diabetes management apart from doctors. This has to be investigated more closely to be able to evaluate the relevance of other HCPs for behavioral empowerment.

Fourthly, due to the sampling method using a cooperation with TOUCH diabetes support in Singapore, the sample mainly included members of support groups. Motivated patients were overrepresented in the sample, and high-risk patients with problematic self-management frequently were not part of support groups. Thus, a certain bias due to the selection of participants through support groups was possible. Additionally, due to the voluntariness of the interview participation, a certain degree of self-selection could not be avoided. However, some patients in the sample represented the problematic target group at risk for diabetes complications. Most research struggles to include hard-to-reach audiences (e.g., unmotivated and uninterested individuals), and the same challenge occurred in this research. Strategies have to be found how to include problematic target audiences into research samples to a larger extent. It is the hard-to-reach audiences who require specific attention, with risk of complications frequently being high in these patient segments.

13.5 Conclusion

The diabetes app user and non-user typology from 21 interviews resulted in two broader diabetes app non-user types and three user types. The differences from the user and non-user typology suggested that diabetes app use differed in groups with differing empowerment levels. This was a first indication of the relevance of empowerment for diabetes app use. The results revealed that very complex relationships between empowerment, diabetes self-management, and app use for self-management were likely, with several influencing factors relevant to this relationship. Moreover, the interviews showed a general trend that the majority of the empowered and motivated patients managed diabetes well, had a favorable attitude towards self-management, and were using apps as additional tools for self-management (apart from the group of non-users without interest). Shared health decision-making, close relationships with specialist doctors and/or participation in specific diabetes programs that included online media seemed to enhance diabetes app usage.

Overall, Study 2, prepared the foundation for more detailed analyses in Study 3, and delivered detailed knowledge on diabetes app use as part of diabetes self-management, as well as on app user and non-user differences. From Study 2 results, specific hypotheses were developed to be tested in Study 3 in a larger sample, using statistical analysis methods. Study 2 delivered results from exploratory analyses and thus did not allow final conclusions on relationships (i.e., causal relationships).

14 Study 3 – An Online Survey on Empowerment as an Antecedent of Diabetes App Use

First results from Study 2 face-to-face interviews implied a relationship between empowerment and diabetes app use, and showed that empowerment was likely an antecedent of diabetes app use. However, due to the exploratory character of Study 2 and the outlined study limitations (Chapter 13.4), further research was required that added statistical analysis for result confirmation. Therefore, based on Study 2 results, Study 3 further investigated if empowerment could be considered a relevant antecedent of diabetes app use in addition to other influencing technology adoption and self-management factors, and aimed at (1) testing if the diabetes app user and non-user typology results from Study 2 in Table 18 and in Table 7 in the Appendix could be statistically confirmed with a different sample to be able to answer *RQ 2* on (non-) user differences (Table 4), (2) testing the hypotheses about specific relationships between variables derived from Study 2 (*H 1* to *H 15*, Table 19), as well as (3) testing the more general hypotheses derived from theory (*H I* to *H III*, Table 4). For a better overview, Figure 5 graphically displays the hypotheses *H I* to *H III* and *H 1* to *H 15* on the processes between empowerment, other influencing factors and diabetes app use (similar to Figure 2, but dropping the aspects that were not focused on in the hypotheses).

14.1 Method

Study 3 included a standardized online survey with all types of diabetes patients (T1DM and T2DM) to collect information about diabetes self-management, app use, empowerment, and other influencing factors. With the main focus on patients using online media and apps for self-management, online data collection offered advantages over offline face-to-face or paper-and-pencil self-administration. It was expected that diabetes patients using apps would be reached most efficiently through online media, and participation would increase if access to the questionnaire was location independent.

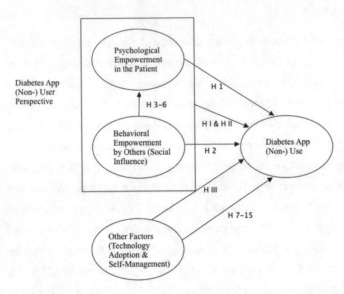

Figure 5. Hypotheses on empowerment as an antecedent of diabetes app use in addition to other anteceding factors (Study 3).

Notes. *H I-III* from theory, *H 1-15* from Study 2 results, positive relationships are hypothesized (apart from *H 6*); other factors include: HCP type (*H 7 & 8*), diabetes program participation (*H 9*), perceived diabetes knowledge (*H 10*), tech. experience (*H 11*), perceived severity of health condition (*H 12*), general attitudes (*H 13*), perceived app potential (performance expectancy, *H 14*), health status and demographics (*H 15*).

With Singaporean diabetes patients mostly leading a busy lifestyle as shown in Study 2, access to the questionnaire was provided from any device anywhere in Singapore (e.g., the participants could fill the questionnaire on their way home from work using public transport). Furthermore, Wright (2006) pointed out that online surveys are especially appropriate when aiming at populations suffering from diseases that are difficult to reach offline, possibly due to stigmatization in society. An online survey "enables communication among people who may be hesitant to meet face-to-face" (Wright, 2006, access to unique populations). With diabetes being a sensitive topic to talk about, participation was expected to be higher in an anonymous online questionnaire than in a face-to-face survey.

The final online questionnaire included questions on the following topics: 1) diabetes background, 2) self-management behaviors, 3) empowerment, 4) mHealth, 5) general attitudes and feelings, 6) demography, and 7) lottery participation. At the beginning and at the end of the survey questions on general diabetes self-care and diabetes background were included to embed the questions on mHealth and on empowerment in a more general frame. The online survey questionnaire can be found in Chapter 3.1 in the Appendix.

14.1.1 Operationalization

Based on the theoretical background on empowerment and app use in Chapter 7, the Study 1 app review results in Chapter 12 and the Study 2 face-to-face interview results in Chapter 13, survey variables were collected for testing the hypotheses *H I-III* in Table 4 and *H 1-15* in Table 19. The variables were operationalized using existing measures and scales, or creating items where scales were not available. Existing scales were selected according to their validity and reliability (see Appendix Chapter 3.3 on scales).

To measure diabetes app use as a dependent variable, previous diabetes app use or non-use, as well as the length and frequency of the previous app use were included as main variables following Study 2 results (Table 15) and based on the National Survey on Health App Use (Krebs & Duncan, 2015).

Psychological empowerment with its four indicators relevance, competence, self-determination and impact was measured with the EMPOWER project scale (Lamprinos et al., 2016; Mantwill et al., 2015) in the same way as in the Study 2 background information questionnaire ($M = 3.87$, $SD = .26$, $\alpha = .957$). For additional validation of the empowerment scale (Mantwill et al., 2015), a second diabetes empowerment scale was added for comparison. Higher empowerment values on the EMPOWER project scale were expected to correlate positively with results from other psychological diabetes empowerment scales. The short form of the Diabetes Empowerment Scale (DES-SF, R. M. Anderson et al., 2003) was chosen ($M = 3.59$, $SD = .15$, $\alpha = .929$) due to its specific focus on diabetes, its recognition in diabetes research, its frequent use (compare citation numbers for R. M. Anderson et al., 2000), and its documented reliability and validity (R. M. Anderson et al., 2003).[15]

Following theoretical explanations on behavioral empowerment in Chapter 7.1.2 and scales used in the Study 2 background information questionnaire, decision-making styles as an indicator of behavior empowerment were measured using the Provider Participatory Decision-making Style Scale by Heisler et al. (2002) (PDMstyle, $M =$ 3.25, $SD = .08$, $\alpha = .943$). Moreover, the Provider Communication Scale (Heisler et al., 2002) was used to assess HCP-patient communication as another behavioral empowerment indicator (PCOM, see theoretical chapters; $M = 3.50$, $SD = .37$, $\alpha = .919$). With the interviews in Study 2 confirming the relevance of social support by private social networks for the behavioral empowerment concept, a scale was added that measured social support by the family and by friends (Diabetes Care Profile DCP, section V, Fitzgerald et al., 1996b, $M = 3.29$, $SD = .19$, $\alpha = .931$). Specific behavioral empowerment scales were not available, thus the mentioned scales were selected to use indicators of behavioral empowerment.

The operationalization of factors from the UTAUT, of inhibiting factors (usage barriers) and of diabetes self-management factors was equally based on Study 2 results (Table 16). Suitable scales were looked for to measure aspects that had been found in Study 2 interview data representing the theoretical factors (Table 16). The UTAUT factors and usage barriers were partly based on the items from the Diabetes Care Profile (Fitzgerald et al., 1996b) and the National Survey on Health App Use (Krebs & Duncan, 2015) as shown in Table 11 in the Appendix. Self-management was based on

---

[15] In contrast to the empowerment scale by Mantwill et al. (2015) which includes perceived competence (self-efficacy) as one indicator out of four (based on Schulz & Nakamoto, 2013), the DES defines and operationalizes psychological empowerment as diabetes-related psychosocial self-efficacy (R. M. Anderson et al., 2003; R. M. Anderson et al., 1995; R. M. Anderson et al., 2000). The authors of the DES state that the DES measures three "related but separate domains of psychosocial self-efficacy" (R. M. Anderson et al., 2000, p. 741). These three resulting subscales are "managing the psychosocial aspects of diabetes", "assessing dissatisfaction and readiness to change", and "setting and achieving diabetes goals". All three subscales assess perceived abilities for performing various behaviors related to diabetes self-management (1. social support obtainability, stress management, self-motivation, decision-making, 2. identification of dissatisfaction, changes in self-management plans, 3. goal-setting, barrier management, goal-achieving, R. M. Anderson et al., 2000). In Chapter 7.1 it was explained that measuring psychological empowerment with self-efficacy is questionable. Thus, the downside of the DES was its limitation of self-efficacy, not paying attention to other empowerment dimensions that were suggested by research groups in other fields. Therefore, although the DES is very specific for the diabetes context, it might capture the empowerment construct in a way that is too narrow. Therefore, the DES-SF was only used for validation purposes.

items from an adapted version of the Summary of Diabetes Self-Care Activities (SDSCA, Toobert et al., 2000, $M = 4.19$, $SD = 1.25$, $\alpha = .576$). As previously discussed in Chapter 13.1.1 (study 2), Cronbach's alpha was low for the SDSCA, and therefore single items were used where needed.

Items for diabetes background were taken and adapted from items from the Diabetes Care Profile (Fitzgerald et al., 1996b) and the National Survey on Health App Use (Krebs & Duncan, 2015). General attitudes (pessimism and optimism) had been found as a relevant factor in Study 2 interviews, and thus were included using a scale on pessimism and optimism from the Life Orientation Test (LOT-R, Scheier, Carver, & Bridges, 1994, without filler items, $M = 3.17$, $SD = .32$, $\alpha = .473$). Cronbach's alpha was low for the LOT-R after removal of the filler items. However, this scale was of minor importance and thus the low alpha value did not pose a major problem. Moreover, psychological aspects had been mentioned as important in Study 2 interviews, and thus feelings towards diabetes were additionally measured with the Problem Areas in Diabetes Scale which assesses diabetes distress (PAID, Welch, Jacobson, & Polonsky, 1997, $M = 2.42$, $SD = .37$, $\alpha = .955$).

Table 11 in the Appendix summarizes Study 3 operationalization. Additionally, scale information, adaptions and validity information for all included scales can be found in Chapter 3.3 in the Appendix.

14.1.2 Pretest and Sampling

A pretest was undertaken with the survey draft to receive feedback on the survey questions, the layout, spelling mistakes, and potential problematic aspects. To include both professional and non-professional feedback, pretest participants were chosen from three specific groups: (health) communication professionals from academia providing feedback on professional survey design; diabetes professionals delivering feedback from the medical diabetes perspective; and diabetes patients providing feedback from the patient perspective. Sixteen participants took part in the pretest which was an equivalent to 25% of the final survey sample of $N = 65$. The pretest required approximately 30 minutes completion time for a patient of higher age. For this reason, the questionnaire was further shortened to decrease the time needed to answer all questions, and to reduce dropout rates. Based on the pretest feedback, the order of the questions was changed for better structure, the introduction text was written more clearly, cash incentives were offered instead of vouchers, participants without diabetes were directed to the end of the survey right at the beginning of the questionnaire, and education and marital status were adapted for Singaporean characteristics. Apart from these changes, the questionnaire did not show any major problems in the pretest.

Official support for a representative sample could neither be achieved by diabetes care organizations nor by hospitals or doctors in Singapore, due to strict IRB study regulations in the medical sector in Singapore (no separate IRB application for Study 3 had been planned to avoid delays in data collection) and due to the large number of studies conducted with diabetes patients with increased funding for studies as part of the proclaimed "war on diabetes" by the Singaporean government (Ministry of Health, 2017). Alternatively, a snowball sampling method had to be used. The link to the online survey was sent to previous face-to-face interview participants to spread the link to other patients. Additionally, social media and support groups were used to reach Singaporean diabetes patients. To increase participation, a lottery participation with cash incentives (three times 100 SGD) was optionally offered at the end of the questionnaire. The applied sampling method resulted in higher self-selection and a small study sample. Major efforts were undertaken to increase the sample size, including an extension of the field phase (to almost one year), contacting other researchers who had conducted studies with similar samples, seeking contact with official care organizations to spread the survey link, seeking cooperation with endocrinologists, and sending survey participation invitations to support groups and online communities several times. Despite these efforts over several weeks, people suffering from diabetes were extremely hesitant to participate in the study, and the study sample remained smaller than expected. The aim was a minimum of 200 participants, and the sample resulted in 65 completed questionnaires after exclusion of incomplete questionnaires (also see Study 3 limitations, Chapter 14.4).

14.1.3   Data Analysis

The data analysis was conducted using IBM SPSS version 25, with statistical analysis applied to the online survey data.

Cluster Analysis

Hierarchical cluster analysis was applied to the study sample to test if the typology resulting from Study 2 (Table 18) could be confirmed in a different sample. Hierarchical cluster analysis was used to compare clusters, without a preliminary cluster specification needed (as in partition clustering, e.g., k-means). Separate clustering was conducted for users and non-users of diabetes apps because clustering variables had to be differentiated for these two groups to be able not just to compare users and non-users on a very general level, but also to compare subgroups within the two groups for usage and non-usage characteristics. For example, the length of the previous app use could only be used as a clustering variable for users while it was not applicable to non-users. A previous hierarchical clustering had shown that a joint analysis for users and non-users did not deliver promising results. Preconditions for cluster analysis were checked, including a check of collinearity among clustering variables, data quality (no missing values), and the sample size in relation to the number of clustering variables. Results on collinearity are presented in Chapter 14.2.3 on results. To guarantee high data quality, after exclusion of cases with missing values for clustering variables, the sample size was reduced from originally $N = 79$ to $N = 65$ with $n = 31$ for diabetes app users and $n = 34$ for diabetes app non-users. Regarding the number of clustering variables, Formann (1984) recommends a minimum sample size of 2^m with m being the number of clustering variables. In the resulting sample of $N = 65$, the maximum recommendable number of clustering variables was six variables ($2^6 = 64$). However, since cluster analysis was conducted for users and non-users separately with $n = 31$ for users and $n = 34$ for non-users, only four clustering variables were used ($2^4 = 16$). Study 2 results had indicated the most relevant factors for diabetes app use found in the data (Chapter 13.2.4.2). Apart from psychological and behavioral empowerment, this included the type/specialty of the supervising doctor (in combination with the decision-making style as indicator of behavioral empowerment), the participation in dia-

betes programs, diabetes knowledge, the severity of the health condition, general attitudes towards life (optimism and pessimism), age, technological experience, and the
perceived usefulness/potential of diabetes apps. From these factors, four selected factors were used as clustering variables for hierarchical cluster analysis. The clustering
variables were selected based on theory, previous Study 2 typology results, and the
best clustering results achieved. Based on theory and the research questions (RQ 2a-d,
Table 4), clustering variables were aimed at including both app (non-) usage variables,
empowerment, and other potentially influencing factors. All remaining factors were
used as explanatory variables to describe the clusters. With Study 2 results indicating
that diabetes app users could be especially distinguished in the length of previous app
use, the perceived app usefulness, and the age of the app users (see Study 2 typology
results, Table 18), these variables were used as clustering variables in addition to empowerment as the main theoretical concept. Thus, for the diabetes app users the final
four clustering variables included the length of the previous diabetes app use, the perceived app usefulness, empowerment, and age. For non-users of diabetes apps the
clustering variables differed due to lack of previous usage. Here, parallel to diabetes
app users and based on Study 2 results, clustering variables included the perceived
diabetes app potential for self-management (i.e., perceived usefulness), empowerment,
and age (best clustering results). For the non-users the perceived diabetes app potential was used instead of perceived app usefulness, with no perceived usefulness of
apps available in non-users of diabetes apps. Non-users of apps could not rate perceived app usefulness without a previous usage of diabetes apps as they lacked insight
into these diabetes apps. However, they could generally give their opinion about the
potential of diabetes apps for self-management. Perceived potential of diabetes apps
was also available for users, but was not used in the user cluster analysis due to significant correlation with the length of the app use ($r = .388$, $p < .05$, Table 22).

Hierarchical cluster analysis was run with the original metric variables[16]. Due to metric scale level, the squared Euclidean distance measure, Ward's method, and z-

---

[16] For comparison, hierarchical clustering was also run using binary variables (0-1, converted from the original
variables with different scales and scale levels). Outliers could be avoided using binary variables, and thus did
not pose a problem for the clustering. Due to the conversion of all variables to binary variables, z-

standardization due to different scales were applied. The dendrogram and the elbow criterion were used for finding the best number of clusters achieved with hierarchical cluster analysis.

After the most appropriate cluster solution had been selected, different (dis)similarity measures were applied to the hierarchical cluster analysis, and the order of objects was re-arranged to test the result for stability. Cluster centroids were compared using T-Tests/ANOVAs to test if clusters differed from one another, and criterion validity was checked for the clusters by checking differences in additional criterion variables (Sarstedt & Mooi, 2014). Additional relevant variables deriving from Study 2 interview results were used as explanatory variables to test if these variables similarly distinguished the clusters resulting from the analysis. Finally, the final cluster solution was compared with the Study 2 result on types of diabetes app users and non-users.

Due to the small sample size(s) hierarchical cluster analysis was manageable, despite being computationally more demanding than partitioning methods. Partitioning cluster analysis (k-means) was not applied to the data due to the need to pre-specify a number of clusters at the beginning of the partitioning procedure. Moreover, hierarchical clustering was chosen because it is applicable to all scale levels (to be able to compare a binary variable solution to a metric variable solution; partitioning clustering is just applicable to metric data).

Binary Logistic Regression

For testing the hypotheses *H 1-15* derived from Study 2 as shown in Table 19, diabetes app user and non-user group differences were analyzed using independent T-Tests and one way ANOVAs. Pearson correlations were used where general relationships between variables were examined.

---

standardization of the data was not needed. Due to nominal scale level of the resulting variables, similarity measures were used (simple matching coefficient), as well as single linkage method. In contrast to Ward's method, single linkage tends to form one large cluster, but Ward's method did not result in an interpretable cluster solution using binary variables (Sarstedt & Mooi, 2014). For several versions of binary clustering variables the hierarchical clustering did not achieve an acceptable solution. This was explicable due to downscaling of variables when converting them to binary format.

To compare the strength of the influence of all empowerment dimensions and other relevant factors on diabetes app use, binary logistic regression was used (enter, blockwise). Psychological and behavioral empowerment dimensions were entered in binary logistic regression as independent factors, as well as technology adoption and self-management factors derived from theory (see Table 11 in Appendix). It was tested if these factors influenced the probability that diabetes apps were used (binary variable of use = 1, non-use = 0). The strength of the influence of the independent factors was then compared. All independent variables were metric or coded as dummy variables. Only factors from theory were entered in binary logistic regression that included data from both app users and non-users. Variables that were relevant for only one group (diabetes app users or non-users) were excluded from the analysis (including the following variables for users: perceived app usefulness, extrinsic motivation for app use, the reasons for starting/stopping an app use; and the following variable for non-users: reasons for not using diabetes apps). From several variables representing a factor (see Table 11 in Appendix), the most important variables were included in regression analysis to limit the number of variables to a manageable amount. For example, due to a low Cronbach's alpha of the SDSCA scale ($\alpha = .576$) only BG testing was used for previous self-management activities, with BG-testing being the most representative behavior for diabetes self-management.

Significant models with the best model fit, best prediction success, and significant predictors were looked for. Starting with all factors from theory, factors were removed in each step to compare models.

14.2 Results

14.2.1 Sample Description

The study sample ($N = 65$ after removal of incomplete questionnaires) included T1DM (20%) and T2DM participants (77%, 3% pre-diabetes) between 20 and 70 years of age (Table 20). The study sample was mainly well educated (75% college or higher), full- or part-time working (71%), and held Singaporean passports (88%). More than 70% did not use health insurance or used health insurance without chronic disease coverage. The use of oral diabetes medication (e.g., Metformin) was reported by 79% of the study participants, while 39% injected insulin (syringe or insulin pump). Similar to Study 2, not just T1DM but also T2DM patients injected insulin, and some T2DM patients used insulin injections and oral medication in parallel.

Diabetes diagnosis ranged from less than one year ago to being diagnosed up to 36 years ago. The majority of the sample said they had a diabetes family history (77%), and 77% had received diabetes education and diabetes management training. Almost the entire sample reported participation in offline or online diabetes support groups (94%), while only 11% were part of a specific diabetes program (e.g., DAFNE). On average, the sample reported minor psychological problems coping with their diabetes condition ($M = 2.42$, $SD = .86$, 5-point scale, Table 20).

Overall, rather well educated patients, T2DM patients, and support group members were overrepresented in the sample. Due to the age groups included in the sample (20 to 70 years of age) married patients and patients working full-time were also more present than other groups. Men and women were equally part of the sample.

The overall sample displayed medium to high psychological empowerment ($M = 3.87$, $SD = .83$ on a 5-point scale with higher scores displaying higher empowerment) and medium behavioral empowerment (average scores between $M = 3.25$ and $M = 3.50$ on 5-point scales for decision-making, HCP-patient communication and support by social private networks, see Table 20).[17]

Looking at the included psychological empowerment scales, both the DES-SF (R. M. Anderson et al., 2003) and the EMPOWER project scale (Mantwill et al., 2015) displayed similar results (Table 20) and correlated positively and significantly with $r = .33$, $p < .01$ ($N = 65$). The similarity of the scale results delivered an additional validation of the EMPOWER project scale as mentioned in Chapter 14.1.1.

---

[17] To facilitate a comparison of empowerment levels in various groups, and for better interpretation, 5-point scale results were split into three equal segments: low, medium, and high empowerment. With the group of low empowerment hardly including any participants when splitting the 5-point scale into three equal segments ($\leq$ 1.67 low, > 1.67 < 3.34 medium, $\geq$ 3.34 high), the segments were used as following: $\leq$ 2.50 low, > 2.50 < 3.50 medium, $\geq$ 3.50 high.

Table 20. Sample Description (Study 3)

Variable	n	% of N	M	SD	Min	Max
Age (in years)			49.74	14.67	20.00	70.00
Education						
MA graduate or higher	15	23.1				
BA graduate/college graduate	22	33.8				
Some college	12	18.5				
High school graduate	12	18.5				
Some high school	3	4.6				
Other education level	1	1.5				
Employment						
Full- time working	34	52.3				
Part-time working	12	18.5				
Retired	7	10.8				
Unemployed	6	9.3				
Student	5	7.7				
Homemaker	1	1.5				
Family status						
Married	32	49.2				
Never married & single	18	27.7				
Divorced	7	10.8				
Never married & relationship	4	6.2				
Widowed	4	6.2				
Gender						
Women	33	50.8				
Men	32	49.2				
Insurance						
Insurance without diabetes coverage	31	47.7				
No health insurance	15	23.1				
Insurance with limited diabetes coverage	12	18.5				
Insurance with full diabetes coverage	3	4.6				
Other	4	6.2				
Nationality						
Singaporean	57	87.7				
Malaysian	4	6.2				
Other	4	6.2				
Diabetes and health background						
Body Mass Index (BMI)			24.80	5.75	15.38	48.07
Diabetes family history	50	76.9				
Diabetes Type						
T2DM	50	76.9				
T1DM	13	20.0				
Pre-diabetes	2	3.1				
Education on diabetes (received)	50	76.9				
Length of diabetes (in years)			13.73	9.81	.00	36.00

Variable	n	% of N	M	SD	Min	Max
Medication						
Oral diabetes medication	51	78.5				
Insulin injection (syringe & pump)	25	38.5				
(Self-) Management						
Diabetes app use						
Never used diabetes apps	34	52.3				
Diabetes app previous use	17	26.2				
Diabetes app current use	14	21.5				
Online health information seeking (days per week)			2.70	2.27	.00	7.00
Part of offline support group	42	64.6				
Part of online support group	19	29.2				
Part of diabetes program	7	10.8				
Empowerment						
Psychological empowerment (EMPOWER)[a]			3.87	.83	1.00	5.00
Relevance			4.15	.77	1.00	5.00
Competence			3.72	.90	1.00	5.00
Self-determination			3.89	.96	1.00	5.00
Impact			3.72	.94	1.00	5.00
Psychological diabetes empowerment (DES-SF)[a]			3.59	.81	1.00	5.00
Behavioral empowerment						
Decision-making style (PDMstyle)[b]			3.25	1.29	1.00	5.00
HCP-patient communication (PCOM)[c]			3.50	1.10	1.40	5.00
Support by private social networks (family/friends; DCP)[a]			3.29	1.19	1.00	5.00
Emotional distress (PAID)[d]			2.42	.86	1.00	4.85
General attitudes: optimism/pessimism (LOT-R)[a]			3.17	.53	1.83	5.00

Notes. N = 65, Diabetes Empowerment Scale Short Form, DES-SF (R. M. Anderson et al., 2003), Diabetes Care Profile, DCP, section V, Q2 (Fitzgerald et al., 1996b), EMPOWER project scale (EMPOWER, Mantwill et al., 2015), Life Orientation Test, LOT-R without filler items (Scheier et al., 1994), Participatory Decision-Making Style, PDMstyle and Provider Communication, PCOM (Heisler et al., 2002), Problem Areas in Diabetes, PAID (Welch et al., 1997)
[a]5-point scale from 1 = strongly disagree to 5 = strongly agree
[b]5-point scale from 1 = none of the time to 5 = all of the time
[c]5-point scale from 1 = poor to 5 = excellent
[d]5-point scale from 1 = not a problem to 5 = serious problem

14.2.2   Diabetes App Use

On average, the sample (*N* = 65) searched for health information online on three days per week. Half of the sample had never used diabetes apps for self-management before (*n* = 34; 52%), while half either had previously used diabetes apps or were using them at the time of data collection (*n* = 31; 48%). From 31 diabetes app users, 14 used diabetes apps at time of data collection and 17 had used diabetes apps but had stopped using them (Table 20). The mentioned diabetes apps almost exclusively related to diary/logbook apps ($n = 20$). A few mentioned diabetes nutrition apps ($n = 1$), did not remember or mention the app name ($n = 6$), or mentioned other apps ($n = 4$). Table 21 displays the diabetes apps mentioned in the Study 3 sample.

Table 21. Diabetes Apps in the Sample (Study 3)

App name	n
Blood Glucose Tracker	3
Bodycloud	1
DAFNE Online Diary	3
Diabetes App	1
Diabetes Zap	1
EasyDiabetes	1
GLA	1
Glooko	2
Glucose	1
Glyco (Leap)	8
MySugr (Logbook)	3
MyHemoglobin	1
One Drop	1
Other	8
Total	35

Note. From $n = 31$ diabetes app users, 4 mentioned more than one app.

The longest period of diabetes app use was from 2 days to 3.29 years. On average the app users used their apps $M = 4.69$ days per week ($SD = 2.84$). Thirty-two percent of app users had shared health information with their HCPs through apps.

In app users ($n = 31$) reasons to start diabetes app use especially included expected usefulness of diabetes apps (55% of users), an expected improvement of self-management by using diabetes apps (32%), the expected ease of use of apps (32%), own knowledge about apps (23%), recommendations by other patients and support groups (19%), doctors' recommendations (13%), incentives (13%), or other reasons (13%). Here, in contrast to Study 2 results, apps being part of programs, HCP offerings, advertising, or family/friend recommendations were less relevant.

From non-users of diabetes apps ($n = 34$), five patients said they didn't use a smart device (15% of non-users). Other reasons for non-usage of diabetes apps especially included never being told about app options (29%), problems in choosing an app

(29%), and lacking app knowledge (24%). None of the non-users said that the app use was too expensive for them. Reasons for stopping an app use ($n = 17$) especially included lacking tailoring of diabetes apps (24%), the time-consuming app use (18%), and varying other reasons (35%).

The perceived importance of app features in both app users and non-users showed that features to stay in touch with other users and features that support own decision-making (e.g., explaining treatment alternatives) were least important, while all other features were perceived as equally important (HCP feedback features, log features, tailoring features, learning features, analysis features).

In the following, before testing the hypotheses and looking at the strength of factors influencing diabetes app use, a test was carried out to establish if the (non-) user typology from Study 2 could be statistically confirmed with data from Study 3 to answer *RQ 2* conclusively on user and non-user differences regarding empowerment and other influencing factors. (Table 4). The typology was a foundation for the hypotheses and a check was required to test if this typology could be (statistically) replicated in a different sample.

14.2.3 Types of Diabetes App (Non-) Users – Results from Hierarchical Cluster Analysis

Preconditions – Collinearity

Regarding collinearity among clustering variables, it was confirmed that the variables correlated neither significantly nor highly (low collinearity among variables, Table 22). Only the perceived app potential and the length of the app use in app users correlated significantly on a moderate level ($r = .388$, $p < .05$, Table 22), but neither variable was used in parallel in the same cluster analysis. Thus, collinearity among the clustering variables could be avoided.

Resulting Clusters for Diabetes App Users

Hierarchical cluster analysis based on the four metric variables *length of the previous app use*, *perceived app usefulness*, *empowerment*, and *age* suggested either a two clus-

Table 22. Pearson Correlation for Clustering Variables (Study 3)

		Overall em-powerment	Age	App potential for self-management	Length of app use	Perceived app usefulness
Overall empower-ment		1	.078	-.015	-.216	-.201
	N	65	65	65	31	31
Age		.078	1	.038	-.082	-.153
	N	65	65	65	31	31
App potential for self-management		-.015	.038	1	.388*	.163
	N	65	65	65	31	31
Length of app use		-.216	-.082	.388*	1	.255
	N	31	31	31	31	31
Perceived app use-fulness		-.201	-.153	.163	.255	1
	N	31	31	31	31	31

Notes. $N = 65$, diabetes app users $n = 31$, bivariate two-tailed correlations, overall empowerment results based on combination of psychological and behavioral empowerment results.
*$p < .05$

ter solution, or a four cluster solution ($n = 31$, Ward's method, squared Euclidean distance, Figure 6 and Figure 7).

The two cluster results displayed significant mean group differences regarding the length of previous diabetes app use, the perceived usefulness of diabetes apps, and overall empowerment. The difference regarding age was shown not to be significant (Table 23).

Cluster 1 could be described as the short-term diabetes app users with an average of $M = 105.31$ days of usage ($SD = 115.62$). This group showed rather low to medium perceived usefulness of diabetes apps ($M = 2.75$, $SD = 1.00$), relatively high empowerment ($M = 3.94$, $SD = .60$, including both psychological and behavioral dimensions), and an average age of $M = 51.31$ years ($SD = 16.13$, Table 23).

In contrast, cluster 2 could be described as long-term diabetes app users with an average of $M = 379.93$ days of usage ($SD = 366.73$). This group reported high perceived usefulness of diabetes apps ($M = 4.13$ on a 5-point scale, $SD = .74$), medium overall empowerment ($M = 3.33$, $SD = .46$), and an average age of $M = 42.20$ years ($SD = 11.99$, Table 23).

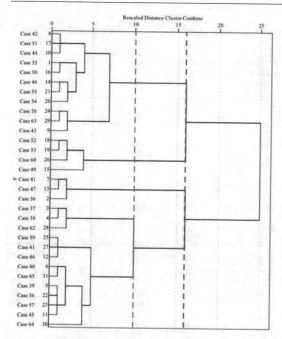

Figure 6. Dendrogram using Ward Linkage – hierarchical cluster analysis for app users (Study 3).

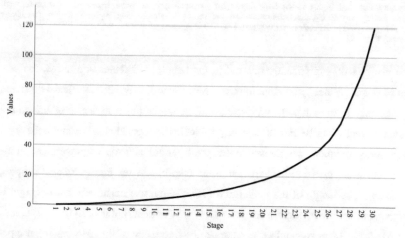

Figure 7. Elbow criterion – hierarchical cluster analysis for app users (Study 3).

Table 23. Two-Cluster Result for Diabetes App Users – Mean Group Differences (Study 3)

Clustering Variables	Cluster 1: short-term diabetes app users ($n = 16$)		Cluster 2: long-term diabetes app users ($n = 15$)					
	M	SD	M	SD	N	df	T	p
Length app use (days)	105.31	115.62	379.93	366.73	31	16.596[a]	2.774	.013*
Perceived app usefulness[b]	2.75	1.00	4.13	.74	31	29	4.347	.000**
Overall empowerment	3.94	.60	3.33	.46	31	29	-3.125	.004**
Behav. empowerment	3.69	.84	2.99	1.02	31	29	-2.099	.045*
Family/friend support (DCP)[b]	3.38	1.16	2.56	1.05	31	29	-2.057	.049*
HCP-patient communication (PCOM)[b]	3.86	1.23	3.45	1.03	31	29	-1.001	.325
Decision-making style (PDMstyle)[b]	3.83	1.23	2.95	1.43	31	29	-1.836	.077
Psych. empowerment[b]	4.18	.58	3.67	1.00	31	29	-1.755	.090
Age	51.31	16.13	42.20	11.99	31	29	-1.776	.086
Explanatory variables								
Average BG values	2.80	1.01	2.25	1.42	27	25	-1.173	.252
Body mass index (BMI)	23.70	2.63	24.75	4.49	30	28	.781	.442
Disease length (in years)	14.13	9.23	14.87	1.56	31	29	.209	.836
Education/schooling	4.50	1.26	5.00	.93	31	29	1.249	.222
Health info seeking online (days per week)	3.19	2.37	3.20	2.31	31	29	.015	.988
Optimism/pessimism (LOT-R)[b]	3.33	.35	3.04	.57	31	29	-1.702	.100
Perceived diabetes knowledge	3.69	.70	3.73	.59	31	29	.195	.847
Psychological distress (PAID)[b]	2.13	.59	2.73	.93	31	29	2.138	.041*
Self-management summary (days per week)	4.58	.99	4.15	.76	30	28	-1.312	.200

Notes. Ward method, independent samples t-tests.
[a] Equal variances not assumed
[b] 5-point scales, with higher values displaying higher perceived app usefulness, higher psych. empowerment, higher participatory HCP-patient communication and shared decision-making, higher optimism, and higher psychological distress, for scales see Chapters 3.1 and 3.3 in Appendix.
*$p < .05$, **$p < .01$

The two clusters significantly differed in the length of diabetes app usage, the perceived app usefulness, and empowerment. More specifically, the two clusters differed significantly in the support by private social networks as an indicator of behavioral empowerment (Family/friends' support, Table 23). All psychological and behavioral empowerment dimensions showed lower results, and thus lower empowerment, in the long-term users than in the short-term users (significant for family/friends' support, Table 23). The length of the period of a diabetes app use negatively but not significantly correlated with empowerment on all empowerment dimensions ($r = -.216$, n.s., $n = 31$, Table 12 in Appendix). In contrast, the frequency of the diabetes app use per week correlated positively with psychological empowerment in diabetes app users (r

= .282, n.s., n = 29), with the empowerment indicator perceived relevance of diabetes self-management significantly and positively correlated with the frequency of the app use (r = .377, p < .05, n = 29). Behavioral empowerment did not correlate with the frequency of the diabetes app use (none of the behavioral empowerment indicators, r = -.057, n.s., n = 29, Table 12 in Appendix).

Looking at additional explanatory variables (especially other relevant factors suggested from Study 2 interviews), psychological distress was significantly shown to be higher in long-term users (M = 2.73 on a 5-point scale, SD = .93) than in short-term users (M = 2.13, SD = .59, $t(29)$ = 2.138, p < .050).

Both groups did not differ significantly in their self-management, with relatively frequent average self-management activities per week (on 4-5 days per week), and their BG ranging between 5.60 to 7.90 mmol/l (categorized as pre-diabetes or non high-risk diabetes range by American Diabetes Association, 2016). High education (some college or undergraduate degree), good perceived diabetes knowledge, a diabetes diagnosis 14-15 years ago, neither very optimistic nor pessimistic attitudes, and an average of three days per week looking for health information online characterized both groups equally (Table 23, additionally see scale information in Chapter 3 in Appendix). Moreover, there were no significant differences in both diabetes app user groups regarding medication (long-term users: 20% insulin injections, 33% oral medication, 47% both; short-term users: 25% insulin injections, 50% oral medication, 19% both, n = 31), HCP types (the majority used diabetes specialists, 80% of long-term users and 67% of short-term users, n = 30), marital status (47% of long-term users married, 38% of short-term users married, n = 31), gender (53% of long-term users female, 50% of short-term users female, n = 31), employment (67% of long-term users working full-time, 56% of short-term users, n = 31), or diabetes program or support group participation (87% of long-term users participating, and 88% of short-term users, n = 31).

In addition, a four cluster solution was compared with the two cluster solution for diabetes app users. However, it did not add much value, but split cluster 1 (short-term users) into younger short-term users and older short-term users, and cluster 2 (long-term users) into two groups of medium to long-term users (see Table 13 in Appendix). The two-cluster solution was preferred with two clusters being very small in a four cluster solution, and the value added being relatively low compared with increased complexity with a higher number of clusters (Table 13 in Appendix).

Resulting Clusters for Non-Users of Diabetes Apps

For non-users of diabetes apps, hierarchical cluster analysis based on the three metric variables *perceived app potential for self-management*, *empowerment*, and *age* suggested a two cluster solution, or a three cluster solution as shown in Figure 8 and in Figure 9 (n = 34, Ward's method, squared Euclidean distance).

In a two-cluster solution, cluster 1 could be described as the diabetes app non-users who evaluated the potential of diabetes apps for self-management as rather low (to medium) with $M = 2.67$ (5-point scales, $SD = .62$). Here, overall empowerment was rather high ($M = 3.78$, $SD = .52$), with high values for all empowerment dimension apart from HCP decision-making (which showed a tendency for a medium level, Table 24). This group reported an average age of $M = 55.87$ years ($SD = 12.68$).

Cluster 2 included diabetes app non-users who perceived the potential of diabetes apps for self-management as very high ($M = 4.68$, $SD = .48$). Here, overall empowerment was on a medium level on all dimensions, apart from psychological empowerment with slightly higher values ($M = 3.74$, $SD = .80$). Average age in this group was $M = 50.32$ years ($SD = 15.47$, Table 24).

The two cluster result for diabetes app non-users displayed significant mean group differences regarding the perceived diabetes app potential for self-management, and the support by family and friends (social network support) as an indicator of behavioral empowerment. The difference regarding age was not shown to be significant (Table 24). All psychological and behavioral empowerment dimensions showed lower results, and thus lower empowerment, in the diabetes app non-users who perceived the app potential as high (cluster 2) than in the ones perceiving the app potential as lower (cluster 1) Especially in family and friends' support this difference was significant between the two clusters with $t(32) = 2.210, p < .05$ (Table 24).

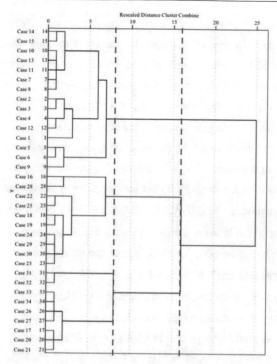

Figure 8. Dendrogram using Ward Linkage – hierarchical cluster analysis for app non-users (Study 3).

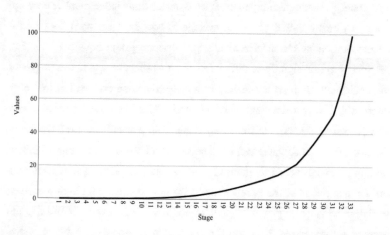

Figure 9. Elbow criterion – hierarchical cluster analysis for app non-users (Study 3).

In relation to additional explanatory variables, both diabetes non-user groups differed significantly in the length of their diabetes since diagnosis. The app non-users who perceived the app potential as high showed significantly longer diabetes experience than the ones who reported lower perceived app potential (cluster 1, $M = 9.33$, $SD = 5.67$; cluster 2, $M = 16.11$, $SD = 11.78$; $t(25.371) = -2.159$, $p < .050$, Table 24).

Apart from the length of diabetes since diagnosis, none of the other explanatory variables significantly differed in the two clusters. However, there were non-significant tendencies. For example, 67% of non-users with lower perceived app potential reported consulting GPs, while 65% of non-users with higher perceived app potential reported consulting diabetes specialists (χ^2 $(1, N = 29) = 2.773$, $p = .096$). Moreover, only 53% of non-users with perceived lower app potential participated in programs or support groups, while 84% of non-users with perceived higher app potential participated in programs or support groups (χ^2 $(2, N = 29) = 6.058$, $p < .050$) (Table 24).

Neither group significantly differed in their self-management, with self-management activities reported on four days per week on average, and relatively low psychological distress with minor to moderate problems reported. In both groups, BG values were reported to range between 7.00 and 7.90 mmol/l on average (categorized as non high-risk diabetes range by American Diabetes Association, 2016). Relatively high education (some college), medium to high perceived diabetes knowledge, neither very optimistic nor pessimistic attitudes, and an average of two days per week looking for health information online characterized both app non-user groups equally (Table 24). Moreover, there were no significant differences in either diabetes app non-user groups regarding medication. Both groups mainly included patients on oral medication (67% of non-users with low perceived app potential, and 75% of non-users with high perceived app potential, $n = 34$). Neither group differed in marital status (60% of non-users with low perceived app potential were married, and 50% of non-users with high perceived app potential were also married, $n = 34$), gender (47% of non-users with low perceived app potential were female, and 53% of non-users with high perceived app potential, $n = 34$), or employment (40% of non-users with low perceived app potential worked full-time, and 27% part-time, and 47% of non-users with high perceived app potential worked full-time, and 21% part-time, $n = 34$, Table 24).

Table 24. Two Cluster Result for Diabetes App Non-Users – Mean Group Differences (Study 3)

Clustering Variables	Cluster 1: diabetes app non-users perceiving the app potential as low (to medium) ($n = 15$)		Cluster 2: diabetes app non-users perceiving the app potential as high ($n = 19$)					
	M	SD	M	SD	N	df	T	p
Perceived app potential[b]	2.67	.62	4.68	.48	34	32	-10.755	.000**
Overall empowerment	3.78	.52	3.42	.74	34	32	1.608	.118
Behav. empowerment	3.66	.86	3.10	.87	34	32	1.866	.071
Family/friend support (DCP)[b]	4.03	.94	3.20	1.19	34	32	2.210	.034*
HCP-patient communication (PCOM)[b]	3.63	1.09	3.14	1.02	34	32	1.354	.185
Decision-making style (PDMstyle)[b]	3.32	1.20	2.96	1.21	34	32	.858	.397
Psych. empowerment[b]	3.91	.88	3.74	.80	34	32	.567	.575
Age	54.87	12.68	50.32	15.47	34	32	.920	.364
Explanatory variables								
Average BG values	2.93	1.21	2.94	1.18	30	28	-.020	.984
Body mass index (BMI)	26.24	8.13	24.55	6.40	33	31	.669	.509
Disease length (in years)	9.33	5.67	16.11	11.78	33	25.371[a]	-2.159	.040*
Education/schooling	4.29	1.14	4.37	1.30	33	31	-.190	.850
Health info seeking online (days per week)	2.20	1.66	2.28	2.56	33	31	-.101	.920
Optimism/pessimism (LOT-R)[b]	3.27	.64	3.06	.50	34	32	1.054	.300
Perceived diabetes knowledge	3.73	.80	3.42	.90	34	32	1.054	.300
Psychological distress (PAID)[b]	2.12	.72	2.67	.98	34	32	-1.813	.079
Self-management summary (days per week)	4.06	1.25	4.01	1.42	34	32	.107	.916

Notes. Ward method, independent samples t-tests.
[a] Equal variances not assumed
[b] 5-point scales, with higher values displaying higher perceived app potential, higher psych. empowerment, higher participatory HCP-patient communication and shared decision-making, higher optimism, and higher psychological distress, for scales see Chapters 3.1. and 3.3 in Appendix.
*$p < .05$, **$p < .01$

As in the diabetes app users, the two cluster result was compared with an alternative cluster result, here including three clusters. Again the cluster solution with more clusters did not add much value, but split cluster 2 of diabetes app non-users reporting higher perceived app potential in one group of younger patients and one group of older patients (Table 14 in Appendix). The three cluster solution showed significant less frequent self-management activities in younger diabetes app non-users with higher perceived app potential than in older non-users with higher perceived app potential (average self management activities on three days per week in younger non-users, M = 3.26, SD = 1.36; average self-management activities on five days per week in older participants, $M = 4.84$, $SD = .99$; $F(2, 31) = 3.984$, $p < .05$).

Stability Tests and Comparison with Study 2 Results

When the clustering results were tested for stability, the results were the same when the order of the clustering variables was changed. Moreover, similar results were achieved with different (dis)similarity measures (city-block distance and Chebychev distance instead of squared Euclidean distance). Using the city-block distance, the age difference between diabetes app non-users with higher and lower perceived app potential was shown to be clearer in the two cluster solution. Here, the ones with lower perceived app potential and higher empowerment were older (cluster 1) than the ones with higher perceived app potential and lower empowerment (cluster 2). This result resembled the three cluster solution for non-users.

For a better overview of the clustering results, Table 25 generalizes and summarizes the results from hierarchical cluster analysis, in order to compare the results with Study 2 interviews and to answer *RQ 2*. Aspects differing from Study 2 interview results are highlighted in Table 25.

The data in Table 25 shows that the results of Study 2 interview typology and Study 3 cluster analysis overlapped to a large percentage and that results on *RQ 2* were quite consistent in both Study 2 and Study 3 samples.

A few major differences were noted between both study results: Firstly, the Study 3 cluster analyses could not confirm that non-users of diabetes apps perceiving the app potential as high were completely identical with interested non-users of diabetes apps in Study 2. This is because perceiving an app potential as high is not necessarily identical to showing high interest in diabetes apps. One could perceive the diabetes app potential as high but still show little interest in diabetes apps.

Secondly, the Study 3 non-users of diabetes apps perceiving the app potential as high could not be confirmed to be equally a group at high risk for diabetes complications as found in the interested non-users in Study 2 typology. This could at least partly be explained by the fact that high-risk patients were underrepresented in Study 3 online survey to a large extent ($n = 8$; operationalized as high BG values in combination with lack of BG testing as the most convincing indicator for poor self-management, also see next chapter).

Table 25. Summarized Results from Hierarchical Cluster Analysis (Study 3)

		Non-User of Diabetes Apps		Diabetes App User	
		The diabetes app non-user perceiving the app potential as low (cluster 1)	The diabetes app non-user perceiving the app potential as high (cluster 2)	The short-term diabetes app user (cluster 1)	The long-term diabetes app user (cluster 2)
Em-power-ment	Psych. Emp.[a]	High[c]	Medium to high	High	Medium to high*
	Behav. Emp.[b]	PDM: medium, PCOM: medium to high*, private network: high**	PDM: medium* PCOM: medium, private network: medium**	PDM & PCOM: medium to high, private network: medium**	PDM & PCOM: medium*, private network: low to medium**
UTAUT	Perceived app usefulness/ potential	Low to medium perceived app potential	High perceived app potential	Limited perceived usefulness	High perceived usefulness
	Previous diab. app use	No diabetes apps used	No diabetes apps used	Short-term diabetes app use (around 3 months)	Long-term diabetes app use (> 1 year)
	Online health info seeking HISc	Online HIS (2 days per week on average)	Online HIS (2 days per week on average)*	Online HIS (3 days per week on average)	Online HIS (3 days per week on average)
Personal factors	Age	Older participants (60+)	Middle aged (around 40)	Middle aged to higher age (around 50)	Middle aged (around 40)*
	Education	Some college**	Some college**	Some college or undergraduate degree**	Some college or undergraduate degree**
	Medication	Predominantly oral medication (T2DM)	Predominantly oral medication (T2DM)	Insulin injection, oral medication, or both	Insulin injection, oral medication, or both
	Diagnosis	Mainly diagnosed around 10 years ago	Mainly diagnosed around 16 years ago	Mainly diagnosed around 14-15 years ago	Mainly diagnosed around 14-15 years ago*
	Risk group/ average BG values plus self-management	7.0-7.9 mmol/l – no risk group	7.0-7.9 mmol/l – no risk group*	5.6-7.9 mmol/l – no risk group	5.6-7.9 mmol/l – no risk group
	Perceived diab. knowledge	Good perceived knowledge	Sufficient perceived knowledge*	Good perceived knowledge	Good perceived knowledge
	Self-management	Activities around 4 days per week	Activities around 4 days per week*	Activities around 4-5 days per week	Activities around 4-5 days per week
	Psychological problems (PAID)	Low distress, minor problems**	Moderate problems**	Low distress, minor problems**	Moderate problems**
Provider factors	HCP types	GP	Specialist doctor*	Specialist doctor	Specialist doctor
	Support group/ program	Around 50% in program or support group*	Around 80% in program or support group*	More than 80% in program or support group	More than 80% in program or support group

Notes. Study 3 survey data; abbreviations: GP = general practitioner, HIS = online health information seeking, HCP = healthcare professional, BG = blood glucose
* Marked results differing from Study 2 interview typology results.
** No comparable data from Study 2
[a] Psychological empowerment results from EMPOWER project scale (Mantwill et al., 2015)

[b] Behavioral empowerment result from summary of family/friends support (Fitzgerald et al., 1996b), PDMstyle & PCOM (Heisler et al., 2002)
[c] To facilitate a comparison of empowerment levels in various groups, and for better interpretation, 5-point scale results were split into three equal segments: low, medium, and high empowerment. With the group of low empowerment hardly including any participants when splitting the 5-point scale into three equal segments (≤ 1.67 low, $> 1.67 < 3.34$ medium, ≥ 3.34 high), the segments were used as following: ≤ 2.50 low, $> 2.50 < 3.50$ medium, ≥ 3.50 high.

Additionally, after using average mean values in Study 3, extremes (high BG values, poor self-management) were not fully visible anymore. As a potential result of both (underrepresentation, average means), the non-users perceiving the app potential as high appeared as a group with rather good average self-management, sufficient diabetes knowledge, and BG values in the normal diabetes range and not at high risk for complications. In contrast to Study 2 interested non-users this group also used specialist doctors and support groups, and searched for online health information.

However, some Study 3 results pointed in a similar direction as found in Study 2 interested high-risk non-users of diabetes apps. It was found that lack of self-management motivation significantly related to interest in diabetes innovations in the overall sample ($r = .256, p < .05, N = 65$), that the perceived diabetes app potential for self-management significantly and positively correlated with payment problems in diabetes care ($r = .334, p < .01, N = 65$), and that non-users who perceived the app potential as higher showed lower empowerment than the group perceiving the app potential as lower (Table 24). Study 2 had shown that unmotivated patients at risk of complications seemed to see potential in technology possibly due to their critical health conditions, for example to compensate for their insufficient self-management, or because diabetes apps were cheap and easy to use tools for self-management (in Study 2 see factor severity of the health condition in Chapter 13.2.4.2, also see "interested non-users of diabetes apps" in Study 2 typology). Because of the underrepresentation of high-risk patients in Study 3 sample (operationalized as high BG values in combination with lacking BG testing as the most convincing indicator for poor self-management, $n = 8$), a separate analysis of the high-risk group did not deliver meaningful results (tendencies suggested high-risk patients as being non-users of diabetes apps in 75%, and without online health information seeking behaviors in 63%).

Thirdly, in the diabetes app long-term users Study 3 results indicated a medium level of both psychological and behavioral empowerment, while the Study 2 typology attributed high empowerment levels to this group (all dimensions). Moreover, in Study 3 the long-term users were middle aged and diagnosed around 15 years ago, while Study 2 indicated long-term users belonging to all age groups, and being diagnosed more than 20 years ago.

Other than these differences, differences between Study 2 and Study 3 results were minor, and results of Study 3 mainly confirmed Study 2 interview results. Overall, the cluster analysis was able to confirm most differences within diabetes app user and non-user groups regarding the included factors.

The following chapter is dedicated to the test of the hypotheses derived from Study 2 interview results in Table 19, and takes a closer look at diabetes app user and non-user differences.

14.2.4   Differences between Diabetes App Users and Non-Users – Hypotheses

Differences concerning empowerment and other factors between diabetes app users and non-users were analyzed along the hypotheses *H 1-15* derived from Study 2 (Table 27).

Results could confirm that some aspects of psychological empowerment were significantly and positively related to diabetes app use (*H 1*). The frequency of the diabetes app use (days per week) for example significantly and positively correlated with the psychological empowerment indicator perceived relevance on a moderate level (*H 1, r* = .377, *p* < .050, Table 12 in Appendix). The perceived app potential for self-management was significantly higher in diabetes app users than non-users (*H 14, p* = .040, Table 26), and correlated significantly and positively with the psychological empowerment indicator self-determination (*H 1, r* = .262, *p* < .05, *N* = 65, see Table 12 in Appendix). For other aspects of psychological empowerment, despite similar tendencies, no significant results could be found (e.g., *H 1*, diabetes app users showing higher overall psychological empowerment than app non-users, Table 26).

An analysis of behavioral empowerment (*H 2*) showed that diabetes app users significantly differed from non-users in the support from family and friends (*H 2c*). Here, in contrast to HCP decision-making and HCP-patient communication ($H\ 2\ a/b$, there was only a non-significant tendency for diabetes app users to report more shared decision-making and better HCP-patient communication than non-users), app users showed significantly lower family or friend support than non-users ($p = .044$, Table 26). The perceived app potential for self-management was significantly higher in diabetes app users than non-users ($H\ 14$, $p = .040$, Table 26), and correlated significantly and negatively with the support of private social networks ($H\ 2$, $r = -.398$, $p < .01$, $N = 65$; no correlations for the other behavioral empowerment indicators, Table 12 in Appendix). An additional result indicated that diabetes app users and non-users significantly differed in the type of HCP (medical specialty) consulted for diabetes management ($H\ 8$), with a larger percentage of users consulting diabetes specialists, and a larger percentage of diabetes app non-users consulting GPs ($p = .028$, Table 26). Diabetes specialists significantly showed more shared decision-making and better HCP-patient communication than GPs (PDMstyle: specialists: $M = 3.72$, $SD = 1.16$, $n = 37$, GPs: $M = 2.65$, $SD = 1.30$, $n = 22$; $t(57) = -3.275$, $p < .01$, $N = 59$; PCOM: specialists: $M = 3.82$, $SD = 1.01$, $n = 37$, GPs: $M = 3.13$, $SD = 1.09$, $n = 22$; $t(57) = -2.472$, $p < .05$, $N = 59$, here unrelated to diabetes app use).

Relationships between psychological empowerment indicators (perceived relevance, competence, self-determination, impact) and behavioral empowerment indicators (decision-making, HCP-patient communication, support by private social networks, $H\ 3$ to $H\ 6$) showed significant positive relationships for non-users (perceived competence and support by private social networks $r = .347$, $p < .050$, $n = 34$; perceived impact and support by private social networks $r = .399$, $p < .050$, $n = 34$; other indicators similar but non-significant), while there were only non-significant weak tendencies of negative relationships found in users (e.g., perceived relevance related to decision-making with $r = -.134$, $p = .473$, $n = 31$, other indicators similar). This means that lower behavioral empowerment went along with lower psychological empowerment in patients not using diabetes apps for self-management, while lower behavioral empowerment could potentially still go along with higher psychological empowerment in diabetes app users.

Table 26. Mean Diabetes App User and Non-User Group Differences (Study 3)

	Non-Users of Diabetes Apps (n = 34)		Diabetes App Users (n = 31)					
	M	SD	M	SD	N	df	T	p
Psych. empowerment[b]	3.81	.83	3.94	.84	65	63	-.588	.558
Perceived relevance	4.17	.74	4.14	.81	65	63	.139	.890
Perceived competence	3.71	.90	3.74	.91	65	63	-.160	.873
Self-determination	3.79	1.00	4.00	.92	65	63	-.861	.393
Perceived impact	3.59	.97	3.86	.90	65	63	-1.169	.247
Behav. empowerment	3.35	.90	3.35	.98	65	63	-.010	.992
Decision-making style (PDMstyle)[b]	3.12	1.20	3.40	1.38	65	63	-.892	.376
HCP-patient communication (PCOM)[b]	3.35	1.06	3.66	1.14	65	63	-1.143	.258
Family/friend support (DCP)[b]	3.57	1.15	2.98	1.17	65	63	2.051	.044*
Average BG values	2.93	1.17	2.56	1.22	57	55	1.192	.238
Body mass index (BMI)	25.32	7.17	24.23	3.65	63	48.517[a]	.770	.445
Diabetes Specialist (dummy)	.44	.50	.71	.46	65	62.998[a]	-2.242	.028*
Disease length (in years)	13.03	9.98	14.48	9.74	64	62	-.589	.558
GP (dummy)	.53	.51	.39	.50	65	63	1.143	.257
Health info seeking online (days per week)	2.24	2.17	3.19	2.30	64	62	-1.704	.093
Interest in diabetes innovations[b]	4.09	1.14	4.42	.96	65	63	-1.262	.211
Optimism/pessimism (LOT-R)[b]	3.15	.56	3.19	.49	65	63	-.317	.753
Paying for my diabetes is a problem[b]	3.38	1.16	3.35	1.20	65	63	.094	.925
Perceived app potential for self-management[b]	3.79	1.15	4.35	.98	65	63	-2.103	.040*
Perceived diabetes knowledge[b]	3.56	.86	3.71	.64	65	60.747[a]	-.806	.424
Perceived health status[b]	2.44	.79	3.03	.80	65	63	-3.012	.004**
Psychological distress (PAID)[b]	2.42	.91	2.42	.82	65	63	.019	.985
Self-management summary (days per weeks)[b]	4.03	1.33	4.38	.90	64	58.326[a]	-1.251	.216
Age	52.32	14.28	46.90	14.78	65	63	1.503	.138
Education/schooling	4.33	1.22	4.74	1.12	64	62	-1.393	.169

Notes. Ward method, independent samples t-tests
[a] Equal variances not assumed
[b] 5-point scales, for scales see Chapters 3.1 and 3.3 in Appendix.
*p < .05, **p < .01

However, a result on high-risk non-users could not be achieved due to underrepresentation of this group, and a positive relationship of empowerment dimensions could therefore not be confirmed here (negative tendencies, Table 27). Overall, the results led to a preliminary rejection of the hypotheses as formulated in *H 3*, *H 5*, and *H 6*, assuming a positive relationship between psychological and behavioral empowerment for app users in *H 3*, a similar positive relationship in app non-users at risk in *H 5*, and a negative relationship for older non-users in *H 6* (see Table 19 and Table 27). Study 3 results rather indicated the opposite directions. Further confirmation of these results is needed using a larger sample. Lack of significance might result from the small sample size. The results partly confirmed Study 2 results that had found positive relationships between psychological and behavioral empowerment with the exceptions of some app switchers and older non-users without interest in apps who had shown high psychological empowerment despite low behavioral empowerment, but with high independence in self-management (see typology, Table 18). Study 3 results repeated the Study 2 tendencies of a negative relationship of empowerment dimensions shown in some app switchers/users.

Looking at other influencing factors apart from empowerment, paternalistic decision-making related to lower perceived diabetes knowledge in non-users of diabetes apps (*H 10*, $r = .442$, $p < .010$, $n = 34$), while this was not the case for app users (no relationship found, Table 27). Further non-significant tendencies, pointing in similar directions, showed that self-management activities as well as online health information seeking were slightly more frequent in diabetes app users, disease length and education higher, and age lower than in diabetes app non-users (Table 26).

Moreover, diabetes app users significantly reported a better *perceived health status* (good health status, *H 15*) than diabetes app non-users (fair health status, $p = .004$, Table 26). The better perceived health status in diabetes app users was mirrored by slightly lower BG values and lower Body Mass Index (BMI) results in diabetes app users than in non-users (Table 26).

Table 27 summarizes all results on the hypotheses that were tested in Study 3 (*H I* to *H III* from theory, and *H 1* to *H 15* from Study 2). Additionally, Figure 10 graphically displays the hypotheses' results related to the overall process between empowerment and diabetes app use. A general Study 3 result summary can be found in Chapter 15.1.

14.2.5   Most Relevant Factors' Strength of Influence on Diabetes App Use

To draw final conclusions for *H III* (Table 4) as the main summarizing hypothesis – hypothesizing that empowerment as an antecedent of diabetes app use is complementing other anteceding factors from technology adoption and self-management theory –

empowerment was entered in binary logistic regression, as well as technology adoption and self-management factors derived from theory (Table 11 in Appendix).

Checking for autocorrelation of all independent variables, the psychological empowerment indicators highly correlated, as well as the behavioral empowerment indicators HCP decision-making and HCP-patient communication with $r = .772$, $p < .01$ (Table 12 in Appendix). Therefore, psychological empowerment was used as one factor, and HCP decision-making and HCP-patient communication were recoded into one variable "HCP-patient relationship".

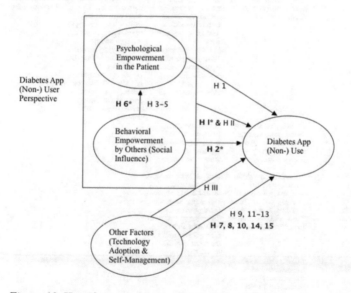

Figure 10. Hypotheses results regarding the process between empowerment and diabetes app use (Study 3).

Notes. Hypotheses confirmed by significant results marked in bold, positive relationships hypothesized (except of *H 6*); hypotheses marked with * show significant reverse or partly reverse results as hypothesized;

For psychological empowerment indicators positive relationship with app use found (*H I*), for behavioral empowerment negative relationship with app use for the support by private social networks found (*H 2*); positive relationship between support by private social networks and perceived impact in older diabetes app non-users found (*H 6*); specialist doctors showed more shared decision-making and app users consulted specialists to a larger extent than non-users (HCP type) (*H 7 & 8*); perceived knowledge (*H 10*), perceived app potential (*H 14*), and perceived health status (*H 15*) positively related to app use.

Table 27. Summary of Hypotheses Testing Results (Study 3)

Theory	Factor	No.	Hypotheses	Significant results	Other non-significant results	Data
		I	Psychological empowerment is positively related to diabetes app use.	Yes, frequency app use positively related to perceived relevance (weak/moderate, sig.) (Additional performance expectancy: perceived app potential positively related to self-determination, weak, sig.)	Difference in previous app use/non-use for self-determination and impact (n.s., higher in users, no differences for relevance and competence) Frequency of app use positively related to competence, self-determination, impact (weak, n.s.) Length of app use negatively related to psych. emp. (weak, n.s.)	Table 26, Table 12 in Appendix
			Behavioral empowerment is positively related to diabetes app use.	Partly reverse, difference in previous app use/non-use for support by private social networks (sig., less support in users) (Additional performance expectancy: perceived app potential negatively related to private network support, weak/moderate, sig.)	Difference in previous app use/non-use for HCP decision-making and HCP-patient comm. (n.s., more info and decision sharing in users) Frequency app use not related to behav. emp. (for all indicators) Length app use negatively related to all behav. emp. indicators (weak, n.s., apart from HCP-patient comm. showing no relationship)	Table 26, Table 12 in Appendix
		II	Psychological and behavioral empowerment are antecedents of diabetes app use for self-management.	The results deliver a first confirmation, further research needed regarding testing for causal relationship	-	
		III	Empowerment as a motivational antecedent of diabetes app use is complementing other anteceding factors from Unified Theory of Acceptance and Use of Technology.	First results confirm the hypothesis, relationships found between empowerment (esp. support by social private network), diabetes app use & other influencing factors, e.g., the medical specialty of the supervising HCP & the health status	-	
Psych. emp.		1	Diabetes app users show higher psychological empowerment than non-users of diabetes apps.	-	Yes (n.s.)	Table 26
	Relevance		a) Diabetes app users show higher perceived relevance of self-management than non-users of diabetes apps.	-	No difference found	Table 26
	Competence		b) Diabetes app users show higher perceived competence for self-management than non-users of diabetes apps.	-	No/marginal difference found (n.s.)	Table 26
	Self-determination		c) Diabetes app users show higher perceived independence in self-management than non-users of diabetes apps.	-	Yes (n.s.)	Table 26
	Impact		d) Diabetes app users show higher perceived impact on self-management outcomes than app non-users.	-	Yes (n.s.)	Table 26

Theory	Factor	No.	Hypotheses	Significant results	Other non-significant results	Data
Behav. emp.		2	Diabetes app users show higher behavioral empowerment than non-users of diabetes apps.	Reverse for behavioral empowerment by private social networks (sig.)	Yes, for behavioral empowerment by HCPs (n.s.)	Table 26
	Health decision-making		a) Diabetes app users report more shared HCP decision-making than non-users of diabetes apps who report more paternalistic decision-making.	-	Yes (n.s.)	Table 26
	HCP-patient communication		b) Diabetes app users report more better and more participatory HCP-patient communication than non-users of diabetes apps.	-	Yes (n.s.)	Table 26
	Support by social networks		c) Diabetes app non-users show less support from private social networks than diabetes app users (family support and support group participation).	Reverse (sig.)	-	Table 26
Psych. & behav. emp.		3	Psychological empowerment positively relates to behavioral empowerment in diabetes app users.	(only for non-users: perceived competence and perceived impact positively related to support by private social networks (moderate, sig.), other indicators similar but non-significant)	Reverse, negative very weak relationships found for all emp. indicators in users (n.s.)	Various; non-users: perceived competence & support by private social networks r = .347, p < .050, n = 34; perceived impact & support by private social networks r = .399, p < .050, n = 34
		4	Shared decision-making results in higher psychological empowerment than paternalistic decision-making in both diabetes app users and non-users.	-	Only in non-users (weak, n.s., no relationship in users found)	Non-users: PDMstyle – psych. emp.: r = .176, p = .320, n = 34
		5	Psychological empowerment positively relates to behavioral empowerment in diabetes app non-users at risk for complications.	-	No valid result due to underrepresentation of risk group. Tendency hints towards negative relationship for all empowerment dimensions in non-users at risk of complications	r = -.389, n.s., n = 6, (similar for separate behav. emp. indicators)
		6	Psychological empowerment negatively relates to behavioral empowerment in older diabetes app non-users above 60 years of age.	Reverse, perceived impact on self-management positively relates to support by social networks in older app non-users (moderate, sig.), for all non-users: perceived competence and perceived impact positively relate to support by private social networks (moderate, sig.)	Reverse, positive relationship between psychological and behavioral emp. in older non-users (weak, n.s.)	Perceived impact – social networks support: r = .533, p < .050, n = 14 Psych. – behav. emp.: r = .160, p = .584, n = 14

Theory	Factor	No.	Hypotheses	Significant results	Other non-significant results	Data
UTAUT & self-manage-ment	Facilitating conditions/social influence/provider factors	7	The type/medical specialty of the supervising HCP relates to decision-making styles and to quality of HCP-patient communication in both user and non-user groups.	Yes, diabetes specialists show more shared decision-making and better communication than GPs (sig.)	-	PDMstyle: specialists: $M = 3.72$, $SD = 1.16$, $n = 37$, GPs: $M = 2.65$, $SD = 1.30$, $n = 22$; $t(57) = -3.275$, $p < .01$, $N = 59$; PCOM: specialists: $M = 3.82$, $SD = 1.01$, $n = 37$, GPs: $M = 3.13$, $SD = 1.09$, $n = 22$; $t(57) = -2.472$, $p < .05$, $N = 59$.
		8	Diabetes app users consult diabetes specialists while non-users consult general practitioners.	Yes, diabetes app users consult specialists to a larger extent than non-users (sig.)	Yes, Non-users of diabetes apps consult GPs to a larger extent than users (n.s.)	Table 26
		9	Participation in diabetes programs relates to longer diabetes app use.	-	Yes (n.s.)	Program attendees: $M = 276.67$, $SD = 453.28$, $n = 6$, non-attendees: $M = 238.21$, $SD = 261.90$, $n = 24$, $t(28) = .276$, $p = .784$
	Experience/knowledge/skill	10	Lack of diabetes knowledge relates to dependence in decision-making, and to the non-use of diabetes apps.	Yes, paternalistic decision-making relates to lower perceived diabetes knowledge in all participants (weak, sig.), similar in non-users (moderate, sig.), in users no relationship found	Yes, less perceived diabetes knowledge in non-users than in users (n.s.)	Table 26, PDMstyle – knowledge overall sample: $r = .267$, $p < .050$, $N = 65$ Non-users: PDMstyle – knowledge: $r = .442$, $p < .010$, $n = 34$
		11	Lack of technological skill and experience relates to the non-use of diabetes apps.	-	Yes, less health info seeking online and less interest in tech. diabetes innovations in non-users (n.s.)	Table 26
	Health condition	12	The higher the (perceived) severity of the health condition the higher the perceived potential of diabetes apps for self-management.	-	No relationship found for perceived health status, tendency of weak negative relationship between BMI and perceived app potential (n.s.)	BMI – app potential: $r = -.133$, $p = .299$
	Attitudes	13	General negative attitudes towards life relate to the non-use of diabetes apps, while general positive attitudes relate to the use of diabetes apps.	-	No difference found	Table 26
	Performance & effort expectancy: perceived app potential	14	Diabetes users report higher perceived app potential for self-management than non-users.	Yes (sig.)	-	Table 26

Theory	Factor	No.	Hypotheses	Significant results	Other non-significant results	Data
	Demogra-phy	15	Diabetes app users and non-users differ in de-mographics and health status.	Yes, diabetes app users report better perceived health status than non-users (sig.)	Yes, diabetes app users report lower BG values and lower BMI than non-users (n.s.), app users are younger, report better education (n.s.), no differ-ence in gender and other demographics found	Table 26

Notes. *H I-III* deriving from theory (Table 4), *H 1-15* from Study 2 (Table 19); Pearson correlations interpreted following Hinkle, Wiersma, and Jurs (2003): weak $r \geq .300$, moderate $r \geq .500$, strong $r \geq .700$.

All other significant correlations of independent factors were on a low or moderate level, and thus acceptable. Table 15 in the Appendix displays the autocorrelation of all independent factors used in binary logistic regression.

A model including all independent factors as shown in Table 11 in the Appendix did not significantly predict diabetes app use. A model with good fit included the factors *psychological empowerment, behavioral empowerment by HCPs and by private social networks*, as well as the UTAUT factors' *perceived app potential* (performance and effort expectancy), *previous health information seeking online* (technological experi-ence), and *age*; and the self-management factors *type of diabetes, length of diabetes, perceived health status, payment problems* and *insurance coverage* (practical socioec-onomic), *BG testing* (self-management behaviors), *interest in innovation* (attitudes), *perceived diabetes knowledge, HCP type*, and *program or support group participation*. The test of this model against the constant only model was statistically significant, indicating that the predictors as a set reliably distinguished between diabetes app use and non-use ($\chi^2(16) = 26.752$, $p < .05$). Nagelkerke's $R^2 = .656$ indicated a high rela-tionship between prediction and grouping (goodness of fit). Prediction success overall was 90% (80% for app non-use and 96% for app use). The Wald criterion demonstrat-ed that only the support by private social networks as an indicator of behavioral em-powerment (*Wald*(1) = 5.315, $p = .021$) and the consulted HCP type (dummy GP or specialist, *Wald*(1) = 4.014, $p = .045$) made a significant contribution to the prediction of diabetes app adoption and use. In contrast, the remaining empowerment aspects psychological empowerment and HCP-patient relationship were not found to be sig-nificant predictors. The *Exp(β)* value indicated that when the support by private social networks was increased, the relative probability (odds ratio) that diabetes apps were adopted and used decreased with $Exp(\beta) = .044$, $\beta = -3.131$. The $Exp(\beta)$ value indicated that when the patients were supervised by specialist doctors the relative probability (odds ratio) that diabetes apps were adopted and used increased with $Exp(\beta) = 9460.805$, $\beta = 9.155$.

A model resulting after the removal of the factors *interest in innovation*, *insurance coverage*, and *program or support group participation* (due to lacking significance) showed a slightly lower prediction success with 75% (70% for app non-use and 79% for app use), but overall model significance with $\chi^2(13) = 26.936$, $p < .05$, and a moderate to high relationship between prediction and grouping (goodness of fit) with Nagelkerke's $R^2 = .509$. In this model, the Wald criterion demonstrated that the support by private social networks as an indicator of behavioral empowerment ($Wald(1) = 6.617$, $p = .010$) and the perceived health status ($Wald(1) = 7.839$, $p = .005$) made a significant contribution to the prediction of diabetes app adoption and use. Again, the $Exp(\beta)$ value showed that when support by private social networks was increased, the relative probability (odds ratio) that diabetes apps were adopted and used decreased with $Exp(\beta) = .283$, $\beta = -1.261$. The $Exp(\beta)$ value also indicated that when the perceived health status was improved the relative probability (odds ratio) that diabetes apps were adopted and used increased with $Exp(\beta) = 8.030$, $\beta = 2.083$.

Further reducing the independent factors, the models showed similar results to the last model, resulting in support by private social networks and the perceived health status being significant predictors of diabetes app use (e.g., empowerment factors, HCP type, perceived diabetes knowledge, perceived health status, and perceived diabetes app potential for self-management, $\chi^2(7) = 19.794$, $p < .01$, Nagelkerke's $R^2 = .380$, overall prediction success of 80%, with 79% for app non-use and 80% for app use; $Wald(1) = 5.427$, $p = .020$, $Exp(\beta) = .444$, $\beta = -.811$ for support by private social networks and $Wald(1) = 8.250$, $p = .004$, $Exp(\beta) = 4.481$, $\beta = 1.500$ for perceived health status). A further reduction of factors decreased the model fit, yet the HCP type nearly reached significance again (e.g., in a model only including support by private social networks, HCP type and perceived health status).

Overall, after testing various models, only the support by private social networks, the HCP type and the perceived health status significantly predicted diabetes app use.

Less support by private social networks was likely leading to a higher chance of diabetes app use, while the use of diabetes specialists and a better perceived health status increased the chance of app use for self-management.

14.3 Discussion

Study 3 tested hypotheses deriving from theory and from Study 2, and looked for factors best predicting diabetes app use.

Empowerment as an Antecedent of Diabetes App Use

Looking into empowerment as an antecedent of diabetes app use, Study 3 results indicated that a lack of self-management support by family and friends influenced diabetes app use positively (possibly a higher perceived need for additional self-management tools), or that high support by family and friends influenced the app use negatively (possibly no need for apps). Previous research found that unsupportive behaviors by relatives and friends could influence diabetes self-management in a negative way (Bennich et al., 2017; Grant & Schmittdiel, 2013; Helgeson et al., 2016). Talukder and Quazi (2011) found significant peer and social network influences on attitudes to technological innovation, as well as to innovation adoption behaviors. The results led to the conclusion that lack of support by private social networks might not just hinder self-management, but could also lead to diabetes patients looking for alternative (technological) means of self-management support.

In addition to the lack of support from private social networks, diabetes app users showed a higher chance of supervision by diabetes specialists than non-users, and diabetes specialists were shown to provide more shared decision-making than GPs (Table 26 and Table 27). Results allowed a first conclusion that higher shared decision-making and better HCP-patient communication were related to a higher chance of previous diabetes app use. The relation between shared decision-making and health app use was previously discussed in Abbasgholizadeh Rahimi, Menear, Robitaille, and Legare (2017), who stated that previous studies had shown that mHealth apps do liver potential to promote patient participation in shared health decision-making, but that studies also had shown disadvantages of mHealth use for shared decision-making, like security concerns or increased patient anxiety. The authors did not discuss shared decision-making as a possible precondition of app use, not addressing the possibility that patients supported in a participatory way might turn to apps more frequently than other patients.

Study 3 data showed that indicators of behavioral empowerment positively related to indicators of psychological empowerment in the majority of non-users of diabetes apps, while other tendencies implied possible negative relationships in diabetes app users (Table 27). Similar results were found for some Study 2 app switchers and non-users without interest in diabetes apps. Both Study 2 and Study 3 results showed that several interpretations were possible regarding the result that some participants showed high psychological empowerment despite low behavioral empowerment.

Firstly, low support by HCPs and private social networks could still go along with high psychological empowerment if patients managed very independently as shown in Study 2 (e.g., app switchers). Independent self-management could lead to a higher chance of diabetes app adoption and use if there were no other hindering factors (e.g., in group of older non-users without interest in Study 2). Study 2 showed that patients managing independently were motivated, and knew about or tried various technological tools for self-management (not necessarily diabetes apps only, see non-users without interest in diabetes apps). This could deliver one explanation for short-term use of diabetes apps and switching behaviors in independent patients showing high psychological and low behavioral empowerment (compare independent app switchers in Study 2).

Secondly, despite not examining empowerment as an outcome of diabetes app use in this research, it should be examined if the negative tendencies between empowerment dimensions suggest potential influences of diabetes app use on empowerment levels when looking at empowerment as an outcome of diabetes app usage (compare Figure 2). Diabetes apps could be used to compensate for low self-management support by HCPs and by the social private network. The resulting app use might influence psychological empowerment as assumed in Figure 2, leading to high psychological empowerment despite low behavioral empowerment in app users. In non-users of diabetes apps this effect was not found in Study 3, with lower behavioral empowerment going along with lower psychological empowerment. Further research is urgently necessary for examination of the causal relationships in both directions as suggested in Figure 2 (empowerment influencing diabetes app use, and diabetes app use influencing empowerment). So far, research has mainly focused on empowerment as an outcome of mHealth use, as explained in Chapter 7.3.1. Abbasgholizadeh Rahimi et al. (2017) summarize that "recent studies suggest that mHealth apps can empower patients" (p. 39). However, the overall process has to be examined with empowerment as an antecedent of diabetes app use, as well as a potential outcome of the app use (Figure 2).

Empowerment Operationalization

Study 3 also delivered information about the operationalization of empowerment with its psychological and behavioral dimensions. Cluster analysis used empowerment as one factor (summarizing psychological and behavioral dimensions) to reduce the number of clustering variables. Later results showed differences between psychological empowerment and behavioral empowerment by the HCPs, and behavioral empowerment by private social networks with only weak to moderate correlations between these three aspects (Table 12 and Table 15 in Appendix). In the analysis, behavioral empowerment was measured using three scales on HCP decision-making (Heisler et al., 2002), HCP-patient communication (Heisler et al., 2002), and the support by private social networks (Fitzgerald et al., 1996a). Psychological empowerment was measured with the EMPOWER project scale (Mantwill et al., 2015). The overall study results indicated that empowerment should not be summarized as one single factor, but used as a multi-dimensional construct including the separate dimensions of psychological and behavioral empowerment, to account for differences in these dimensions (as used in binary logistic regression analysis in Chapter 14.2.5). Continued discussion on this aspect can be found in Chapter 15.4.

Health Status Influencing App Use – the Discrepancy between Usage Intention and Use

In relation to other antecedent UTAUT and self-management factors apart from empowerment, a particularly relevant factor for diabetes app use was the perceived health status, found as a significant predictor in the logistic regression model. A higher perceived health status increased the chance of diabetes app adoption and use. This was in line with previous study results showing that health app download or use was more likely among those with reported good health than those with reported poor health (Robbins, Krebs, Jagannathan, Jean-Louis, & Duncan, 2017). Furthermore, these results also confirmed Study 2 results that indicated that diabetes app non-users at high risk of complications reported interest in diabetes apps but did not use diabetes apps due to perceived barriers (see typology). Study 2 results implied a discrepancy between attitudes and diabetes app usage intentions, and actual app adoption and usage in this risk group of patients. Discrepancies between diabetes apps usage intention and actual usage were found in previous studies, with intentions being higher than occurrence of actual usage (Dou et al., 2017; James et al., 2016). Barriers to actual technology usage in contrast to usage intentions were for example lack of ease of use, negative subjective norms, or lack of usage preparation (trainings) in previous studies (James et al., 2016). Study 2 results were confirmed in that Study 3 displayed that for example lack of self-management motivation significantly related to interest in diabetes innovations (but not to use). The hypothesis *H 12* on the severity of the health condition relating to the perceived potential of diabetes apps could not be confirmed in Study 3, probably due to the underrepresentation of high-risk diabetes patients in Study 3.

Discrepancies between usage intentions and actual usage relate to previous criticism of the UTAUT, with the UTAUT factors mainly contributing to an explanation of behavioral intention instead of the behavior itself (Chang, 2012). According to Al-Mamary et al. (2016), the included UTAUT factors might be insufficient predictors of actual technology acceptance and usage behaviors. These limitations of the UTAUT have to be kept in mind when looking at Study 3 results. The UTAUT limitations might be an explanation for the Study 3 result that the included technology adoption and self-management factors apart from the perceived health status did not significantly predict diabetes app use. This might point to possibly low relevance of these factors for actual diabetes app use. Other explanations for the lack of significant prediction of diabetes app use by other factors from theory in Study 3 could be the specific operationalization of the factors used in Study 3 (see Table 11 in Appendix), the sample used, or the combination of factors with the influence of several factors cancelling each other out. The operationalization of the factors from the UTAUT might be responsible for lacking significant relationships because the UTAUT factors were operationalized in a very study-specific way, for example using perceived usefulness of diabetes apps to measure performance expectancy, with perceived usefulness being a root construct of performance expectancy in Venkatesh et al. (2003) (also compare Table 2). Other operationalization of the UTAUT factors might lead to different results.

To summarize, findings in Venkatesh et al. (2003) on UTAUT factors did not fully recur in the current study. Follow-up studies should look into the UTAUT and self-management factors predicting diabetes app use in a larger sample, and should compare results based on diverse factor operationalization, as well as based on differing theoretical models.

App Features Influencing Diabetes App Use

An examination of diabetes app use in the Study 3 sample showed a higher percentage of diabetes patients who previously had used diabetes apps (almost 50%) as compared with a study by L. Boyle et al. (2017). The survey on diabetes patients in New Zealand by L. Boyle et al. (2017) showed that only 20% of the study participants had used diabetes apps. Diabetes app users were younger than non-users in L. Boyle et al. (2017) and predominantly suffered from T1DM in comparison with other forms of diabetes mellitus. The majority of T1DM were app users in Study 3, while the majority of T2DM were non-users (69% of T1DM were users, 44% of T2DM were users). However, overall there were more T2DM in the sample, and of all app users the majority were T2DM (71%). The age tendency from the previous study could be equally confirmed in Study 3.

In line with the study results from New Zealand, as well as Study 1 results, Study 3 found that diabetes apps used were almost exclusively limited to diary apps (logbooks). Study 1 showed that only three percent of the examined 121 apps were community apps or apps similar to a patient forum while 62% were logbook apps. Only less than 10% of all 121 examined diabetes apps included features to communicate with private social networks, with other app users, or provided advisory functions or therapy support by HCPs (Table 8). Despite not all apps mentioned by study participants in studies 2 and 3 being part of Study 1, approximately half of the apps overlapped (three out of six mentioned app names in Study 2 which were part of Study 1, and six out of 13 mentioned app names in Study 3 that were part of Study 1; compare Tables 3 and 9 in Appendix on Study 1 and Study 2 apps, and Table 21 on Study 3 apps). This also means that the logbook apps used by the participants in studies 2 and 3 that appeared in Study 1 mostly did not include advanced features to communicate with HCPs, other app users, or private social networks (following Study 1 results). Study 3 results showed that social support by private patient networks negatively related to diabetes app use. Even though support by private social networks measured in Study 3 did not specifically refer to online social support but to support on a general level (see questionnaire in Chapter 3.1 in Appendix), the results on a negative relationship between the support by private social networks and app use might additionally be influenced by lack of included communication features in the apps (Figure 2). It could be hypothesized that the lack of communication features in diabetes apps influences lower support by private social networks in diabetes app users than in nonusers. However, it also has to be kept in mind that Study 2 displayed that most diabetes app users additionally used other non-diabetes-specific apps as part of their self-management (Study 2 participants especially mentioned WhatsApp to communicate with other patients, see results in Chapter 13.2.2). Moreover, Study 2 also showed that independence of patients in their self-management (HCPs just as advisors, decisions mainly taken by the patient) was a factor that could explain less support by private social networks, with patients managing their condition all by themselves. To conclude from the study results, diabetes app characteristics are possibly one factor of several factors influencing diabetes app use as shown in Figure 2. Studies have to triangulate results further between app analyses and patient assessments to draw more specific conclusions about the influence of app features on usage outcomes.

14.4 Study Limitations

The method of using an online survey had some potential disadvantages over face-to-face or paper-and-pencil data collection (Wright, 2006). The downsides of an online questionnaire had to be kept in mind when analyzing the survey results. According to Wright (2006), an online questionnaire is fully self-reported, and the correctness of demographic, disease, or other data cannot be guaranteed. Self-selection bias is another major disadvantage of online survey research, and could not be fully avoided using the sampling method described.

As a result of the snowball sampling method – a representative study sample could not be achieved despite efforts undertaken to have a representative sample at hand – patients at high risk of complications were underrepresented in the study sample. Thus, it was difficult to test results on the high-risk group found in the Study 2 user typology (interested non-users of diabetes apps). Larger variation in patients regarding their diabetes management, their motivation and their health status would be helpful to differentiate more clearly between patients at high risk for complications and patients at normal risk. Especially with diabetes being a common subject for research in Singapore due to the proclaimed "war on diabetes" by the Singaporean government (Ministry of Health, 2017), patients tend to receive a large number of invitations for study participation. The willingness to participate in research studies likely decreases with the number of requests received. This was a major problem for response rates in the survey, and led to a smaller sample size than strived for. Despite repeated efforts to increase the sample size as explained in Chapter 14.1.2 on the sampling procedure, the sample size could not sufficiently be improved. The small sample size had consequences for data analysis, with limited multivariate analysis being applicable. Furthermore, using lottery incentives to increase response rates in the online surveys could have decreased the survey credibility, and might have led to decreased participation rates, or to a bias in answers given. Some participants might have participated in the survey only to take part in the lottery without giving serious answers to survey questions. Other individuals invited for the survey might have considered invitation emails or posts in online communities as spam, which could have decreased their willingness to participate.

Weaknesses regarding the operationalization in Study 3 included – similar to Study 2 – that behavioral empowerment didn't consider differences between HCPs in detail. The PDMstyle and PCOM scale subsumed both doctors and other HCPs as part of the same scales. Thus, no distinction could be drawn between empowering behaviors by doctors and by other HCPs (like diabetes nurse educators, DNEs, or dieticians). The answer to the scales most likely mainly referred to doctors with the doctor being mentioned first. Research is necessary looking into behavioral empowerment specifically by nurses and dieticians, and their role in the overall diabetes self-management. First results in Study 2 indicated that the role of nurses and dieticians varied largely in patients.

Similarly, empowerment by other patients through support groups was underexposed in the online survey. Study 2 results showed that other patients and support groups (DSS/Diabetes Singapore or TOUCH support group) played a major role in the empowerment of diabetes patients because they provided support in various ways, comprising educational support, financial support, or emotional and motivational support. This is in line with research increasingly supporting a social model of care instead of a mere medical care model (see more on this in Chapter 15.2.2; Disability Nottinghamshire, 2018; Shakespeare & Watson, 2002). Thus, a stronger focus should be put on behavioral empowerment by other patients and support groups in future research in addition to HCP and family/friends' support (more on this aspect see Chapter 15.4).

Regarding the operationalization of diabetes app use, Study 3 failed to measure explicitly interest in diabetes apps. To shorten the online questionnaire, the item was removed from the survey, and the relevance of the item for data analysis just revealed in the course of Study 3 analyses. The perceived diabetes app potential for self-management had to be used as an alternative variable in app non-users for analysis. Study 2 additionally showed that the interest in diabetes apps was a relevant aspect in non-users of diabetes apps (typology).

14.5 Conclusion

Study 3 was able to confirm Study 2 typology results to a large extent, as well as the validity of the psychological empowerment scale, and outlined the need for behavioral empowerment scales that distinguish between indicators of support by HCPs and by private social networks (family, friends, other patients). Study 3 results indicated that psychological empowerment, behavioral empowerment by HCPs and behavioral empowerment by patient's private social networks were at least partly related to diabetes app use. Behavioral empowerment by private social networks was able to predict diabetes app use in addition to the perceived health status and the type/medical specialty of the supervising HCP. Thus, it could be confirmed that aspects of empowerment should be considered antecedents of diabetes app use in addition to other influencing factors. Future research should aim at confirming Study 3 results, and at examining relationships that could not be fully confirmed in Study 3 (non-significant tendencies). Moreover, research accounting for causal relationships has to be added.

15 Discussion and Deriving Research Gaps

15.1 Summary on Study Results from Studies 1 to 3

The research interest focused on examining empowerment as an antecedent of diabetes app use in addition to other influencing factors. Empowerment was defined as including both a psychological and a behavioral component, and as a unique motivational approach it was especially relevant in a diabetes self-management context. Psychological empowerment included the indicators *perceived relevance*, *perceived competence*, *self-determination*, and *perceived impact*, while behavioral empowerment comprised the indicators *HCP-decision-making*, *HCP-patient communication*, and *support by private social networks*. It was argued that characteristics of diabetes apps (*RQ 1*), as well as the psychological empowerment in the patient and the behavioral empowerment in terms of social influence by others could potentially influence diabetes app use (*H II*), and that empowerment as a motivational antecedent of app use complements other antecedent factors from technology adoption theory (UTAUT) and from self-management theory (*H III*, Table 4).

To answer research questions and to test hypotheses, Study 1 explored diabetes app characteristics, while Studies 2 and 3 used interview and survey research to examine the patient perspective on diabetes app (non-) use, and to evaluate relationships between empowerment, previous diabetes app (non-) use and other influencing factors. The following paragraphs deliver details of the respective studies, and summarize study results:

Study 1

The first study looked into 121 diabetes apps for self-management and their features to get an update on diabetes apps available in Singapore and to evaluate how app characteristics promoted the potential of diabetes apps for empowered self-management, as well as the likelihood of maintained app use.

N. Brew-Sam, *App Use and Patient Empowerment in Diabetes Self-Management*, https://doi.org/10.1007/978-3-658-29357-4_15

App quality was analyzed, as well as how features of diabetes apps corresponded with theoretical indicators of empowerment. The study results from this app analysis indicated insufficient diabetes app quality and a narrow range of features supporting indicators of psychological and behavioral empowerment in the majority of the free-to-download apps. Most apps offered simple diabetes diaries or logbooks for health data recording, or databases informing about food content (carbohydrates etc.). Despite limited app types, insufficient app quality, and the limited potential of most apps, some advanced app series (e.g., MySugr Apps) were found that could serve as exemplary interactive, innovative, and empowering mobile platforms for the support of diabetes self-management. These app series included health data recording and analysis, diabetes information, entertainment, and HCP feedback to provide a foundation for improved BG monitoring, diet and exercise. They provided promising tools to improve adherence to and structuring of diabetes self-management. Moreover, they delivered a platform to enhance online immediate and location independent empowering support by diabetes supervisors.

Overall, Study 1 delivered a first step towards relating app features to the theoretical approach of empowerment, as well as to a patient perspective on diabetes app use in Studies 2 and 3. App reviews can be improved by using theoretical approaches as a foundation for empirical app assessment tools. Study 1 was the first study connecting app review methodology with the concept of empowerment to evaluate apps for self-management. Study 1 also prepared the foundation for examining the influence of diabetes app characteristics on actual diabetes app use. App characteristics were summarized as one potential factor influencing diabetes app adoption and use as shown in Figure 2 and in addition to other anteceding factors, like psychological empowerment in the patient, and social support by others (behavioral empowerment). Finally, Study 1 used an adapted version of the Mobile App Rating Scale that might be of higher practicability than the original lengthy scale.

Study 2

Study 2 added interview research to the previous Study 1 app review and delivered basic information on diabetes app (non-) use in a study sample of 21 T1DM and

T2DM patients, background on empowerment, as well as background on diabetes and self-management behaviors. The Study 1 app review results were confirmed by Study 2 (face-to-face) interviewees who commented on the perceived usefulness of diabetes apps for self-management. In line with results on diabetes apps in Study 1 and in line with previous study results on diabetes apps (Chapter 3.3) some patients in Study 2 reported that they either did not use diabetes apps because of lacking perceived app usefulness, or that they had stopped diabetes app use because diabetes apps didn't provide reliable tools for self-management with problems inherent in the apps. These patients mentioned being dissatisfied with the state of diabetes apps for self-management due to insufficient app reliability, poor app design, few app features, or the lack of compatibility with other devices like BG meters. Especially young patients wished for more advanced apps including a larger variation of interactive features for the support of self-management. In line with lacking features corresponding to theoretical indicators of empowerment in Study 1, the patients in Study 2 only attributed a limited potential for self-management to diabetes apps. Study 2 results in combination with Study 1 results delivered first indications that characteristics of diabetes apps, including lack of app quality, lack of app features, or insufficient app reliability were possibly influencing app adoption and use negatively (compare Figure 2, and dissatisfied app adopters in Study 2 typology).

Based on diabetes app usage characteristics, the interview results revealed four types of diabetes app users and non-users. First, patients at high risk of complications showing interest in diabetes apps but who had never used diabetes apps before due to lack of knowledge about app options or high barriers to app use. The second group included older diabetes app non-users with no interest in diabetes apps. The third group of short-term diabetes app users either included young app adopters or experienced app switchers, while the fourth group included diabetes app long-term users mostly part of diabetes programs. Differences in the (non-) user groups regarding psychological and behavioral empowerment were analyzed and hypotheses on differences were developed from the results.

In contrast to all other (non-) user groups who displayed high psychological empowerment, only the interested non-users at high risk of complications reported lower psychological empowerment. Looking at behavioral empowerment, all diabetes app non-user groups reported lower behavioral empowerment than diabetes app users (apart from some diabetes app switchers who reported lower behavioral empowerment as well). As concluded from the results, with differences in groups found, empowerment was likely related to diabetes app use.

As an indicator of behavioral empowerment, Study 2 emphasized the relevance of support by private social networks for diabetes self-management. It could be shown that non-professionals (other patients, friends, family) empowered patients in addition to HCPs, or when empowerment by HCPs was weak. Study 2 participants stressed the importance of support groups, and interaction with other patients for their own empowerment for diabetes self-management. For example, interaction with other patients in support groups delivered positive motivation to improve own self-management behaviors, provided diabetes information (learning), and enhanced the feeling of competence.

Yet, it could be confirmed that empowerment was likely not the only relevant antecedent factor for app use, with other technology adoption and self-management factors relevant as well. The type/medical specialty of the supervising doctor was especially likely to influence diabetes app use. Diabetes app users reported using diabetes specialists to a larger extent than diabetes app non-users, with diabetes specialists reported to follow shared decision-making to a larger extent than GPs. GPs were reported to be partly unsupportive, to offer short consultations, to lack diabetes knowledge, and never to recommend diabetes apps. In addition to the type of HCP (medical specialty) and the style of decision-making, the participation in diabetes programs, diabetes knowledge, technological experience, the severity of the health condition, general optimistic attitudes, lower age, and the perceived diabetes app usefulness and potential were found likely to influence diabetes app adoption and use. In some app users high psychological empowerment was found despite low behavioral empowerment by GPs. Independence in self-management was used as a potential explanatory factor.

Study 3

Study 3 used cluster analysis to test the Study 2 diabetes app user and non-user typology in a sample of 65 diabetes patients. The Study 2 typology with interested and non-interested non-users, and short-term and long-term users could largely be confirmed using statistical analysis. As compared with Study 2, some (minor) differences occurred in Study 3. Due to an underrepresentation of high-risk patients found in Study 3, it could not be confirmed if non-users contained one subgroup of diabetes patients at risk for complications as suggested in Study 2. Moreover, interest in diabetes apps was not available in Study 3, but perceived diabetes app potential was used as a variable instead. Study 3 at least partly confirmed the Study 2 result that unmotivated patients were mostly part of non-users of diabetes apps. In Study 2, the high-risk group showed interest in diabetes apps, but diabetes app use did not take place in this group due to high barriers to the apps' use and general diabetes self-management. This implied discrepancies between usage intentions and actual usage in risk groups as found in previous research.

Apart from the typology, Study 3 tested hypotheses deriving from both theory and Study 2, examining the relationship between diabetes app use and empowerment as an antecedent factor, as well as other technology adoption and self-management factors. For psychological empowerment, only specific indicators were significantly related to aspects of app use (the perceived relevance was significantly and positively related to the frequency of the app use, as well as self-determination of the perceived app potential). Moreover, psychological empowerment could not be confirmed as a significant predictor of app use in the logistic regression analysis. As a result, the hypothesis assuming a positive relationship between psychological empowerment and diabetes app use could only partly be confirmed (*H 1*, Table 4).

As part of behavioral empowerment by HCPs, diabetes app users showed a significantly higher likelihood of supervision by diabetes specialists instead of GPs (Table 26), and specialists were reported to provide more shared decision-making than GPs. The type of HCP used for supervision was a significant predictor of diabetes app use in the logistic regression analysis. Regarding behavioral empowerment by private social networks, higher family and friend support was significantly related to a lower chance of previous diabetes app use, and to lower perceived app potential for self-management (Table 26, Table 12 in Appendix). Diabetes app users reported lower support by the social private network than non-users. In binary logistic regression, from all empowerment dimensions, only the support by private social networks could be confirmed to be a significant predictor of diabetes app use. Less support from private social networks increased the chance of diabetes app adoption and use (or reverse). With significant results on support by the social private network, Study 3 was able to clarify results on social support that Study 2 had left unclear. The hypothesis assuming a positive relationship between behavioral empowerment and diabetes app use could be rejected in regard to support by private social networks, with a negative relationship proven instead ($H1$, Table 4).

To summarize, Study 3 results indicated that app users generally showed some aspects of better psychological empowerment (but longer users showed lower psychological empowerment again), more shared decision-making and better HCP-patient communication (diabetes specialists) but less support by private social networks than non-users.

The results on empowerment further indicated that lower behavioral empowerment significantly related to lower psychological empowerment in diabetes patients not using apps for self-management, while lower behavioral empowerment potentially related to higher psychological empowerment in diabetes app users (Table 27). Similar to Study 2, independence of patients was discussed as a potential explanation of negative relationship tendencies between psychological and behavioral empowerment in users (high psychological empowerment despite a lack of social support).

Considering other influencing technology adoption and self-management factors, apart from significant results confirming that diabetes app users showed a higher chance of supervision by diabetes specialists than non-users (provider factors), users also displayed a better perceived health status than non-users (severity of the health condition), and a higher perceived app potential than non-users (performance expectancy). Yet, only the perceived health status and the type of HCP (medical specialty) were found to be significant predictors of diabetes app use in different logistic regression models. A lower perceived health status decreased the chance of diabetes app adoption and use (or reverse), while supervision by diabetes specialists increased the chance for app use (as compared to GPs).

From Study 2 and Study 3 results, it could be summarized that only specific empowerment dimensions (support by private social networks as an indicator of behavioral empowerment) could be confirmed as significant antecedents of diabetes app use (*H II*, Table 4), and in addition to specific other technology adoption and diabetes self-management factors (e.g., perceived health status, type of HCP, *H III*). With both specific (behavioral) empowerment indicators and other factors confirmed to be predictors of app use, a first limited confirmation of the hypothesis was delivered that specific empowerment aspects complement other influencing factors from technology adoption or self-management theory (*H III*, Table 4). Moreover, the results of all three studies suggested an additional influence of diabetes app characteristics on diabetes app use (e.g., app quality). However, the results also indicated that relationships between empowerment dimensions, other influencing factors and diabetes app use were more complex than shown in Figure 2. Tests for causal relationships are required in follow-up research to be able to confirm the current results.

After summarizing the main results, it is discussed what empowerment actually explained in the context of diabetes app use. Based on this, the value of empowerment for mHealth research is discussed. Moreover, based on the study results the operationalization of empowerment is reconsidered.

15.2 What does Empowerment Explain?

15.2.1 Empowerment and Diabetes App Use

Looking back at the theoretical model in Figure 2 and the study results, it could be discussed what empowerment actually explained in the studies. From there, some first conclusions could be drawn about the value of an empowerment approach for mHealth research, as well as its barriers.

It was hypothesized that psychological empowerment and behavioral empowerment, (as well as characteristics of the diabetes apps, technological aspects) and other factors influenced the use of diabetes apps. Following the process perspective in Figure 2, successful app use could then lead to improved self-management behaviors and improved health outcomes, that could enhance empowerment in return.

The focus was on antecedents of diabetes app use, with study results presenting that certain empowerment indicators explained diabetes app use to a certain extent, especially the support by private social networks. These results are in keeping with previous study findings as shown in Chapter 14.3. However, the prediction of diabetes app use just included aspects of app usage such as previous diabetes app use or non-use, as well as the length and frequency of previous app use (see Study 3 operationalization). Study 2 added some results that suggested levels of motivation, empowerment, and self-management attitudes/behaviors influencing a general adoption or rejection of the app use, the interest in diabetes apps, or health information sharing with HCPs based on app data. However, diabetes app use is much more complex, considering the app use behaviors in everyday life, and the inclusion of app use in the overall diabetes self-management. It has to be further investigated how the app use is integrated in daily self-management activities (Wirth et al., 2008), how the technology use replaces or complements other self-management behaviors, and how this relates to general psychological empowerment, to HCP support and to support by the private social patient network. Previous research has suggested a move away from a simple app adoption or rejection perspective, to digging further into the complexity of everyday mobile technology use, including various usage and meaning patterns on individual and social levels (Wirth et al., 2008). Thus, only very particular aspects of empowerment could explain very particular aspects of diabetes app use in the conducted studies, and an extension to a broader understanding of app use is needed.

Looking at the second part in Figure 2, the studies conducted did not focus on or examined empowerment as an outcome of diabetes app use. However, previous research focused on empowerment as an outcome of mHealth use, and delivered information about this aspect (Bradway et al., 2015; Cumming et al., 2014; Krošel et al., 2016; Li et al., 2013; Omboni et al., 2016; Park, Burford, Lee, et al., 2016; Wiederhold, 2015; Zhang & Ho, 2017). Previous studies delivered initial proof that mHealth use could empower patients (Bradway et al., 2015; Cumming et al., 2014; Krošel et al., 2016; L. M. S. Miller et al., 2017; Park, Burford, Lee, et al., 2016; Zhang & Ho, 2017). Thus, first results from literature are available confirming that successful app use enhances patient empowerment as suggested in Figure 2. Yet, the literature fails to explain details about empowerment resulting from use of a health app (also see Chapter 7.3.1), and more comprehensive explanations and analyses are required, especially in context of diabetes. Further high-quality research is necessary to show convincingly "that empowered self-care does lead to better health outcomes" (Asimakopoulou et al., 2012, p. 282), and more research on empowerment in relation to diabetes app use is needed to test relationships in Figure 2.

15.2.2 Empowerment and Other Influencing Factors

The question if empowerment complements other factors predicting app use from technology adoption models could be answered to a limited extent. In Study 3 it could be shown that empowerment was not the only factor predicting diabetes app use, with support by private social networks as an indicator of behavioral empowerment predicting diabetes app use in addition to the perceived health status and the type/medical specialty of the supervising HCP (Chapter 14.2.5). Other factors from the UTAUT could not be confirmed as predictors.

Structural equation modeling in a larger sample, or mediation and moderation analysis could help understand how other factors mediate or moderate the relationship between empowerment as an antecedent and diabetes app use (Study 3 sample was too small to apply these analyses). Based on theory (moderator-mediator distinction, R. M. Baron & Kenny, 1986) and the study results, it needs to be discussed and examined which factors are likely moderators of a relationship between empowerment and diabetes app use, and which are likely mediators.

Based on the study results, Figure 11 delivers a first suggestion on which factors from UTAUT and from self-management theory could serve as moderators or mediators of the relationship between empowerment as an antecedent and diabetes app use. Some factors are more likely moderators than mediators, like the suggested moderating variables in the UTAUT (voluntariness, experience, and demography, Venkatesh et al., 2003). Study 2 data suggested that there were at least some demographic differences in diabetes app (non-) use (e.g., older versus younger diabetes app users and non-users, see typology results in Table 18), and that demographic aspects might affect the relationship between empowerment and diabetes app (non-) use. Similarly, only non-users of diabetes apps reported no previous experience with eHealth or mHealth, and thus experience might also moderate the relationship between empowerment and app (non-) use.

The UTAUT factors *facilitating conditions* and *social influences* different from the included behavioral empowerment dimensions could be expected to be moderators of a relationship between empowerment and diabetes app use, as well as other self-management factors that generally influence the situation the patient is in, like *physical factors*, *practical factors*, *care access*, and *previous diabetes education* (Figure 11).

The study 2 results for example showed that participation in a diabetes program as a facilitating condition influenced app use, with some program participants using a diabetes app that was part of a program for a long time. Social influences could be shown to affect diabetes app use (e.g., social private patient network, study 3), and other aspects of social influence not included in the behavioral empowerment dimensions might have an impact on the relationship between empowerment and app use, too (e.g., societal expectations). Further, the study 2 data showed that physical factors (e.g., new occurring symptoms like eye problems) could initiate the interest for or use of diabetes apps, and thus be moderating the relationship between empowerment and app use. Socioeconomic (practical) factors were mentioned to be relevant for (technology-supported) self-management in study 2, and thus should be considered a potential moderator. Differences in access to care like the medical specialty of the consulted physician were shown to affect app use in studies 2 and 3, and thus could be moderators of the relationship between empowerment and app use. Initial diabetes education is affecting (technology-supported) diabetes care as shown by previous studies. In the own studies, only app non-users reported a lack of diabetes eductaion (study 2). This might affect empowerment and app use.

The UTAUT factors *performance and effort expectancy* might result from empowerment in addition to information about apps, and lead to app (non-) use, and thus mediate the relationship between empowerment and app use. The perceived usefulness and potential of diabetes apps was reported differently by study participants (study 2), and it could be shown that the perceived usefulness also varied in patient groups with differing empowerment levels (e.g., see typology, Table 18). Thus, it could be hypothesized that empowerment affects perceived usefulness which affects app use in return. Similarly, *attitudes* towards diabetes app use and self-management, as well as other *psychological factors* related to app use (like usage motivation) might result from general psychological and behavioral empowerment, and might influence app use in return (mediators, Figure 11).

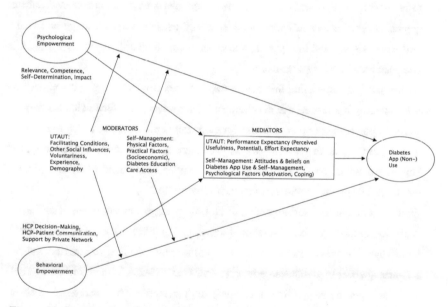

Figure 11. Suggested mediators and moderators of the relationship between empowerment as an antecedent factor and diabetes app use.

Overall, this would mean that other factors are not just influencing diabetes apps use as shown in Figure 2, but rather are mediating or moderating the relationship between empowerment and diabetes app use. Figure 2 included other factors as a generalized influencing aspect. However, the model would have to be specified based on moderation and mediation results, and furnished with specific factors found to be mediators or moderators of the association between empowerment and app use.

Moreover, it also has to be investigated in which cases empowerment is the mediating or moderating variable between other factors and diabetes app use. As shown previously Camerini and Schulz (2012) for example hypothesized that psychological empowerment mediates a relationship between the availability of interactive features on an eHealth application and patients' health outcomes. They did not find any significant impact of interactivity on empowerment, but could show that empowerment indicators positively affected health outcomes. This relates back to the fact that diabetes app characteristics should be included as an influencing factor on usage and health outcomes as suggested in Figure 2, and as shown preliminarily by Study 1 results in combination with Study 2 results.

Factors not just influencing the relationship between empowerment and app use, but also generally influencing the development of empowerment – including barriers towards empowerment or preconditions for empowerment – could be added to the model in Figure 2. The factors knowledge, healthcare system, and culture are discussed here as examples, with these general factors having been found likely to influence empowerment processes (Study 2 results in Chapter 13.2.4.2).

Firstly, according to Asimakopoulou et al. (2012) empowerment is based on having "sufficient knowledge to make rational decisions" (p. 281). Here, perceived diabetes knowledge was operationalized as a factor influencing technology supported diabetes self-management in addition to empowerment (see self-management factors in Table 1). This was based on the theoretical argumentation that perceived diabetes knowledge is not synonymous with perceived competence as an indicator of psychological empowerment (e.g., Glajchen & Bookbinder, 2001). While knowledge relates to aspects of health literacy, with perceived knowledge being the perception of how much the patient feels he or she knows about diabetes, perceived competence relates to perceptions of self-efficacy – the "belief in one's agentive capabilities, that one can produce given levels of attainment" (Bandura, 1997, p. 382). Schulz and Nakamoto (2013) deliver a detailed distinction of the concepts of health literacy and psychological empowerment. Study 2 results indicated that patients with insufficient diabetes knowledge presented lower psychological and behavioral empowerment than other patient groups, and that this was potentially related to poor self-management and a non-use of diabetes apps. Social support from HCPs or other individuals can be expected to enhance diabetes knowledge while knowledge could influence psychological empowerment in return (e.g., perceived competence increasing with more knowledge). A lack of knowledge could pose a barrier to both psychological empowerment and self-management behaviors (Asimakopoulou et al., 2012), and knowledge and literacy are needed as a foundation for eHealth or mHealth use (Camerini & Schulz, 2012). Deeper insights into diabetes knowledge as a precondition for empowerment, and for technology-supported self-management behaviors are needed.

Secondly, as a crucial foundation for empowerment, a healthcare system is necessary that supports participatory health decision-making and acknowledges patient responsibility in diabetes treatment by strengthening diabetes self-management. Only then empowerment for diabetes self-management can be successfully promoted. Health system related barriers to empowered diabetes self-management have to be removed, and attitudes to diabetes as a disease have to be changed. Here diabetes research can learn from research on disability, where researchers are asking for a Social Care Model instead of a Medical Care Model to change basic views of health issues. While the medical model attributes disability to differences or impairments in individuals (what is "wrong" with the patient), the social model rather attributes disability to the way the society looks at disability and how it is organized (what the patient needs; Disability Nottinghamshire, 2018; Shakespeare & Watson, 2002). Only when barriers related to the understanding of the impairment or disease are removed, patients "can be independent and equal in society, with choice and control over their own lives" (Disability Nottinghamshire, 2018). Thus, the social approach is a foundation for improved patient empowerment, coping, and successful self-management. Similar to disability care, in diabetes care the Social Care Model should be promoted, to replace a Medical Care Model. By changing the perceptions of diabetes as a disease inherent in the patient towards how society deals with diabetes patients, barriers to diabetes care and patient-led management can be removed. Only with changed perceptions towards diabetes, cooperative HCP-patient relationships are promoted, and a foundation for behavioral empowerment by HCPs is provided, potentially positively influencing psychological empowerment. This can pave the way for improved self-determined (technology-supported) management of diabetes by the patients themselves.

An example as to why the medical care approach has to be replaced with a social care approach is psychological support. The medical care approach disregards the relevance of psychological support in diabetes care to a large extent by mainly offering medical solutions for health problems (e.g., medication). Psychological support is still largely underrepresented in medical diabetes care. Singaporean Study 2 participants mentioned that the Singaporean diabetes care system did not yet include professional psychological support in treatment and diabetes care, even though patients considered psychological support outstandingly important (see Study 2 interview extracts, Table 6 in Appendix). The relevance of psychosocial problems in diabetes has also been examined in the cross-national DAWN study (Peyrot et al., 2006; Peyrot et al., 2005). The Dawn-Study showed worldwide perceived relevance of professional psychological support in diabetes management. "A satisfactory account of diabetes care would pay attention to the 'inner' world, while acknowledging the social and political conditions in which diabetes-related experiences unfold" (Gomersall et al., 2011, p. 853). A social care approach can deliver a solution to these shortcomings in diabetes care, by focusing on what patients need in a more holistic way, for example including not just medical but also psychological support. Ways to self-manage can then be fully made use of, leading to improved empowerment.

With the consideration of psychological aspects, the social care approach is suitable for psychological research perspectives, as well as for empowerment research, and provides opportunities for mHealth research. This is for example shown in the paper by Chib and Jiang (2014) who suggest an integrated biopsychosocial approach based on a social model for examining experiences with mobile phones in certain (patient) target groups. They argue that mobile phone adoption and use "allowed the management of personal identities and social networks, leading to a sense of empowerment" (p. 1). According to them, mobile phones offer opportunities for empowerment by strengthening social support (behavioral empowerment) and by supporting the development of independence and self-determination (psychological empowerment).

Thirdly, apart from the societal and healthcare system related preconditions for empowered technology-supported self-management, culture is a general fundamental factor that has to be addressed when looking into patient empowerment. Previous research showed that attitudes towards health, disease and disease management strongly vary in cultures, with general norms and values shaping diabetes management attitudes (Naeem, 2016; Shaw, Huebner, Armin, Orzech, & Vivian, 2008). For example, Ahmed et al. (2010) published a study presenting that a considerable number of diabetes patients of a South Asian Muslim community thought that "insulin use would interfere with religious obligations" (p. 169). Specifically for South East Asia (including Singapore), Kesavadev et al. (2014) summarize challenges to diabetes management. For example, the authors mention that "unlike in the Western world, being known as a diabetes patient is a social sigma and poses a huge emotional burden living with the disease and getting married" (p. 600). Cultural background can make empowerment approaches more or less useful for diabetes management, depending on norms and values towards diabetes as a disease and towards the management of this disease. While in some cultures participatory decision-making is already largely supported, other cultures still follow paternalistic decision-making. In cultures where a strong hierarchy of authority prevents shared decision-making in the clinic, it is also less likely that apps for diabetes self-management are recommended by HCPs, used by the patients, or perceived as useful by both groups (Abbasgholizadeh Rahimi et al., 2017; Mead et al., 2013). Attitudes towards diabetes apps for self-management are likely to differ considerably in different cultures. Cultural background has to be taken into consideration when designing diabetes apps for specific target audiences. For example, Study 2 participants frequently reported that diabetes apps coming from an American market were not suitable for Asian diabetes patients due to differences in cultural background (e.g., food databases not tailored for Asian market).

To summarize, the Studies revealed factors likely influencing empowerment considerably, posing barriers to empowerment, or mediating/moderating the relationship between empowerment and diabetes app use and other self-management behaviors. Besides factors influencing diabetes app use in addition to empowerment found in Study 3 (e.g., perceived health status), more general background factors like culture, or the type of healthcare system have to be examined as foundations for empowerment in further research.

15.3 The Value of Empowerment for mHealth Research

From the previous and current study results, a conclusion could be drawn on what an empowerment approach adds in value for mHealth research. Study 1 confirmed that mHealth tools are characterized by content that can be adapted for the user over time based on prior outcome, prior responses, environmental and social context, and other factors (Riley et al., 2011). Addressing the general lack of theory in mHealth research and the dynamic of mobile tools, empowerment can deliver a theoretical approach that is suitable to address dynamic processes in self-management, and adds a relatively new motivational approach to mHealth research that includes both intrinsic and extrinsic motivational aspects. In contrast to empowerment, traditional behavior change models "appear inadequate to answer many of the intervention development questions likely to arise as interventions better leverage the interactive capabilities of mobile technologies.... The development of time-intensive, interactive, and adaptive health behavior interventions via mobile technologies demands more intra-individual dynamic regulatory processes than represented in our current health behavior theories" (Riley et al., 2011, p. 66). The authors attribute a mainly static and linear nature to behavior change theories that are used to study between-person differences, and that don't fit the intra-individual dynamics of mHealth and within-person developments. Empowerment adds a theoretical approach that is suitable for studying processes that focus on within-person developments. As a motivational approach, it delivers a useful approach for technology-supported diabetes care, especially for modern participatory self-care approaches. The approach is suitable to explain the self-determined and self-motivated use of mobile health tools that requires user initiative (apps as "pull" media, patient-led usage). The approach is furthermore suitable for combination with behavior change and technology adoption theories/models, when empowerment is understood as one antecedent factor in addition to other factors from theory.

It could be shown that the empowerment concept is unique due to its combination of psychological empowerment influenced by empowering behaviors of HCPs and other individuals. Thus, looking at empowerment as an antecedent, it delivers a unique approach for explaining diabetes self-management behaviors (Funnell & Anderson, 2003; Tol et al., 2015; Yang et al., 2015), as well as diabetes app use.

With the psychological (feeling) and the behavioral dimensions (social influence), it includes dimensions that focus on social influence as an important aspect of technology-supported diabetes self-management (Grant & Schmittdiel, 2013; Helgeson et al., 2016; A. G. Ramirez & Turner, 2010; Rosland et al., 2008; Veazie et al., 2018). Using behavioral empowerment as a concept including the indicators HCP decision-making, HCP-patient communication and support by the private social patient network delivers advantages over the usage of single aspects of social support (e.g., peer support only) in context of (mobile) technology use as found in previous studies (Talukder & Quazi, 2011, for example only looked at peer and social network support when talking about social influence in relation to innovation adoption). This is because behavioral empowerment combines several research branches on social support (e.g., HCP decision-making, HCP-patient communication, support by private social networks), while most previous studies neither looked at various combined aspects of social support as a precondition for mHealth use for self-management, nor related their findings to theoretical concepts specifically relevant for diabetes self-management, like empowerment. It is helpful to use empowerment as a theoretical foundation when examining the influence of social support on mHealth use to be able to place the findings in a larger self-management context. Empowerment delivers an appropriate framework for locating the relevance of social support for self-management. Moreover, using behavioral empowerment allows comparison of the influence of its various behavioral empowerment indicators on mHealth use for self-management (HCPs versus social patient networks). The Study 3 results for example indicated that especially the support by private social networks was able to predict diabetes app use, while additional Study 2 and Study 3 results showed that HCP types were related to styles of decision-making and HCP-patient communication. Differing HCP types significantly predicted diabetes app use in binary logistic regression (Chapter 14.2.5). The small sample size potentially influenced study outcomes, and it can be expected that more than one behavioral empowerment indicator predicts diabetes app use in samples larger in size and less distorted (risk patients were underrepresented in Study 3). Thus, to summarize, the concept of behavioral empowerment adds value to research on social support in an mHealth context.

Similarly and overall, the empowerment approach combines research that previously either looked at psychological empowerment, or at single indicators of behavioral empowerment (without referral to empowerment). Thus, by using the multi-dimensional empowerment approach with psychological and behavioral dimensions as a theoretical framework as suggested here, knowledge from different research directions is brought together and connected to a theoretical concept, leading to a stronger theoretical and empirical foundation for an explanation of self-management outcomes, as well as of mHealth use as part of diabetes self-management – compared with previous studies focusing on single aspects of empowerment only, and without any relation to the theoretical concept.

15.4 The Operationalization of Empowerment

The operationalization of psychological empowerment was based on previous operationalization including items measuring the four indicators *perceived relevance*, *perceived competence*, *self-determination*, and *perceived impact* (Mantwill et al., 2015; Spreitzer, 1995). The results could not confirm psychological empowerment as a significant predictor of diabetes app use, but app use frequency significantly and positively related to perceived relevance, while the perceived app potential significantly and positively related to self-determination. Based on the distinct results for the four psychological empowerment indicators, and based on some indicators (e.g., impact) mostly not showing significant relationships, while other indicators did, the four-dimensional psychological empowerment model had to be further discussed to make sure the operationalization was valid and reliable. Some research asked for different model versions, Gutschoven and van den Bulck (2006) for example tested the four-dimensional model by Thomas and Velthouse (1990) against a three-dimensional model by Menon (2001, including goal internalization, perceived competence, perceived control) to find the most suitable model with the highest validity. The overlap between both models was found to be high[18], only differing in the three-dimensional model excluding the indicator perceived impact. The authors conclude that both models explain the same amount of total variance, and show a good model fit. Yet, after running confirmatory factor analyses, they suggest that the three-dimensional model was the better alternative with higher parsimony because "the costs associated with the addition of a fourth factor to the construct of psychological health empowerment are not sufficiently compensated by an increase in model fit" (Gutschoven & van den Bulck, 2006, p. 2).

In addition to testing the four-dimensional model, the single indicators of psychological empowerment still further need to be differentiated from related constructs. As explained in Chapter 7, in diabetes research and in early psychological approaches psychological empowerment was understood as perceived self-efficacy (R. M. Anderson et al., 1995; Conger & Kanungo, 1988). In the four-dimensional model self-efficacy was then included as one of four indicators of psychological empowerment, and was used synonymously with perceived competence (Schulz & Nakamoto, 2013). Yet, some authors argue that self-efficacy and perceived competence can be distinguished even though frequently used interchangeably (Rodgers, Markland, Selzler, Murray, & Wilson, 2014). Rodgers et al. (2014) classify perceived competence as conceived in SDT, and self-efficacy as conceived in social-cognitive theory. Other authors fully separate self-efficacy from empowerment (Moattari et al., 2012). The outcomes in this research could not further clarify the differentiation between the concepts, potentially influencing some study outcomes based on a certain operationalization chosen (results might look different with differing operationalization). Follow-up research should further differentiate the psychological empowerment indicators from

---

[18] *Perceived competence* and *control* are similar to the psychological empowerment indicators *competence* and *choice/self-determination* in the four-dimensional psychological empowerment approach (Gutschoven & van den Bulck, 2006). According to Gutschoven and van den Bulck (2006) *goal internalization* is similar to the indicator *meaningfulness/relevance*. Goal internalization defines the individual's identification with health policy and health system goals. Internalized goals become valued goals that lead to the desired health behavior, e.g., leading a healthy lifestyle (Menon, 2002).

related concepts, and examine which concepts exactly are indicators of empowerment, and which are not. Research about the theoretical concept of psychological empowerment is still confusing, and clarification is urgently needed.

Concerning behavioral empowerment, this aspect was operationalized by using items measuring HCP decision-making, HCP-patient communication, and support by private social networks. As argued before, support by both HCPs and private social networks (family, friends, other patients) has frequently been discussed and examined in diabetes research (e.g., Armour et al., 2005; Bennich et al., 2017; Grant & Schmittdiel, 2013; Kaselitz et al., 2018; Rosland et al., 2008), yet without specifically relating these aspects to behavioral empowerment. Despite the definition of empowerment by M. Lee and Koh (2001) limiting the behavioral aspects of empowerment to behaviors of (medical) supervisors, and thus implying a professional hierarchy between empowering and empowered individuals, Chapter 7.1.2 supported an inclusion of behaviors by private social networks as an indicator of behavioral empowerment, with previous literature showing the relevance of social support by family and peers for diabetes self-management and diabetes outcomes. Study 2 showed that especially "peer" patients (A. G. Ramirez & Turner, 2010) played an important role as sources of information and of empowerment for patients, confirming previous research on the relevance of peer support for diabetes self-management (Heisler et al., 2010; Kaselitz et al., 2018; Kowitt et al., 2017; Litchman et al., 2018; A. G. Ramirez & Turner, 2010). In Study 3, social support by private patient networks was shown to be a relevant aspect of behavioral empowerment that related to other behavioral empowerment indicators like HCP decision-making and HCP-patient communication and to indicators of psychological empowerment (Table 12 in Appendix), confirming previous research (Oh & Lee, 2012). Support by private social networks could be shown to be one of the strongest predictors of diabetes app use for self-management in Study 3. To conclude, social support could be confirmed to be a relevant aspect of behavioral empowerment in addition to HCP support in the conducted studies. Behavioral empowerment should not just focus on empowerment by medical supervisors, but should also include empowerment by private social networks. Follow-up studies are needed for further confirmation of the current results, as well as research comparing the relevance of HCP support with the relevance of support by private social networks, and studies testing if HCP decision-making, HCP-patient communication, and social support are valid and exhaustive indicators of behavioral empowerment. Reliable and valid measurement of behavioral empowerment has to be found, with scales on this aspect lacking in empowerment research.

In relation to the operationalization of the overall empowerment concept (including both psychological and behavioral dimensions), implications derived from the study outcomes showed heterogeneous results for empowerment dimensions. Study 3 showed that psychological and behavioral empowerment dimensions differed in their relationship with diabetes app use. Results varied for the four psychological empowerment indicators, as well as the three behavioral empowerment indicators. These results emphasized that the measurement of empowerment needs to pay attention to its multi-dimensionality. A clear distinction of the dimensions and their measurement is needed, while taking both psychological and behavioral empowerment into account. Study results should always be presented for psychological and behavioral empowerment separately, to account for differences in the dimensions (as mentioned in Study 3 discussion in Chapter 14.3). This avoids an over-generalization of study results on empowerment. By just measuring single aspects of empowerment, previous studies indirectly paid attention to differences in empowerment dimensions (e.g., Zoffmann & Kirkevold, 2012). However, they did not relate their results to the theoretical concept of empowerment (Aljasem, Peyrot, Wissow, & Rubin, 2001; Krichbaum, Aarestad, & Buethe, 2003), and/or did not refer to other dimensions of the concept (e.g., limitation to psychological empowerment in Schulz & Nakamoto, 2013). Thus, this research adds value to previous research by including the measurement of both psychological and behavioral empowerment dimensions in one research approach, but by separating the outcomes of the different dimensions.

Generally, problems of operationalization and the measurement of empowerment need to be addressed, arising from unclear theoretical concept definitions, and a variety of interpretations in a large number of diverse empowerment publications (Asimakopoulou et al., 2012). Concept ideas and definitions of empowerment are constantly changing, for example with a paternalistic approach giving way to active patient participation (Chin, 2002), leaving an unclear notion about their meaning. This research tried to address these problems by defining in detail the underlying empowerment concept that was used for the research.

After discussing the main research results, as well as the operationalization used in the research, the implications for other health domains and for practical diabetes care are discussed, based on the results of this research.

16 Learning from Research Results – Implications for Research and Diabetes Care Practice

16.1 Implications for Other Health Domains

Even though the research looked into diabetes apps and the relevance of empowerment for diabetes app use, the study results can at least partly be applied to other health domains in which self-management plays a crucial role. Diabetes is a precedent for chronic disease self-management. However, other chronic diseases require similar patient initiative and self-determination. Empowerment is relevant for self-management not just in diabetes, but for all chronic diseases that require patient self-care in addition to traditional medical care. Thus, other health domains can learn from studies on diabetes self-management, and the results can be used to inform both research and app design for other chronic diseases, including heart diseases, obesity, asthma, stroke, cancer, arthritis, COPD, hypertension, multiple sclerosis, etc. (Centers for Disease Control and Prevention, 2017; Council for Medical Schemes, 2018). For example, cancer is categorized as a chronic condition with individuals suffering from cancer frequently surviving long-term (Hammer et al., 2015). Thus, cancer requires medical care on the one hand, and patient self-management on the other hand, including for example the management of chemotherapy-related or disease-related symptoms, problem solving, uncertainty management, healthy lifestyles (diet, exercise), or stress management (McCorkle et al., 2011). "The expectation for cancer patients to participate in their care and manage treatment effects between visits emerged as a demand that could no longer be ignored by oncology health care professionals" (McCorkle et al., 2011, p. 54). Disease management of all chronic diseases takes place within patient-HCPs relationships, at least partly involves family members and relatives, and includes psychosocial challenges for patients.

Both psychological empowerment and social support by HCPs, families and other relevant individuals is equally needed e.g., for cancer self-management as it is for diabetes self-management.

Depending on self-management activities at the center of the respective disease, smart device apps will differ in their content and their main purpose from diabetes apps. However, mHealth studies on apps for other chronic diseases can learn from studies conducted on diabetes apps for self-management. The general lack of theory in mHealth research and the shortcomings of theory applied to mHealth research (Chapter 4.2.2) are equally relevant for other health domains, and not limited to diabetes. And with the general relevance of empowerment for disease self-management, both psychological and behavioral empowerment can similarly be expected to be anteceding factors of an app use for self-management in cancer or other chronic disease contexts.

16.2 Advancing Methodology

The results of this research showed that triangulation between technological app reviews and app (non-) user perception assessments is required to be able to evaluate comprehensively aspects of diabetes app characteristics and diabetes app usage, as well as factors influencing diabetes app use and usage outcomes. Study 1 included both an app feature and an app quality assessment, using previous app assessment instruments (Stoyanov et al., 2015), and developing these instruments further to achieve improved practicability of the existing scales (shortened MARS version). To advance health app review methodology, a app quality assessment tool that proved to be of high quality itself was selected, and was combined with an app feature analysis based on a theoretical (empowerment) approach. The results of the app assessment were then connected to (non-) user perspectives on diabetes app use. Moreover, some of the main methodological challenges appearing in this app analysis were made transparent in Chapter 12.4. Previous research, as well as Study 1 demonstrated that app quality assessments are essential for app evaluations, and validated and reliable quality assessment tools should be used for evaluating apps.

The analysis results of Study 1 in this research demonstrated that app assessments face many methodological challenges that have to be addressed, including valid quality assessments, the interactive nature of diabetes apps, and the technological developments leading to merging online cloud-based platforms that are independent of end-user devices. Grundy et al. (2016) pointed out that research on health app quality has to be advanced, with the majority of app quality assessment studies falsely claiming "to have performed an exhaustive, replicable, and systematic search and data extraction" (p. 1051). According to the authors, outcome evaluations and evidence-based studies are more common than theory-based and validated quality assessment tools. Some previous app assessment studies did not use theoretical foundation for their analysis, but rather used practical guidelines as a foundation instead (e.g., Brzan et al., 2016; Chomutare et al., 2011). Theoretical approaches can give empirical instruments a much stronger study foundation (Riley et al., 2011). Apart from quality assessments, user evaluations need to be included in an assessment of health apps and their features, to be able to evaluate usability, feasibility and other relevant aspects from a user perspective. Some app assessment (review) studies have already started assessing apps from a user perspective (Khalid et al., 2015), and general user evaluations of mHealth apps are available in literature to a large extent (e.g., Garcia-Zapirain, de la Torre Diez, Sainz de Abajo, & Lopez-Coronado, 2016; Palazuelos et al., 2013; Smahel, Elavsky, & Machackova, 2017). However, a user-based app evaluation has to be further connected to theoretical approaches and existing app assessment tools as available in the literature (e.g., app quality rating scales) to be able to comprehensively evaluate health apps.

16.3 Implications for Diabetes Care – The Practical Value of Diabetes Apps

After introducing a theoretical empowerment approach to better understand diabetes app use, the question remains what practical value diabetes apps add for overall diabetes self-management, and what their relevance in self-management is. Conclusions could be drawn from the conducted studies.

Due to the fact that the potential of the included diabetes apps for empowered self-management was interpreted as rather low in Study 1, and low app quality was found in a majority of the examined apps, there is urgent need for improvement of diabetes apps for self-management. A similar overall conclusion was reported by Zaires et al. (2017) who asked for "improvement in order to approach a holistic manageme[ne]nt point-of-view from an mHealth perspective" (p. 177). Complementing Study 1 results on diabetes apps, Study 2 showed that the relevance of diabetes apps for self-management should not be overestimated. Study 2 showed that patients did not only use diabetes apps for their diabetes self-management. They used their mobile smart devices much more broadly by combining the use of diabetes apps with other non-diabetes specific apps and channels. Some patients reported a preference for other mobile apps and channels and considered diabetes apps of limited usefulness for various reasons (Table 7 in Appendix). In Study 2, some patients reported using app logbooks for recording BG values and other health data, searching for carbohydrate contents in food through general online search engines (to adjust insulin to food consumption), having step counters connected to fitness apps on mobile devices, communicating with HCPs via email or through instant messengers, and with other patients through instant messenger chat groups (e.g., WhatsApp). Some still used printouts to show BG developments to HCPs, e.g., Excel lists, or sent graphic app outputs to their HCPs through email. Some used online clouds to collect and store their health data, and to make the data accessible to their HCPs (see interview extract examples in Table 6 in Appendix). Overall, technology-supported diabetes self-management was found to be much more holistic than limited to the use of diabetes apps.

One Study 2 participant called diabetes app "just another tool" (Jie, age 64, T1DM), which summarizes that diabetes apps were perceived as not powerful enough to replace other traditional care and self-management strategies, but rather add potential for improved diabetes self-management in combination with traditional tools and strategies. Studies 2 and 3 further confirmed that diabetes app use doesn't work independently from the overall diabetes self-management process (Brahmbhatt et al., 2017). Handing an app to a diabetes patient and leaving it without support of HCPs or integration into the traditional diabetes care process is likely to reduce the app use effectiveness (Katz et al., 2012). "The cell phone alone is not sufficient to make a difference. A successful mHealth... system requires attention to all of the links in the chain of chronic care" (Katz et al., 2012, p. 71). Only with additional HCP support, diabetes app use could be found to result in improved health outcomes in previous research (Veazie et al., 2018). This emphasizes the relevance of an inclusion of diabetes apps in the HCP-patient relationship, as well as the relevance of social support in self-management (behavioral empowerment). Study 1 showed that improved apps should be included in diabetes programs to a larger extent, making the app use more likely and efficient. As part of a diabetes program, an appropriate app selection and effective use could be taught by diabetes educators as part of the overall diabetes education. Moreover, available data from the apps (e.g., logbooks) could be used by the cooperating HCPs for improved feedback on BG results and improved data monitoring adherence. Results from the app use could be discussed in the care program and appropriate feedback could be given. Both patients and HCPs could benefit from data collected through diabetes apps for self-management. For patients, apps could provide improved feedback, and for HCPs, apps could provide better data overviews, as well as time-saving technology-supported feedback procedures.

Abbasgholizadeh Rahimi et al. (2017) discussed whether mHealth applications are useful for supporting shared decision-making in diagnostic and treatment decisions. According to them, mobile health applications generally offer improved opportunities for and greater participation in shared decision-making. mHealth tools are attributed with better accessibility than web-based applications, cost efficiency, extensibility, better visualization, an enhancement of HCP efficiency (saving time), real-time connectivity and collaborative decision-making. Moreover, smart applications can support patient decisions remotely, especially relevant for areas without easy access to medical centers (Abbasgholizadeh Rahimi et al., 2017). On the other hand, disadvantages of mHealth for supporting shared decision-making include a potential overuse of mHealth apps if HCPs replace face-to-face consultation with online feedback, diminishing the quality of HCP-patient interaction (Abbasgholizadeh Rahimi et al., 2017). Moreover, health disparities might be increased when vulnerable populations lack skills for mHealth app usage or access to mHealth apps. Additionally, there is lacking regulation around mHealth apps, leading to poor app quality, that might affect patient decisions and health outcomes negatively when incorrect information is misleading. It is discussed if apps could increase patient anxiety, and concern about patient data is expressed that might reduce usefulness of apps for shared decision-making (Abbasgholizadeh Rahimi et al., 2017).

In addition to the need for inclusion of diabetes apps in an HCP-patient context, selected diabetes apps should be promoted by the government. HCPs and patients can rely on good app quality when apps are officially tested and promoted by the government (in Singapore: health promotion board). An official approval makes it easier for HCPs to recommend apps to their patients. With more frequent recommendation by the doctors, app use is likely to increase, and data from the apps can be used more efficiently in cooperation between patient and HCPs.

16.4 Designing Diabetes Apps for Specific Target Groups

Previous studies as well as Study 2 interviews showed that diabetes apps work only for specific *segments* of the diabetes target population. Study 2 participants reported that diabetes apps were not suitable for older patients or patients with poor self-management, lacking basic diabetes knowledge or lacking self-motivation. In Study 2 older patients were reported to be partly unable to handle mobile technology, or to be unable to self-manage their disease like patients in nursing homes, or highly aged patients. Scheibe et al. (2015) found that older diabetes patients lacked acceptance of diabetes app usage due to a perceived lack of benefits and ease of use. Gao, Zhou, Liu, Wang, and Bowers (2017) found in an app review of 71 diabetes apps that the "features of most apps failed to include content areas of known importance for managing diabetes in older adults" (p. 68).

Similarly, following previous research, resource-poor patients might perceive barriers to diabetes app use as high. Katz et al. (2012) showed that the dropout rate in a type 2 mHealth diabetes program was about 50% because patients could not afford low-cost mobile phone services. Patients who cannot afford even the cheapest mobile phone services are likely to fail in using apps for diabetes self-management (El-Gayar et al., 2013).

Another problematic target group in Study 2 for diabetes apps was found to be patients with poor self-management and poorly controlled diabetes. Patients with poor diabetes self-management could be found to show low self-management motivation in Study 2. Diabetes app use requires a certain amount of self-initiative and motivation for self-care (Chapter 3.1). Following the differentiation of push and pull healthcare marketing in Kingsley (1987), diabetes apps are categorized as "pull" media. Without motivation for self-management the adoption and use of diabetes apps is rather unlikely (Studies 2 and 3), even though there might be general interest in diabetes apps (Study 2). A gap between attitudes towards mHealth usage, usage intentions, general interest in mHealth, and the actual mHealth adoption and use has been shown in previous studies (Dou et al., 2017; James et al., 2016).

In contrast, Studies 2 and 3 found that segments of the diabetes patient population who might gain profit from diabetes apps mostly comprised those patients who were already unproblematic, who brought along high motivation for self-management and good ability to care for themselves. Study 2 participants recommended younger motivated patients as a target group that could be addressed with diabetes apps. However, Study 2 results also displayed that another challenge came with this group of patients because it could be shown that young diabetes patients were not satisfied with the available diabetes apps for self-management. From Study 2 and 3 results, young patients with high psychological empowerment, independence in their health decision-making, and high interest in technological innovation expressed the need for advanced mobile tools with a variety of innovative and interactive app features, and an attractive app design.

These examples and previous studies (Scheibe et al., 2015) show that patients suffering from diabetes are not a homogeneous group that can be addressed with one diabetes app for all patients. Instead, subgroups have to be built based on segmentation principles (Donovan & Henley, 2003) and have to be addressed specifically based on their characteristics and needs. Factors influencing diabetes app use have to be considered when tailoring diabetes apps. For example, while young diabetes app users requested innovative and interactive diabetes apps in Study 2, older patients or high-risk groups lacking diabetes knowledge were found to require minimalist and simplified diabetes apps to structure basic diabetes self-management (mostly simple diabetes logbooks). Patients switching apps and parallel using several apps preferred dynamic apps that can be easily synchronized with other apps and devices, to be always "up-to-date" in the latest technology. Long-term users of diabetes apps especially expressed the need for reliable apps they can trust over a longer period of time. In addition to fitness apps, health information apps and connected external devices (meters, step counters, etc.), patients injecting insulin showed interest in diabetes logbooks and food content databases in Study 2, while patients on oral diabetes medication used logbooks only (also compare Study 2 typology).

In addition, it has to be kept in mind that preferences are individual even in homogeneous subgroups (Scheibe et al., 2015). Thus, there should always be further diabetes app tailoring options and feature choices left to the individual patient. Scheibe et al. (2015) suggest that diabetes apps should be individually adaptable to meet patient needs in subgroups that appear homogeneous but actually are less homogeneous than assumed. Apps are taking a first step towards individual "app packages" that can be combined following individual preferences. For example, the described MySugr app series (https://mysugr.com) offered a number of apps that could be used in any combination (Chapter 12.2.5). However, the idea of combined apps has to be taken one step further with giving a choice to patients in selecting the app features individually that are relevant to them. Moreover, lack of app quality has to be addressed, by providing apps that fulfill high quality standards that are made transparent to the user.

Overall, practice has to be sensitized for the importance to consider theoretical and empirical research when designing health apps (Pereira-Azevedo et al., 2016), to increase usage effectiveness, and to enhance the diabetes app potential for self-management.

17 Summarizing Research Limitations

Study limitations were included in the respective study chapters. This chapter additionally summarizes the three main research limitations of the overall research, including all three conducted studies.

Firstly, the studies took a step towards investigating empowerment as an antecedent of diabetes app use. Yet, the study design did not allow final conclusions on causality to be drawn, and the results could be interpreted only as a first indication of empowerment being an antecedent of diabetes app use. Research suitable for examining causal relationships has to be added in follow-up research to finalize conclusions about relationships between diabetes apps use, empowerment, and other involved factors. Here, especially experimental study design is needed that compares the influence of different levels of empowerment on diabetes app use. Moreover, longitudinal study design is required, to be able to measure changes in empowerment before, during, and after diabetes app use, in order to draw conclusions about the overall empowerment process in relation to diabetes app use.

Secondly, a triangulation between Study 1 on the one hand and studies 2 and 3 on the other was limited, with Study 1 not investigating all apps mentioned by study participants in studies 2 and 3 (or reverse). Study 2 used one selected app from Study 1, and asked the participants for their previous use of diabetes apps, as well as their opinions about those apps and their experiences with them. Study 3 asked the survey participants about their previous diabetes app use. However, not all the mentioned apps in studies 2 and 3 were examined in the Study 1 app feature analysis. As a result, app characteristics could not be included as an influencing factor on diabetes app use in Study 3 as suggested in Figure 2. This resulted in a limitation of possible conclusions about the relationship between app characteristics (e.g., app quality) and diabetes app use. A better fit between the app analysis in Study 1 and the user perspective in studies 2 and 3 could have been achieved if the app feature analysis in Study 1 had been added after the user perspective assessment in studies 2 and 3, to be able to examine all the apps mentioned by the study participants for their features and quality. In this way, the triangulation between the studies and the fit between app characteristics and the perception of diabetes app (non-) users about the respective apps could have been improved.

Thirdly, the sampling methods in studies 2 and 3 led to some insufficiencies in the resulting study samples. Specific groups including motivated support group members were overrepresented, and at risk patients were underrepresented in both samples, due to the use of support groups for recruitment of participants, as well as snowball sampling methods. Moreover, the sampling led to difficulties when trying to increase the Study 3 sample size, resulting in the sample being much smaller than planned. This also had consequences for data analysis, with complex multivariate analysis (like structural equation modeling) not being applicable to the data. As a rule of thumb 10 to 20 times as many cases as variables are suggested for structural equation modeling, but most researchers prefer a sample of 200 to 400 cases for 10 to 15 included variables (Statistics Solutions, 2018). For further analysis with the sample, including mediation and moderation analysis, the sample size should be increased (applicable analysis for small samples could be discussed, e.g., PROCESS analysis, Hayes, 2017).

18 Conclusion

Overall, research on relationships between empowerment and mHealth use is scarce, and research needs to be added on empowerment processes in relation to mHealth, empowerment as an antecedent of mHealth use, as well as empowerment as an outcome of mHealth use. Both researchers and practitioners need to find ways to step out of the never ending circle of poorly designed mHealth tools and weak effect studies showing hardly any outcomes of mHealth use in self-management processes. Theoretical approaches like the empowerment approach, a "patient-centered, collaborative approach tailored to match the fundamental realities of diabetes care" (Chen & Li, 2009, abstract), can be used to understand anteceding factors of health app use, and can deliver a useful foundation for tailoring and designing apps for specific target groups. This also includes the consideration of an adaption of apps for specific cultural backgrounds, as well as for resource-poor populations.

At the same time, the focus has to be extended from diabetes apps, and research examining the combination of all relevant online and offline (mobile) channels used by diabetes patients is needed to inform practice about ways to actively reach patients, and to improve technology-supported and empowered self-management. It could be shown that patient empowerment is able to improve health outcomes, yet "for many policy makers it seems clear that the primary driver is the potential to control healthcare costs" (Lucas, 2015, p. 150). According to The Lancet (2012), "in countries such as China and India, health systems will only be able to cope with the onslaught of chronic disease with patient empowerment" (p. 1677). Thus, potential in mobile tools for self-management is especially seen in an automatization of patient data, and an improvement of self-managed diabetes with close monitoring by HCPs, to finally reduce costs associated with diabetes care.

> It has... been suggested that a move to greater self-management supported by... smart phone technology could improve the treatment of many millions of patients with chronic diseases in low and middle income economies that are also confronting the potential cost implications of epidemiological and demographic transitions, combined with the higher expectations of a more educated and knowledgeable population. (Lucas, 2015, p. 145)

Despite resting hope in mobile smart diabetes tools, many challenges and barriers to mHealth use have still to be recognized to be able to achieve improvements in technology-supported diabetes self-management (Fatehi, Gray, & Russell, 2017).

References

Abbasgholizadeh Rahimi, S., Menear, M., Robitaille, H., & Legare, F. (2017). Are mobile health applications useful for supporting shared decision making in diagnostic and treatment decisions? *Global Health Action, 10*(sup3), 1332259. doi: 10.1080/16549716.2017.1332259

Agarwal, R., & Prasad, J. (1998). The antecedents and consequents of user perceptions in information technology adoption. *Decision Support Systems, 22*(1), 15-29. doi: 10.1016/S0167-9236(97)00006-7

Ahmed, U. S., Junaidi, B., Ali, A. W., Akhter, O., Salahuddin, M., & Akhter, J. (2010). Barriers in initiating insulin therapy in a South Asian muslim community. *Diabetic Medicine, 27*(2), 169-174. doi: 10.1111/j.1464-5491.2009.02904.x

Ahola, A. J., & Groop, P. H. (2013). Barriers to self-management of diabetes. *Diabetic Medicine, 30*(4), 413-420. doi: 10.1111/dme.12105

Ajzen, I. (1991). The theory of planned behavior. *Organizational Behavior and Human Decision Processes, 50*(2), 179-211. doi: 10.1016/0749-5978(91)90020-t

Al-Mamary, Y. H., Al-Nashmi, M., Hassan, Y. A. G., & Shamsuddin, A. (2016). A critical review of models and theories in field of individual acceptance of technology. *International Journal of Hybrid Information Technology, 9*(6), 143-158. doi: 10.14257/ijhit.2016.9.6.13

Alanzi, T. M., Bah, S., Jaber, F., Alshammari, S., & Alzahrani, S. (2016). *Evaluation of a mobile social networking application for glycaemic control and diabetes knowledge in patients with type 2 diabetes: A randomized controlled trial using whatsapp.* Paper presented at the Qatar Foundation Annual Research Conference.

Aljasem, L. I., Peyrot, M., Wissow, L., & Rubin, R. R. (2001). The impact of barriers and self-efficacy on self-care behaviors in type 2 diabetes. *The Diabetes Educator, 27*(3), 393-404. doi: 10.1177/014572170102700309

Alsop, R., & Heinsohn, N. (2005). *Measuring empowerment in practice: Structuring analysis and framing indicators.* Washington, DC: World Bank.

American Association of Diabetes Educators, AADE. (2016). Quantity of diabetes apps makes it tough to determine quality. Retrieved 09/21/2017, from http://www.aademeeting.org/quantity-of-diabetes-apps-makes-it-tough-to-determine-quality/

American Association of Diabetes Educators, AADE. (2017). AADE7 self-care behaviors™. Retrieved 08/02/2017, from http://www.diabeteseducator.org/patient-resources/aade7-self-care-behaviors

American Diabetes Association, ADA. (2010). Diagnosis and classification of diabetes mellitus. *Diabetes Care, 33*(Supp. 1), 62-69. doi: 10.2337/dc10-S062

American Diabetes Association, ADA. (2014). Standards of medical care in diabetes 2014. *Diabetes Care, 37*(Supp. 1), 14-80. doi: 10.2337/dc14-S014

American Diabetes Association, ADA. (2015). Living with diabetes: Complications. Retrieved 02/21/2015, from http://www.diabetes.org/living-with-diabetes/complications/

American Diabetes Association, ADA. (2016). Diagnosing diabetes and learning about prediabetes. Retrieved 12/16/2016, from http://www.diabetes.org/diabetes-basics/diagnosis/

American Medical Association, AMA. (1847). AMA code of medical ethics. Retrieved 07/13/2015, from http://www.ama-assn.org/resources/doc/ethics/x-pub/1847code.pdf

American Medical Association, AMA. (2015). AMA's code of medical ethics.   Retrieved 07/13/2015, from http://www.ama-assn.org/ama/pub/physician-resources/medical-ethics/code-medical-ethics.page?

Anderson, K., Burford, O., & Emmerton, L. (2016). App chronic disease checklist: Protocol to evaluate mobile apps for chronic disease self-management. *JMIR Research Protocols, 5*(4), e204. doi: 10.2196/resprot.6194

Anderson, R. M., Fitzgerald, J. T., Gruppen, L. D., Funnell, M. M., & Oh, M. S. (2003). The diabetes empowerment scale-short form (DES-SF). *Diabetes Care, 26*(5), 1641-1642. doi: 10.2337/diacare.26.5.1641-a

Anderson, R. M., & Funnell, M. M. (2010). Patient empowerment: Myths and misconceptions. *Patient Education and Counseling, 79*(3), 277-282. doi: 10.1016/j.pec.2009.07.025

Anderson, R. M., Funnell, M. M., Aikens, J. E., Krein, S. L., Fitzgerald, J. T., Nwankwo, R., . . . Tang, T. S. (2009). Evaluating the efficacy of an empowerment-based self-management consultant intervention: Results of a two-year randomized controlled trial. *The Patient Educator, 1*(1), 3-11. doi: 10.1051/tpe/2009002

Anderson, R. M., Funnell, M. M., Butler, P. M., Arnold, M. S., Fitzgerald, J. T., & Feste, C. C. (1995). Patient empowerment: Results of a randomized controlled trial. *Diabetes Care, 18*(7), 943-949. doi: 10.2337/diacare.18.7.943

Anderson, R. M., Funnell, M. M., Fitzgerald, J. T., & Marrero, D. G. (2000). The diabetes empowerment scale: A measure of psychosocial self-efficacy. *Diabetes Care, 23*(6), 739-743. doi: 10.2337/diacare.23.6.739

Anshari, M., & Almunawar, M. N. (2015). mHealth technology implication: Shifting the role of patients from recipients to partners of care. In S. Adibi (Ed.), *mHealth multidisciplinary verticals*. Boca Raton, London, New York: CRC Press, Taylor & Francis Group.

Anshari, M., & Almunawar, M. N. (2016). Mobile health (mHealth) services and online health educators. *Biomedical Informatics Insights, 8*, 19-27. doi: 10.4137/BII.S35388

Anshari, M., Almunawar, M. N., Low, P. K., & Al-Mudimigh, A. S. (2012). Empowering clients through e-health in healthcare services: Case Brunei. *International Quarterly of Community Health Education, 33*(2), 189-219. doi: 10.2190/IQ.33.2.g

Armour, T. A., Norris, S. L., Jack, L., Jr., Zhang, X., & Fisher, L. (2005). The effectiveness of family interventions in people with diabetes mellitus: A systematic review. *Diabetic Medicine, 22*(10), 1295-1305. doi: 10.1111/j.1464-5491.2005.01618.x

Arnhold, M., Quade, M., & Kirch, W. (2014). Mobile applications for diabetics: A systematic review and expert-based usability evaluation considering the special requirements of diabetes patients age 50 years or older. *Journal of Medical Internet Research, 16*(4), e104. doi: 10.2196/jmir.2968

Årsand, E., Frøisland, D. H., Skrøvseth, S. O., Chomutare, T., Tatara, N., Hartvigsen, G., & Tufano, J. T. . (2012). Mobile health applications to assist patients with diabetes: Lessons learned and design implications. *Journal of Diabetes Science and Technology, 6*(5), 1197-1206.

Asimakopoulou, K., Gilbert, D., Newton, P., & Scambler, S. (2012). Back to basics: Re-examining the role of patient empowerment in diabetes. *Patient Education and Counseling, 86*(3), 281-283. doi: 10.1016/j.pec.2011.03.017

Austin, S., Senécal, C., Guay, F., & Nouwen, A. (2011). Effects of gender, age, and diabetes duration on dietary self-care in adolescents with type 1 diabetes: A self-determination theory perspective. *Jounral of Health Psychology, 16*(6), 917-928. doi: 10.1177/135910531039639

Avers, D., Brown, M., Chui, K. K., Wong, R. A., & Lusardi, M. (2011). Editor's message: Use of the term "elderly". *Journal of Geriatric Physical Therapy, 34*(4), 153-154. doi: 10.1519/JPT.0b013e31823ab7ec

Azhar, F. A. B., & Dhillon, J. S. (2016). *A systematic review of factors influencing the effective use of mHealth apps for self-care.* Paper presented at the 3rd International Conference on Computer and Information Sciences (ICCOINS), Kuala Lumpur.

Bagozzi, R.P. (2007). The legacy of the technology acceptance model and a proposal for a paradigm shift. *Journal of the Association for Information Systems, 8*(4), 244-254.

Bainbridge Frymier, A. (1994). A model of immediacy in the classroom. *Communication Quarterly, 42*(2), 133-144. doi: 10.1080/01463379409369922

Bandura, A. (1977). Self-efficacy: Toward a unifying theory of behavioral change. *Psychological Review, 84*(2), 191-215.

Bandura, A. (1997). *Self-efficacy: The exercise of control.* New York, NY: Freeman.

Bandura, A. (2002). Social cognitive theory of mass communication. In J. Bryant & M. B. Oliver (Eds.), *Media effects: Advances in theory and research* (pp. 94-124). NY: Routledge.

Barak, A., Boniel-Nissim, M., & Suler, J. (2008). Fostering empowerment in online support groups. *Computers in Human Behavior, 24*(5), 1867-1883. doi: 10.1016/j.chb.2008.02.004

Bardus, M., van Beurden, S. B., Smith, J. R., & Abraham, C. (2016). A review and content analysis of engagement, functionality, aesthetics, information quality, and change techniques in the most popular commercial apps for weight management. *The International Journal of Behavioral Nutrition and Physical Activity, 13*, 35. doi: 10.1186/s12966-016-0359-9

Baron, J., McBain, H., & Newman, S. (2012). The impact of mobile monitoring technologies on glycosylated hemoglobin in diabetes: A systematic review. *Journal of Diabetes Science and Technology, 6*(5), 1185-1196.

Baron, R. M., & Kenny, D. A. (1986). The moderator-mediator variable distinction in social psychological research: Conceptual, strategic, and statistical considerations. *Journal of Personality and Social Psychology, 51*(6), 1173-1182.

Barrera, M. (2006). Social support and social-ecological resources as mediators of lifestyle intervention effects for type 2 diabetes. *Journal of Health Psychology, 11*(3), 483-495. doi: 10.1177/1359105306063321

Bartlett, Y. K., & Coulson, N. S. (2011). An investigation into the empowerment effects of using online support groups and how this affects health professional/patient communication. *Patient Education and Counseling, 83*(1), 113-119. doi: 10.1016/j.pec.2010.05.029

Basilico, A., Marceglia, S., Bonacina, S., & Pinciroli, F. (2016). Advising patients on selecting trustful apps for diabetes self-care. *Computers in Biology and Medicine, 71*, 86-96. doi: 10.1016/j.compbiomed.2016.02.005

Batenburg, A., & Das, E. (2015). Virtual support communities and psychological well-being: The role of optimistic and pessimistic social comparison strategies. *Journal of Computer-Mediated Communication, 20*(6), 585-600. doi: 10.1111/jcc4.12131

Beckman, D., Reehorst, C. M., Henriksen, A., Muzny, M., Årsand, E., & Hartvigsen, G. (2016). Better glucose regulation through enabling group-based motivational mechanisms in cloud-based solutions like Nightscout. *International Journal of Integrated Care, 16*(5), 4. doi: 10.5334/ijic.2548

Benabou, R., & Tirole, J. (2003). Intrinsic and extrinsic motivation. *Review of Economic Studies, 70*(3), 489-520. doi: 10.1111/1467-937x.00253

Bennich, B. B., Roder, M. E., Overgaard, D., Egerod, I., Munch, L., Knop, F. K., . . . Konradsen, H. (2017). Supportive and non-supportive interactions in families with a type 2 diabetes patient: An integrative review. *Diabetology and Metabolic Syndrome, 9*, 57. doi: 10.1186/s13098-017-0256-7

Beratarrechea, A., Diez-Canseco, F., Irazola, V., Miranda, J., Ramirez-Zea, M., & Rubinstein, A. (2016). Use of m-health technology for preventive interventions to tackle cardiometabolic conditions and other non-communicable diseases in Latin America – challenges and opportunities. *Progress in Cardiovascular Diseases, 58*(6), 661-673. doi: 10.1016/j.pcad.2016.03.003

Berelson, B. (1952). *Content analysis in communication research*. Glencoe: Free Press.

Berkowitz, C. M., Zullig, L. L., Koontz, B. F., & Smith, S. K. (2017). Prescribing an app? Oncology providers' views on mobile health apps for cancer care. *JCO Clinical Cancer Informatics, 1*, 1-7. doi: 10.1200/cci.17.00107

Bhattarai, P., Newton-John, T. R. O., & Phillips, J. L. (2018). Quality and usability of arthritic pain self-management apps for older adults: A systematic review. *Pain Medicine, 19*(3), 471-484. doi: 10.1093/pm/pnx090

Biller Krauskopf, P. (2017). Review of American Diabetes Association diabetes care standards and MySugr mobile apps. *The Journal for Nurse Practitioners, 13*(3), e159-e160. doi: 10.1016/j.nurpra.2016.12.005

Bloomfield, G. S., Vedanthan, R., Vasudevan, L., Kithei, A., Were, M., & Velazquez, E. J. (2014). Mobile health for non-communicable diseases in Sub-saharan Africa: A systematic review of the literature and strategic framework for research. *Globalization and Health, 10*(1), 49. doi: 10.1186/1744-8603-10-49

Bohme, C., von Osthoff, M. B., Frey, K., & Hubner, J. (2017). Development of a rating tool for mobile cancer apps: Information analysis and formal and content-related evaluation of selected cancer apps. *Journal of Cancer Education*. doi: 10.1007/s13187-017-1273-9

Bohme, C., von Osthoff, M. B., Frey, K., & Hubner, J. (2018). Qualitative evaluation of mobile cancer apps with particular attention to the target group, content, and advertising. *Journal of Cancer Research and Clinical Oncology, 144*(1), 173-181. doi: 10.1007/s00432-017-2533-0

Booth, A. O., Lowis, C., Dean, M., Hunter, S. J., & McKinley, M. C. (2013). Diet and physical activity in the self-management of type 2 diabetes: Barriers and facilitators identified by patients and health professionals. *Primary Health Care Research and Development, 14*(3), 293-306. doi: 10.1017/S1463423612000412

Boyle, L., Grainger, R., Hall, R. M., & Krebs, J. D. (2017). Use of and beliefs about mobile phone apps for diabetes self-management: Surveys of people in a hospital diabetes clinic and diabetes health professionals in New Zealand. *JMIR mHealth and uHealth, 5*(6), e85. doi: 10.2196/mhealth.7263

Boyle, S. C., Earle, A. M., LaBrie, J. W., & Smith, D. J. (2017). PNF 2.0? Initial evidence that gamification can increase the efficacy of brief, web-based personalized normative feedback alcohol interventions. *Addictive Behaviors, 67*, 8-17. doi: 10.1016/j.addbeh.2016.11.024

Bozan, K., Davey, B., & Parker, K. (2015). Social influence on health it adoption patterns of the elderly: An institutional theory based use behavior approach. *Procedia Computer Science, 63*, 517-523. doi: 10.1016/j.procs.2015.08.378

Bradway, M., Arsand, E., & Grottland, A. (2015). Mobile health: Empowering patients and driving change. *Trends in Endocrinology and Metabolism, 26*(3), 114-117. doi: 10.1016/j.tem.2015.01.001

Brahmbhatt, R., Niakan, S., Saha, N., Tewari, A., Pirani, A., Keshavjee, N., . . . Keshavjee, K. (2017). Diabetes mHealth apps: Designing for greater uptake. In F. Lau, J. Bartle-Clar, G. Bliss, E. Borycki, K. Courtney & A. Kuo (Eds.), *Building capacity for health informatics in the future* (Vol. 234, pp. 49-53). Amsterdam et al.: IOS Press.

Braun, V., & Clarke, V. (2006). Using thematic analysis in psychology. *Qualitative Research in Psychology, 3*(2), 77-101. doi: 10.1191/1478088706qp063oa

Brew-Sam, N. , & Chib, A. (2019). How do smart device apps for diabetes self-management correspond with theoretical indicators of empowerment? An analysis of app features. *International Journal of Technology Assessment in Health Care, 35*(2), 150-159. doi: 10.1017/S0266462319000163

Brew-Sam, N., & Chib, A. (2020, in process). Theoretical advances in mobile health communication research: An empowerment approach to self-management. In J. Kim & H. Song (Eds.), *Technology and health: Promoting attitude and behavior change*: Elsevier.

Brooks, C. F. , & Young, S. L. (2011). Are choice-making opportunities needed in the classroom? Using self-determination theory to consider student motivation and learner empowerment. *International Journal of Teaching and Learning in Higher Education, 23*(1), 48-59.

Browning, A. M. (2013). CNE article: Moral distress and psychological empowerment in critical care nurses caring for adults at end of life. *American Journal of Critical Care, 22*(2), 143-151. doi: 10.4037/ajcc2013437

Bryman, Alan. (2008a). *Social research methods* (3rd ed.). Oxford: Oxford University Press.

Bryman, Alan. (2008b). Thematic analysis. In A. Bryman (Ed.), *Social research methods* (3rd ed., pp. 554-556). Oxford: Oxford University Press.

Brzan, P. P., Rotman, E., Pajnkihar, M., & Klanjsek, P. (2016). Mobile applications for control and self management of diabetes: A systematic review. *Journal of Medical Systems, 40*(9), 210. doi: 10.1007/s10916-016-0564-8

Buhi, E. R., Trudnak, T. E., Martinasek, M. P., Oberne, A. B., Fuhrmann, H. J., & McDermott, R. J. (2013). Mobile phone-based behavioural interventions for health: A systematic review. *Health Education Journal, 72*(5), 564-583. doi: 10.1177/0017896912452071

Burke, S. D., Sherr, D., & Lipman, R. D. (2014). Partnering with diabetes educators to improve patient outcomes. *Diabetes, Metabolic Syndrome and Obesity, 7*, 45-53. doi: 10.2147/DMSO.S40036

Burner, E., Lam, C. N., DeRoss, R., Kagawa-Singer, M., Menchine, M., & Arora, S. (2018). Using mobile health to improve social support for low-income latino patients with diabetes: A mixed-methods analysis of the feasibility trial of TExT-MED + FANS. *Diabetes Technology and Therapeutics, 20*(1), 39-48. doi: 10.1089/dia.2017.0198

Burson, R., & Moran, K. J. (2015). Empowerment and engagement. *Home Healthcare Now, 33*(1), 49-50. doi: 10.1097/NHH.0000000000000178

Camerini, L., & Schulz, P. J. (2012). Effects of functional interactivity on patients' knowledge, empowerment, and health outcomes: An experimental model-driven evaluation of a web-based intervention. *Journal of Medical Internet Research, 14*(4), e105. doi: 10.2196/jmir.1953

Camerini, L., Schulz, P. J., & Nakamoto, K. (2012). Differential effects of health knowledge and health empowerment over patients' self-management and health outcomes: A cross-sectional evaluation. *Patient Education and Counseling, 89*(2), 337-344. doi: 10.1016/j.pec.2012.08.005

Carter-Edwards, L., Skelly, A. H., Cagle, C. S., & Appel, S. J. (2004). "They care but don't understand": Family support of African American women with type 2 diabetes. *Diabetes Educator, 30*(3), 493-501. doi: 10.1177/014572170403000321

Cenfetelli, R. T. (2004). Inhibitors and enablers as dual factor concepts in technology usage. *Journal of the Association for Information Systems, 5*(11), 472-492.

Centers for Disease Control and Prevention, CDC. (2017). Chronic disease overview. Retrieved 09/06/2018, from http://www.cdc.gov/chronicdisease/overview/index.htm

Chang, A. (2012). UTAUT and UTAUT 2: A review and agenda for future research. *The Winners, 13*(2), 10. doi: 10.21512/tw.v13i2.656

Chavez, S., Fedele, D., Guo, Y., Bernier, A., Smith, M., Warnick, J., & Modave, F. (2017). Mobile apps for the management of diabetes. *Diabetes Care, 40*(10), e145-e146. doi: 10.2337/dc17-0853

Chen, Y. C. , & Li, I. C. (2009). Effectiveness of interventions using empowerment concept for patients with chronic disease: A systematic review. *JBI Library of Systematic Reviews, 7*(27), 1179-1233.

Chib, A., & Jiang, Q. (2014). Investigating modern-day talaria: Mobile phones and the mobility-impaired in Singapore. *Journal of Computer-Mediated Communication, 19*(3), 695-711. doi: 10.1111/jcc4.12070

Chib, A., van Velthoven, M. H., & Car, J. (2015). mHealth adoption in low-resource environments: A review of the use of mobile healthcare in developing countries. *Journal of Health Communication, 20*(1), 4-34. doi: 10.1080/10810730.2013.864735

Chib, A., & Lin, S. H. (2018). Theoretical advancements in mHealth: A systematic review of mobile apps. *Journal of Health Communication, 23*(10-11), 909-955. doi: 10.1080/10810730.2018.1544676

Chin, J.J. (2002). Doctor-patient relationship: From medical paternalism to enhanced autonomy. *Singapore Medical Journal, 43*(3), 152-155.

Chomutare, T., Fernandez-Luque, L., Årsand, E., & Hartvigsen, G. (2011). Features of mobile diabetes applications: Review of the literature and analysis of current applications compared against evidence-based guidelines. *Journal of Medical Internet Research, 13*(3), e65. doi: 10.2196/jmir.1874

Cinar, A. B., & Schou, L. (2014). Impact of empowerment on toothbrushing and diabetes management. *Oral Health and Preventive Dentistry, 12*(4), 337-344. doi: 10.3290/j.ohpd.a32130

Clark, N. M., & Houle, C. R. (2009). Theoretical models and strategies for improving disease management by patients. In S. A. Shumaker, J. K. Ockene & K. A. Riekert (Eds.), *The handbook of health behavior change* (3rd ed., pp. 19-38). New York: Springer Pub. Co.

Colman, A. M. (2015). Motivation. In A. M. Colman (Ed.), *Oxford dictionary of psychology* (Vol. 4, pp. 479). Oxford, UK: Oxford University Press.

Conger, J. A., & Kanungo, R. N. (1988). The empowerment process: Integrating theory and practice. *Academy of Management Review, 13*(3), 471-482.

Consumer Barometer. (2014). Google study: Singapore is world's top smartphone market per capita. Press release.   Retrieved 07/03/2017, from http://www.mumbrella.asia/2014/10/google-study-singapore-worlds-top-smartphone-market-per-capita/

Consumer Barometer. (2017). Singapore.   Retrieved 01/10/2017, from http://www.consumerbarometer.com/en/trending/?countryCode=SG&category=TRN-NOFILTER-ALL

Conway, N., Campbell, I., Forbes, P., Cunningham, S., & Wake, D. (2016). mHealth applications for diabetes: User preference and implications for app development. *Health Informatics Journal, 22*(4), 1111-1120. doi: 10.1177/1460458215616265

Cook, D. A., Levinson, A. J., & Garside, S. (2010). Time and learning efficiency in internet-based learning: A systematic review and meta-analysis. *Advances in Health Sciences Education, 15*(5), 755-770. doi: 10.1007/s10459-010-9231-x

Council for Medical Schemes. (2018). Chronic diseases list. Retrieved 09/06/2018, from http://www.medicalschemes.com/medical_schemes_pmb/chronic_disease_list.htm

Cumming, T. M., Strnadová, I., Knox, M., & Parmenter, T. (2014). Mobile technology in inclusive research: Tools of empowerment. *Disability and Society, 29*(7), 999-1012. doi: 10.1080/09687599.2014.886556

Danaher, B. G., Brendryen, H., Seeley, J. R., Tyler, M. S., & Woolley, T. (2015). From black box to toolbox: Outlining device functionality, engagement activities, and the pervasive information architecture of mHealth interventions. *Internet Interventions, 2*(1), 91-101. doi: 10.1016/j.invent.2015.01.002

Davis, F. D. (1985). *A technology acceptance model for empirically testing new end-user information systems – theory and results* (PhD thesis), Massachusetts Inst. of Technology, Massachusetts.

Davis, F. D., Bagozzi, R. P., & Warshaw, P. R. (1989). User acceptance of computer technology: A comparison of two theoretical models. *Management Science, 35*(8), 982-1003. doi: 10.1287/mnsc.35.8.982

Davis, F. D., Bagozzi, R. P., & Warshaw, P. R. (1992). Extrinsic and intrinsic motivation to use computers in the workplace. *Journal of Applied Social Psychology, 22*(14), 1111-1132.

Debussche, X., Besançon, S., Balcou-Debussche, M., Ferdynus, C., Delisle, H., Huiart, L., & Sidibe, A. T. (2018). Structured peer-led diabetes self-management and support in a low-income country: The st2ep randomised controlled trial in Mali. *PLoS ONE, 13*(1), e0191262. doi: 10.1371/journal.pone.0191262

Deci, E. L. (1975). *Intrinsic motivation*. New York: Plenum Press.

Deci, E. L., Koestner, R., & Ryan, R. M. (1999). A meta-analytic review of experiments examining the effects of extrinsic rewards on intrinsic motivation. *Psychological Bulletin, 125*(6), 627-668. doi: 10.1037/0033-2909.125.6.627

Deci, E. L., & Ryan, R. M. (2008). Self-determination theory: A macrotheory of human motivation, development, and health. *Canadian Psychology/Psychologie Canadienne, 49*(3), 182-185. doi: 10.1037/a0012801

Demidowich, A. P., Lu, K., Tamler, R., & Bloomgarden, Z. (2012). An evaluation of diabetes self-management applications for Android smartphones. *Journal of Telemedicine and Telecare, 18*(4), 235-238. doi: 10.1258/jtt.2012.111002

Deng, X., Khuntia, J., & Ghosh, K. (2013). *Psychological empowerment of patients with chronic diseases: The role of digital integration.* Paper presented at the Thirty Fourth International Conference on Information Systems, Milan.

Deng, Z. (2013). Understanding public users' adoption of mobile health service. *International Journal of Mobile Communications, 11*(4), 351-373. doi: 10.1504/IJMC.2013.055748

Department of Statistics Singapore. (2015). General household survey 2015. Singapore: Department of Statistics Singapore.

DeShazo, J., Harris, L., Turner, A., & Pratt, W. (2010). Designing and remotely testing mobile diabetes video games. *Journal of Telemedicine and Telecare, 16*(7), 378-382. doi: 10.1258/jtt.2010.091012

DeSwert, K. (2012). *Calculating inter-coder reliability in media content analysis using Krippendorff's Alpha*. University of Amsterdam. Amsterdam. Retrieved from http://www.polcomm.org/wp-content/uploads/ICR01022012.pdf

Di Iorio, C. T., Carinci, F., & Massi, B. M. (2015). The diabetes challenge: From human and social rights to the empowerment of people with diabetes. In R. A. DeFronzo, E. Ferrannini, K. Alberti, P. Zimmet & G. Alberti (Eds.), *International textbook of diabetes mellitus* (4th ed., Vol. 1, pp. 1103-1112). Oxford: Wiley.

Diabetes Digital Media. (2017). Diabetes types.   Retrieved 09/19/2017, from http://www.diabetes.co.uk/diabetes-types.html

Diabetes Digital Media. (2018). Treatment for diabetes.   Retrieved 08/06/2018, from http://www.diabetes.co.uk/treatment.html

Diabetes Prevention Program Research Group. (2012). The 10-year cost-effectiveness of lifestyle intervention or Metformin for diabetes prevention: An intent-to-treat analysis of the DPP/DPPOS. *Diabetes Care, 35*(4), 723-730. doi: 10.2337/dc11-1468

DiFilippo, K. N., Huang, W., & Chapman-Novakofski, K. M. (2017). A new tool for nutrition app quality evaluation (AQEL): Development, validation, and reliability testing. *JMIR mHealth uHealth, 5*(10), e163. doi: 10.2196/mhealth.7441

Disability Nottinghamshire. (2018). The social model vs the medical model of disability. Retrieved 03/24/2018, from http://www.disabilitynottinghamshire.org.uk/about/social-model-vs-medical-model-of-disability/

Dogruel, L., Joeckel, S., & Bowman, N. D. (2015). Choosing the right app: An exploratory perspective on heuristic decision processes for smartphone app selection. *Mobile Media and Communication, 3*(1), 125-144. doi: 10.1177/2050157914557509

Donovan, R., & Henley, N. (2003). *Social marketing: Principles and practice*. Melbourne: IP Communications.

Dou, K., Yu, P., Deng, N., Liu, F., Guan, Y., Li, Z., . . . Duan, H. (2017). Patients' acceptance of smartphone health technology for chronic disease management: A theoretical model and empirical test. *JMIR mHealth uHealth, 5*(12), e177. doi: 10.2196/mhealth.7886

Drincic, A., Prahalad, P., Greenwood, D., & Klonoff, D. C. (2016). Evidence-based mobile medical applications in diabetes. *Endocrinology and Metabolism Clinics of North America, 45*(4), 943-965. doi: 10.1016/j.ecl.2016.06.001

Dutta, M. J., Pfister, R., & Kosmoski, C. (2010). Consumer evaluation of genetic information online: The role of quality on attitude and behavioral intentions. *Journal of Computer-Mediated Communication, 15*(4), 592-605. doi: 10.1111/j.1083-6101.2009.01504.x

Dwivedi, Y. K., Shareef, M. A., Simintiras, A. C., Lal, B., & Weerakkody, V. (2016). A generalised adoption model for services: A cross-country comparison of mobile health (m-health). *Government Information Quarterly, 33*(1), 174-187. doi: 10.1016/j.giq.2015.06.003

El-Gayar, O., Timsina, P., Nawar, N., & Eid, W. (2013). Mobile applications for diabetes self-management: Status and potential. *Journal of Diabetes Science and Technology, 7*(1), 247-262. doi: 10.1177/193229681300700130

Emanuel, E. J., & Emanuel, L. L. (1992). Four models of the physician-patient relationship. *The Journal of the American Medical Association, JAMA, 267*(16), 2221. doi: 10.1001/jama.1992.03480160079038

Eng, D. S., & Lee, J. M. (2013). The promise and peril of mobile health applications for diabetes and endocrinology. *Pediatric Diabetes, 14*(4), 231-238. doi: 10.1111/pedi.12034

Eyuboglu, E., & Schulz, P. J. (2016). Do health literacy and patient empowerment affect self-care behaviour? A survey study among Turkish patients with diabetes. *BMJ Open, 6*(3), e010186. doi: 10.1136/bmjopen-2015-010186

Fatehi, F., Gray, L. C., & Russell, A. W. (2017). Mobile health (mHealth) for diabetes care: Opportunities and challenges. *Diabetes Technology and Therapeutics, 19*(1), 1-3. doi: 10.1089/dia.2016.0430

Fiore, P. (2017). How to evaluate mobile health applications: A scoping review. In F. Lau, J. Bartle-Clar, G. Bliss, E. Borycki, K. Courtney & A. Kuo (Eds.), *Building capacity for health informatics in the future* (Vol. 234, pp. 109-114). Amsterda et al.: IOS Press.

Fischer, H. H., L., Moore S., D., Ginosar, J., Davidson A., M., Rice-Peterson C., J., Durfee M., & et al. (2012). Care by cell phone: Text messaging for chronic disease management. *American Journal Of Managed Care, 18*(2), e42-e47.

Fitzgerald, J. T., Davis, W. K. , Connell, C. M., Hess, G. E., Funnell, M. M., & Hiss, R. G. (1996a). Diabetes care profile.   Retrieved 04/13/2018, from http://academicdepartments.musc.edu/family_medicine/rcmar/dcp.htm

Fitzgerald, J. T., Davis, W. K., Connell, C. M., Hess, G. E., Funnell, M. M., & Hiss, R. G. (1996b). Development and validation of the diabetes care profile. *Evaluation and the Health Professions, 19*(2), 208-230. doi: 10.1177/016327879601900205

Fook, C. Y., Brinten, L., Sidhu, G. K., & Fooi, F. S. (2011). Relationships between psychological empowerment with work motivation and withdrawal intention among secondary school principals in malaysia. *Procedia – Social and Behavioral Sciences, 15*, 2907-2911. doi: 10.1016/j.sbspro.2011.04.212

Formann, A. K. (1984). *Die Latent-Class-Analyse: Einführung in die Theorie und Anwendung [The latent-class-analysis: Introduction to theory and application]*. Weinheim: Beltz.

Fortmann, A. L., Gallo, L. C., Garcia, M. I., Taleb, M., Euyoque, J. A., Clark, T., . . . Philis-Tsimikas, A. (2017). Dulce Digital: An mHealth SMS-based intervention improves glycemic control in Hispanics with type 2 diabetes. *Diabetes Care*, dc170230. doi: 10.2337/dc17-0230

Fortuna, K. L., DiMilia, P. R., Lohman, M. C. , Bruce, M. L., Zubritsky, C. D., Halaby, M. R., . . . Bartels, S. J. (2018). Feasibility, acceptability, and preliminary effectiveness of a peer-delivered and technology supported self-management intervention for older adults with serious mental illness. *Psychiatric Quarterly, 89*(2), 293-305. doi: 10.1007/s11126-017-9534-7

Free, C., Phillips, G., Galli, L., Watson, L., Felix, L., Edwards, P., . . . Cornford, T. (2013). The effectiveness of mobile-health technology-based health behaviour change or disease management interventions for health care consumers: A systematic review. *PLoS Medicine, 10*(1), e1001362. doi: 10.1371/journal.pmed.1001362

Fu, H., McMahon, S. K., Gross, C. R., Adam, T. J., & Wyman, J. F. (2017). Usability and clinical efficacy of diabetes mobile applications for adults with type 2 diabetes: A systematic review. *Diabetes Research and Clinical Practice, 131*, 70-81. doi: 10.1016/j.diabres.2017.06.016

Funnell, M. M., & Anderson, R. M. (2003). Patient ampowerment: A look back, a look ahead. *The Diabetes Educator, 29*(3), 454-464. doi: 10.1177/014572170302900310

Funnell, M. M., & Anderson, R. M. (2004). Empowerment and self-management of diabetes. *Clinical Diabetes, 22*(3), 123-127. doi: 10.2337/diaclin.22.3.123

Funnell, M. M., Anderson, R. M., Arnold, M. S., Barr, P. A., Donnelly, M., Johnson, P. D., . . . White, N. H. (1991). Empowerment: An idea whose time has come in diabetes education. *The Diabetes Educator, 17*(1), 37-41. doi: 10.1177/014572179101700108

Furner, C. P., Racherla, P., & Babb, J. S. (2016). What we know and do not know about mobile app usage and stickiness. A research agenda. In Information Ressources Management Association (Ed.), *Geospatial research: Concepts, methodologies, tools, and applications* (pp. 117-141). Hershey: Info. Science Reference.

Gagné, M., Senécal, C. B., & Koestner, R. (1997). Proximal job characteristics, feelings of empowerment, and intrinsic motivation: A multidimensional model. *Journal of Applied Social Psychology, 27*(14), 1222-1240. doi: 10.1111/j.1559-1816.1997.tb01803.x

Gallant, M. P. (2003). The influence of social support on chronic illness self-management: A review and directions for research. *Health Education & Behavior, 30*(2), 170-195. doi: 10.1177/1090198102251030

Gao, C., Zhou, L., Liu, Z., Wang, H., & Bowers, B. (2017). Mobile application for diabetes self-management in China: Do they fit for older adults? *International Journal of Medical Informatics, 101*, 68-74. doi: 10.1016/j.ijmedinf.2017.02.005

Garcia-Zapirain, B., de la Torre Diez, I., Sainz de Abajo, B., & Lopez-Coronado, M. (2016). Development, technical, and user evaluation of a web mobile application for self-control of diabetes. *Telemedicine Journal and e-Health, 22*(9), 778-785. doi: 10.1089/tmj.2015.0233

Georgsson, M., & Staggers, N. (2016). An evaluation of patients' experienced usability of a diabetes mHealth system using a multi-method approach. *Journal of Biomedical Informatics, 59*, 115-129. doi: 10.1016/j.jbi.2015.11.008

Georgsson, M., & Staggers, N. (2017). Patients' perceptions and experiences of a mHealth diabetes self-management system. *Computers, Informatics, Nursing, 35*(3), 122-130. doi: 10.1097/CIN.0000000000000296

Glajchen, M., & Bookbinder, M. (2001). Knowledge and perceived competence of home care nurses in pain management. *Journal of Pain and Symptom Management, 21*(4), 307-316. doi: 10.1016/s0885-3924(01)00247-0

Glaser, B. G., & Strauss, A. L. (1967). *The discovery of grounded theory: Strategies for qualitative research*. New Brunswick (US), London: Aldine.

Glasgow, R. E., Toobert, D. J., & Gillette, C. D. (2001). Psychosocial barriers to diabetes self-management and quality of life. *Diabetes Spectrum, 14*(1), 33-41. doi: 10.2337/diaspect.14.1.33

Goh, S. Y., Ang, S. B., Bee, Y. M., Chen, R. Y., Gardner, D., Ho, E., . . . Yap, F. (2014). Ministry of Health clinical practice guidelines: Diabetes mellitus. *Singapore Medical Journal, 55*(6), 334-347. doi: 10.11622/smedj.2014079

Gomersall, T., Madill, A., & Summers, L. K. M. (2011). A metasynthesis of the self-management of type 2 diabetes. *Qualitative Health Research, 21*(6), 853-871. doi: 10.1177/1049732311402096

Gomez-Galvez, P., Suarez Mejias, C., & Fernandez-Luque, L. (2015). Social media for empowering people with diabetes: Current status and future trends. *Conference Proceedings, 37th Annual International Conference of the IEEE, Engineering in Medicine and Biology Society (EMBC), 2015*, 2135-2138. doi: 10.1109/EMBC.2015.7318811

Graf-Vlachy, L, Buhtz, K., & König, A. (2018). Social influence in technology adoption: Taking stock and moving forward. *Management Review Quarterly, 68*(1), 37-76. doi: 10.1007/s11301-017-0133-3

Graffy, J. (2013). Approaches to diabetes: Empowerment, control or both? *Primary Health Care Research and Development, 14*(3), 221-223. doi: 10.1017/S1463423613000236

Grant, R. W., & Schmittdiel, J. A. (2013). Adults with diabetes who perceive family members' behaviour as unsupportive are less adherent to their medication regimen. *Evidence Based Nursing, 16*(1), 15-16. doi: 10.1136/eb-2012-100947

Grundy, Q. H., Wang, Z., & Bero, L. A. (2016). Challenges in assessing mobile health app quality: A systematic review of prevalent and innovative methods. *American Journal of Preventive Medicine, 51*(6), 1051-1059. doi: 10.1016/j.amepre.2016.07.009

Guo, Y., Bian, J., Leavitt, T., Vincent, H. K., Vander Zalm, L., Teurlings, T. L., . . . Modave, F. (2017). Assessing the quality of mobile exercise apps based on the American College of Sports medicine guidelines: A reliable and valid scoring instrument. *Journal of Medical Internet Research, 19*(3), e67. doi: 10.2196/jmir.6976

Gutschoven, K., & van den Bulck, J. (2006). *Towards the measurement of psychological health empowerment in the general public.* Paper presented at the Annual Conference of the International Comm. Association, Dresden, Germany.

Hall, A. K., Cole-Lewis, H., & Bernhardt, J. M. (2015). Mobile text messaging for health: A systematic review of reviews. *Annual Review of Public Health, 36*, 393-415. doi: 10.1146/annurev-publhealth-031914-122855

Hammer, M. J., Ercolano, E. A., Wright, F., Dickson, V. V., Chyun, D., & Melkus, G. D. (2015). Self-management for adult patients with cancer: An integrative review. *Cancer Nursing, 38*(2), E10-26. doi: 10.1097/NCC.0000000000000122

Hao, H., Padman, R., Sun, B., & Telang, R. (2014). *Examining the social influence on information technology sustained use in a community health system: A hierarchical Bayesian learning method analysis.* Paper presented at the 47th Hawaii International Conference on System Science, Hawaii.

Hayes, A. F. (2017). *Introduction to mediation, moderation, and conditional process analysis: A regression-based approach* (2nd ed.). New York: Guilford Press.

Heintzman, N. D. (2016). A digital ecosystem of diabetes data and technology: Services, systems, and tools enabled by wearables, sensors, and apps. *Journal of Diabetes Science and Technology, 10*(1), 35-41. doi: 10.1177/1932296815622453

Heisler, M., Bouknight, R. R., Hayward, R. A., Smith, D. M., & Kerr, E. A. (2002). The relative importance of physician communication, participatory decision making, and patient understanding in diabetes self-management. *Journal of General Internal Medicine, 17*(4), 243-252. doi: 10.1046/j.1525-1497.2002.10905.x

Heisler, M., Vijan, S., Makki, F., & Piette, J. D. (2010). Diabetes control with reciprocal peer support versus nurse care management: A randomized trial. *Annals of Internal Medicine, 153*(8), 507-515. doi: 10.7326/0003-4819-153-8-201010190-00007

Helgeson, V. S., Mascatelli, K., Seltman, H., Korytkowski, M., & Hausmann, L. R. (2016). Implications of supportive and unsupportive behavior for couples with newly diagnosed diabetes. *Health Psychology, 35*(10), 1047-1058. doi: 10.1037/hea0000388

Henke, J., Joeckel, S., & Dogruel, L. (2018). Processing privacy information and decision-making for smartphone apps among young German smartphone users. *Behaviour & Information Technology, 37*(5), 488-501. doi: 10.1080/0144929x.2018.1458902

Henze, N., Pielot, M., Poppinga, B., Schinke, T., & Boll, S. (2011). My app is an experiment: Experience from user studies in mobile app stores. *International Journal of Mobile Human Computer Interaction, 3*(4), 71-91. doi: 10.4018/jmhci.2011100105

Hewson, M. (2010). Agency. In A. Mills, G. Durepos & E. Wiebe (Eds.), *Encyclopedia of case study research* (pp. 13-17). Thousand Oaks, CA: SAGE Publications, Inc.

Hides, L., Kavanagh, D., Stoyanov, S., Zelenko, O., Tjondronegoro, D., & Mani, M. (2014). *Mobile application rating scale (MARS): A new tool for assessing the quality of health mobile applications.* Melbourne: Young and Well Cooperative Research Centre.

Hill, E., & Sibthorp, J. (2006). Autonomy support at diabetes camp: A self-determination theory approach to therapeutic recreation. *Therapeutic Recreation Journal, 40*(2), 107-125.

Hinkle, D. E., Wiersma, W., & Jurs, S. G. (2003). *Applied statistics for the behavioral sciences* (5th ed.). Boston: Houghton Mifflin.

Ho, K., Newton, L., Boothe, A., & Novak-Lauscher, H. (2015). *Mobile digital access to a web-enhanced network (mDAWN): Assessing the feasibility of mobile health tools for self-management of type-2 diabetes.* Paper presented at the AMIA Annual Symposium Proceedings.

Hoan, N. T., Chib, A., & Mahalingham, R. (2016). *Mobile phones and gender empowerment.* Paper presented at the Eighth International Conference on Information and Communication Technologies and Development, Michigan, USA.

Holloway, I. & Todres, L. (2003). The status of method: Flexibility, consistency and coherence. *Qualitative Research, 3*(3), 345-357. doi: 10.1177/1468794103033004

Holsti, O. R. (1969). *Content analysis for the social sciences and humanities.* Reading, MA: Addison-Wesley.

Holtz, B., & Lauckner, C. (2012). Diabetes management via mobile phones: A systematic review. *Telemedicine and e-Health, 18*(3), 175-184. doi: 10.1089/tmj.2011.0119

Holtz, B. E., Murray, K. M., Hershey, D. D., Dunneback, J. K., Cotten, S. R., Holmstrom, A. J., . . . Wood, M. A. (2017). Developing a patient-centered mHealth app: A tool for adolescents with type 1 diabetes and their parents. *JMIR mHealth and uHealth, 5*(4), e53. doi: 10.2196/mhealth.6654

Hoppe, C. D., Cade, J. E., & Carter, M. (2017). An evaluation of diabetes targeted apps for Android smartphone in relation to behaviour change techniques. *Journal of Human Nutrition and Dietetics, 30*(3), 326-338. doi: 10.1111/jhn.12424

Hoque, R., & Sorwar, G. (2017). Understanding factors influencing the adoption of mHealth by the elderly: An extension of the UTAUT model. *International Journal of Medical Informatics, 101*, 75-84. doi: 10.1016/j.ijmedinf.2017.02.002

Howorka, K., Pumprla, J., Wagner-Nosiska, D., Grillmayr, H., Schlusche, C., & Schabmann, A. (2000). Empowering diabetes out-patients with structured education. *Journal of Psychosomatic Research, 48*(1), 37-44. doi: 10.1016/s0022-3999(99)00074-4

Hu, F. B. (2011). Globalization of diabetes: The role of diet, lifestyle, and genes. *Diabetes Care, 34*(6), 1249-1257. doi: 10.2337/dc11-0442

Hu, M.-C. (2012). Antecedents for the adoption of new technology in emerging wireless cities: Comparisons between Singapore and Taipei. *Regional Studies, 48*(4), 665-679. doi: 10.1080/00343404.2012.674638

Huang, J. (2017). The relationship between employee psychological empowerment and proactive behavior: Self-efficacy as mediator. *Social Behavior and Personality, 45*(7), 1157-1166. doi: 10.2224/sbp.6609

Huckvale, K., Adomaviciute, S., Prieto, J. T., Leow, M. K., & Car, J. (2015). Smartphone apps for calculating insulin dose: A systematic assessment. *BMC Medicine, 13*(1), 106. doi: 10.1186/s12916-015-0314-7

Huckvale, K., Prieto, J. T., Tilney, M., Benghozi, P. J., & Car, J. (2015). Unaddressed privacy risks in accredited health and wellness apps: A cross-sectional systematic assessment. *BMC Medicine, 13*, 214. doi: 10.1186/s12916-015-0444-y

Humble, J. R., Tolley, E. A., Krukowski, R. A., Womack, C. R., Motley, T. S., & Bailey, J. E. (2016). Use of and interest in mobile health for diabetes self-care in vulnerable populations. *Journal of Telemedicine and Telecare, 22*(1), 32-38. doi: 10.1177/1357633X15586641

Hunt, C. W. (2015). Technology and diabetes self-management: An integrative review. *World Journal of Diabetes, 6*(2), 225-233. doi: 10.4239/wjd.v6.i2.225

Hunter, C. M. (2016). Understanding diabetes and the role of psychology in its prevention and treatment. *American Psychologist, 71*(7), 515-525. doi: 10.1037/a0040344

Husted, G. R., Weis, J., Teilmann, G., & Castensoe-Seidenfaden, P. (2018). Exploring the influence of a smartphone app (young with diabetes) on young people's self-management: Qualitative study. *JMIR mHealth and uHealth, 6*(2), e43. doi: 10.2196/mhealth.8876

Ibrahim, S., & Alkire, S. (2007). *Agency & empowerment: A proposal for internationally comparable indicators*. OPHI working paper series. Cambridge & Oxford, UK.

Infocomm Media Development Authority Singapore. (2017). Telecommunications – mobile phone penetration rate. Retrieved 08/19/2017, from http://www.imda.gov.sg/industry-development/facts-and-figures/telecommunications-1x

International Data Corporation, IDC. (2015). Smartphone OS market share, Q2 2015. Retrieved 10/22/2015, from http://www.idc.com/prodserv/smartphone-os-market-share.jsp

International Diabetes Federation, IDF. (2010). Diabetes burden shifting to developing countries. Retrieved 03/22/2016, from http://www.idf.org/diabetes-burden-shifting-developing-countries

International Diabetes Federation, IDF. (2014a). About diabetes: Risk factors. Retrieved 02/21/2015, from http://www.idf.org/about-diabetes/risk-factors

International Diabetes Federation, IDF. (2014b). IDF diabetes atlas. Key findings 2014. Retrieved 07/03/2015, from http://www.idf.org/diabetesatlas/update-2014

International Diabetes Federation, IDF. (2015a). Diabetes atlas 2015. In International Diabetes Federation (Ed.), (7th ed.). Brussels, Belgium.

International Diabetes Federation, IDF. (2015b). Singapore. Retrieved 12/16/2015, from http://www.idf.org/membership/wp/singapore

Inukollu, V. N., Keshamon, D. D., Kang, T., & Inukollu, M. (2014). Factors influncing quality of mobile apps: Role of mobile app development life cycle. *International Journal of Software Engineering & Applications, 5*(5), 15-34. doi: 10.5121/ijsea.2014.5502

Isaković, M., Sedlar, U., Volk, M., & Bešter, J. (2016). Usability pitfalls of diabetes mHealth apps for the elderly. *Journal of Diabetes Research, 2016*, 1-9. doi: 10.1155/2016/1604609

Isaksson, G., Lexell, J., & Skär, L. (2007). Social support provides motivation and ability to participate in occupation. *OTJR: Occupation, Participation and Health, 27*(1), 23-30. doi: 10.1177/153944920702700104

Isaksson, U., Hajdarevic, S., Abramsson, M., Stenvall, J., & Hornsten, A. (2015). Diabetes empowerment and needs for self-management support among people with type 2 diabetes in a rural inland community in Northern sweden. *Scandinavian Journal of Caring Sciences, 29*(3), 521-527. doi: 10.1111/scs.12185

Istepanian, R. S. H., Casiglia, D., & Gregory, J. W. (2017). Mobile health (m-health) for diabetes management. *British Journal of Healthcare Management, 23*(3), 102-108. doi: 10.12968/bjhc.2017.23.3.102

Jacques Rose, K., Petrut, C., L'Heveder, R., & de Sabata, S. (2017). IDF Europe position on mobile applications in diabetes. *Diabetes Research and Clinical Practice*. doi: 10.1016/j.diabres.2017.08.020

James, S., Perry, L., Gallagher, R., & Lowe, J. (2016). Diabetes educators' intended and reported use of common diabetes-related technologies: Discrepancies and dissonance.

Journal of Diabetes Science and Technology, 10(6), 1277-1286. doi:
10.1177/1932296816646798

Jansen, J., McCaffery, K. J., Hayen, A., Ma, D., & Reddel, H. K. (2012). Impact of graphic
format on perception of change in biological data: Implications for health monitoring
in conditions such as asthma. *Primary Care Respiratory Journal, 21*(1), 94-100. doi:
10.4104/pcrj.2012.00004

Jindal, D., Jha, D., Gupta, P., Vamadevan, A. S., Roy, A., Venugopal, V., . . . Prabhakaran, D.
(2016). Development of an electronic clinical decision support system: "mWellcare –
an integrated mHealth system for prevention and care of chronic diseases". *Endocrine
Abstracts.* doi: 10.1530/endoabs.43.OC19

Johnson, D., Deterding, S., Kuhn, K.-A., Staneva, A., Stoyanov, S., & Hides, L. (2016).
Gamification for health and wellbeing: A systematic review of the literature. *Internet
Interventions, 6*, 89-106. doi: 10.1016/j.invent.2016.10.002

Jones, K. R., Lekhak, N., & Kaewluang, N. (2014). Using mobile phones and short message
service to deliver self-management interventions for chronic conditions: A meta-
review. *Worldviews on Evidence-Based Nursing, 11*(2), 81-88. doi:
10.1111/wvn.12030

Jones, L. F. (2008). The scope and methods of political science. Block 9 objective 4:
Understanding variables.   Retrieved 12/16/2017, from
http://www.angelo.edu/faculty/ljones/gov3301/block9/objective4.htm

Kamel Boulos, M. N., Brewer, A. C., Karimkhani, C., Buller, D. B., & Dellavalle, R. P.
(2014). Mobile medical and health apps: State of the art, concerns, regulatory control
and certification. *Online Journal of Public Health Informatics, 5*(3). doi:
10.5210/ojphi.v5i3.4814

Kamphoff, C. S., Hutson, B. L., Amundsen, S. A., & Atwood, J. A. (2016). A
motivational/empowerment model applied to students on academic probation. *Journal
of College Student Retention: Research, Theory & Practice, 8*(4), 397-412. doi:
10.2190/9652-8543-3428-1j06

Kao, C. W., Chuang, H. W. , & Chen, T. Y. (2017). The utilization of health-related
applications in chronic disease self-management. *The Journal of Nursing (Hu Li Za
Zhi).* doi: 10.6224/JN.000050

Kaselitz, E., Shah, M., Choi, H., & Heisler, M. (2018). Peer characteristics associated with
improved glycemic control in a randomized controlled trial of a reciprocal peer
support program for diabetes. *Chronic Illness*, 1742395317753884. doi:
10.1177/1742395317753884

Kato, P. M. (2012). Evaluating efficacy and validating games for health. *Games for Health
Journal, 1*(1), 74-76.

Katz, R., Mesfin, T., & Barr, K. (2012). Lessons from a community-based mHealth diabetes
self-management program: "It's not just about the cell phone". *Journal of Health
Communication, 17*(sup1), 67-72. doi: 10.1080/10810730.2012.650613

Kennedy, S., Hardiker, N., & Staniland, K. (2015). Empowerment an essential ingredient in
the clinical environment: A review of the literature. *Nurse Education Today, 35*(3),
487-492. doi: 10.1016/j.nedt.2014.11.014

Kesavadev, J., Sadikot, S. M., Saboo, B., Shrestha, D., Jawad, F., Azad, K., . . . Kalra, S.
(2014). Challenges in type 1 diabetes management in South East Asia: Descriptive
situational assessment. *Indian Journal of Endocrinology and Metabolism, 18*(5), 600-
607. doi: 10.4103/2230-8210.139210

Khalid, H., Shihab, E., Nagappan, M., & Hassan, A. E. (2015). What do mobile app users
complain about? *IEEE Software, 32*(3), 70-77. doi: 10.1109/ms.2014.50

Kingsley, B. R. (1987). Push and pull strategies: Applications for health care marketing. *Health Care Strategic Management, 5*(8), 13-15.

Kirk, C. M., Lewis, R. K., Brown, K., Karibo, B., Scott, A., & Park, E. (2015). The empowering schools project. *Youth & Society, 49*(6), 827-847. doi: 10.1177/0044118x14566118

Kirkman, B. L., & Rosen, B. (1999). Beyond self-management: Antecedents and consequences of team empowerment. *Academy of Management Journal, 42*(1), 58-74. doi: 10.5465/256874

Kitsiou, S., Paré, G., Jaana, M., & Gerber, B. (2017). Effectiveness of mHealth interventions for patients with diabetes: An overview of systematic reviews. *PLoS ONE, 12*(3), e0173160. doi: 10.1371/journal.pone.0173160

Kleier, J. A., & Dittman, P. W. (2014). Attitude and empowerment as predictors of self-reported self-care and A1c values among African Americans with diabetes mellitus. *Nephrology Nursing Journal, 41*(5), 487-493.

Kleine, D. (2010). ICT4what? Using the choice framework to operationalise the capability approach to development. *Journal of International Development, 22*(5), 674-692. doi: 10.1002/jid.1719

Knittle, K., Morrison, L., Inauen, J., Warner, L. M., Kassavou, K., Naughton, F., & Michie, S. (2016). mHealth: Past success, future challenges, and the role of the EHPS. *The European Health Psychologist, 18*(6), 266-272.

Knol, J., & van Linge, R. (2009). Innovative behaviour: The effect of structural and psychological empowerment on nurses. *Journal of Advanced Nursing, 65*(2), 359-370. doi: 10.1111/j.1365-2648.2008.04876.x

Kowitt, S. D., Ayala, G. X., Cherrington, A. L., Horton, L. A., Safford, M. M., Soto, S., . . . Fisher, E. B. (2017). Examining the support peer supporters provide using structural equation modeling: Nondirective and directive support in diabetes management. *Annals of Behavioral Medicine, 51*(6), 810-821. doi: 10.1007/s12160-017-9904-2

Krebs, P., & Duncan, D. T. (2015). Health app use among us mobile phone owners: A national survey. *JMIR mHealth uHealth, 3*(4), e101. doi: 10.2196/mhealth.4924

Kreuter, M. W., & Wray, R. J. (2003). Tailored and targeted health communication: Strategies for enhancing information relevance. *American Journal of Health Behavior, 27*(Supp. 3), 227-232.

Krichbaum, K., Aarestad, V., & Buethe, M. (2003). Exploring the connection between self-efficacy and effective diabetes self-management. *The Diabetes Educator, 29*(4), 653-662. doi: 10.1177/014572170302900411

Krippendorff, K. (1980). *Content analysis: An introduction to its methodology.* Beverly Hills, CA: Sage Publications.

Krošel, M., Švegl, L., Vidmar, L., & Dinevski, D. (2016). Empowering diabetes patients with mobile health technologies. In W. Bonney (Ed.), *Mobile health technologies - theories and applications*: InTech.

Kwong, W. (2015). What is government's role in medical apps? *CMAJ Canadian Medical Association Journal, 187*(11), E339. doi: 10.1503/cmaj.109-5063

Lamprinos, I., Demski, H., Mantwill, S., Kabak, Y., Hildebrand, C., & Ploessnig, M. (2016). Modular ICT-based patient empowerment framework for self-management of diabetes: Design perspectives and validation results. *International Journal of Medical Informatics, 91*, 31-43. doi: 10.1016/j.ijmedinf.2016.04.006

Larco, A., Diaz, E., Yanez, C., & Luján-Mora, S. (2018). Autism and web-based learning: Review and evaluation of web apps. In Á. Rocha, H. Adeli, L. Reis & S. Costanzo (Eds.), *Trends and advances in information systems and technologies.* (Vol. 746, pp. 1434-1443). Cham: Springer.

Lau, P. W. C., Lau, E. Y., Wong, D. P., & Ransdell, L. (2011). A systematic review of information and communication technology-based interventions for promoting physical activity behavior change in children and adolescents. *Journal of Medical Internet Research, 13*(3), e48. doi: 10.2196/jmir.1533

Leasure, J. L., & Jones, M. (2008). Forced and voluntary exercise differentially affect brain and behavior. *Neuroscience, 156*(3), 456-465. doi: 10.1016/j.neuroscience.2008.07.041

Lee, J., & Rho, M. J. (2013). Perception of influencing factors on acceptance of mobile health monitoring service: A comparison between users and non-users. *Healthcare Informatics Research, 19*(3), 167-176. doi: 10.4258/hir.2013.19.3.167

Lee, M., & Koh, J. (2001). Is empowerment really a new concept? *The International Journal of Human Resource Management, 12*(4), 684-695. doi: 10.1080/713769649

Lewis, Z. H., Swartz, M. C., & Lyons, E. J. (2016). What's the point?: A review of reward systems implemented in gamification interventions. *Games for Health Journal, 5*(2), 93-99. doi: 10.1089/g4h.2015.0078

Li, Y., Owen, T., Thimbleby, H., Sun, N., & Rau, P.-L. P. (2013). A design to empower patients in long term wellbeing monitoring and chronic disease management in mHealth. In M.-C. Beuscart-Zéphir, M. Jaspers, C. Kuziemsky, C. Nøhr & J. Aarts (Eds.), *Context sensitive health informatics: Human and sociotechnical approaches* (Vol. 194, pp. 82-87). Amsterdam et al.: IOS Press.

Lin, S.-P. (2011). Determinants of adoption of mobile healthcare service. *International Journal of Mobile Communications, 9*(3). doi: 10.1504/IJMC.2011.040608

Lin, Y., Tudor-Sfetea, C., Siddiqui, S., Sherwani, Y., Ahmed, M., & Eisingerich, A. B. (2018). Effective behavioral changes through a digital mHealth app: Exploring the impact of hedonic well-being, psychological empowerment and inspiration. *JMIR mHealth uHealth, 6*(6), e10024. doi: 10.2196/10024

Lincoln, N. D., Travers, C., Ackers, P., & Wilkinson, A. (2002). The meaning of empowerment: The interdisciplinary etymology of a new management concept. *International Journal of Management Reviews, 4*(3), 271-290. doi: 10.1111/1468-2370.00087

Lister, C., West, J. H., Cannon, B., Sax, T., & Brodegard, D. (2014). Just a fad? Gamification in health and fitness apps. *JMIR Serious Games, 2*(2), e9. doi: 10.2196/games.3413

Litchman, M. L., Rothwell, E., & Edelman, L. S. (2018). The diabetes online community: Older adults supporting self-care through peer health. *Patient Education and Counseling, 101*(3), 518-523. doi: 10.1016/j.pec.2017.08.023

Logan, M. S., & Ganster, D. C. (2007). The effects of empowerment on attitudes and performance: The role of social support and empowerment beliefs. *Journal of Management Studies, 44*(8), 1523-1550. doi: 10.1111/j.1467-6486.2007.00711.x

Lorant, V., & Dauvrin, M. (2012). Ethnicity and socioeconomic status as determinants of health. In D. Ingleby (Ed.), *Cost series on health and diversity* (Vol. 1, pp. 69-78). Antwerpen; Apeldoorn: Garant.

Loy, J. S., Ali, E. E., & Yap, K. Y. (2016). Quality assessment of medical apps that target medication-related problems. *Journal of Managed Care & Specialty Pharmacy, 22*(10), 1124-1140. doi: 10.18553/jmcp.2016.22.10.1124

Lucas, H. (2015). New technology and illness self-management: Potential relevance for resource-poor populations in Asia. *Social Science and Medicine, 145*, 145-153. doi: 10.1016/j.socscimed.2014.11.008

Maki, K. G., & O'Mally, A. K. (2018). Analyzing online social support within the type 1 diabetes community. In S. Sekalala & B. C. Niezgoda (Eds.), *Global perspectives on health communication in the age of social media* (pp. 59-84). Hershey, PA: IGI Global.

Mantwill, S., Fiordelli, M., Ludolph, R., & Schulz, P. J. (2015). Empower – support of patient empowerment by an intelligent self-management pathway for patients: Study protocol. *BMC Medical Informatics and Decision Making, 15*, 18. doi: 10.1186/s12911-015-0142-x

Martin, D., Vicente, O., Vicente, S., Ballesteros, J., & Maynar, M. (2014). *I will prescribe you an app*. Paper presented at the 2014 Summer Simulation Multiconference.

Martinez, K., Frazer, S. F., Dempster, M., Hamill, A., Fleming, H., & McCorry, N. K. (2016). Psychological factors associated with diabetes self-management among adolescents with type 1 diabetes: A systematic review. *Journal of Health Psycholology*. doi: 10.1177/1359105316669580

Masterson Creber, R. M., Maurer, M. S., Reading, M., Hiraldo, G., Hickey, K. T., & Iribarren, S. (2016). Review and analysis of existing mobile phone apps to support heart failure symptom monitoring and self-care management using the mobile application rating scale (MARS). *JMIR mHealth uHealth, 4*(2), e74. doi: 10.2196/mhealth.5882

Mathers, C. D., & Loncar, D. (2006). Projections of global mortality and burden of disease from 2002 to 2030. *PLoS Medicine, 3*(11), e442. doi: 10.1371/journal.pmed.0030442

Mathiesen, A. S., Thomsen, T., Jensen, T., Schiotz, C., Langberg, H., & Egerod, I. (2017). The influence of diabetes distress on digital interventions for diabetes management in vulnerable people with type 2 diabetes: A qualitative study of patient perspectives. *Journal of Clinical & Translational Endocrinology, 9*, 41-47. doi: 10.1016/j.jcte.2017.07.002

Mayberry, L. S., Berg, C. A., Harper, K. J., & Osborn, C. Y. (2016). The design, usability, and feasibility of a family-focused diabetes self-care support mHealth intervention for diverse, low-income adults with type 2 diabetes. *Journal of Diabetes Research, 2016*, 1-13. doi: 10.1155/2016/7586385

Mayberry, L. S., Mulvaney, S. A., Johnson, K. B., & Osborn, C. Y. (2017). The messaging for diabetes intervention reduced barriers to medication adherence among low-income, diverse adults with type 2. *Journal of Diabetes Science and Technology, 11*(1), 92-99. doi: 10.1177/1932296816668374

McCorkle, R., Ercolano, E., Lazenby, M., Schulman-Green, D., Schilling, L. S., Lorig, K., & Wagner, E. H. (2011). Self-management: Enabling and empowering patients living with cancer as a chronic illness. *CA Cancer Journal for Clinicians, 61*(1), 50-62. doi: 10.3322/caac.20093

McLeod, J. (2001). *Qualitative research in counselling and psychotherapy*. London: Sage.

McMillan, B., Hickey, E., Patel, M. G., & Mitchell, C. (2016). Quality assessment of a sample of mobile app-based health behavior change interventions using a tool based on the National Institute of Health and Care Excellence behavior change guidance. *Patient Education and Counseling, 99*(3), 429-435. doi: 10.1016/j.pec.2015.10.023

Mead, E. L., Doorenbos, A. Z., Javid, S. H., Haozous, E. A., Alvord, L. A., Flum, D. R., & Morris, A. M. (2013). Shared decision-making for cancer care among racial and ethnic minorities: A systematic review. *Am Journal of Public Health, 103*(12), e15-29. doi: 10.2105/AJPH.2013.301631

Meer, M. (2015). Empowering patients with diabetes. *British Journal of Nursing, 24*(16), 828. doi: 10.12968/bjon.2015.24.16.828

Menon, S. T. (2001). Employee empowerment: An integrative psychological approach. *Applied Psychology, 50*(1), 153-180. doi: 10.1111/1464-0597.00052

Menon, S. T. (2002). Toward a model of psychological health empowerment: Implications
for health care in multicultural communities. *Nurse Education Today, 22*(1), 28-43.
doi: 10.1054/nedt.2001.0721

Middelweerd, A., Mollee, J. S., van der Wal, C. N., Brug, J., & te Velde, S. J. (2014). Apps
to promote physical activity among adults: A review and content analysis.
International Journal of Behavioral Nutrition and Physical Activity, 11(1). doi:
10.1186/s12966-014-0097-9

Miller, A. S., Cafazzo, J. A., & Seto, E. (2016). A game plan: Gamification design principles
in mHealth applications for chronic disease management. *Health Informatics Journal,
22*(2), 184-193. doi: 10.1177/1460458214537511

Miller, K. H., Ziegler, C., Greenberg, R., Patel, P. D., & Carter, M. B. (2012). Why
physicians should share PDA/smartphone findings with their patients: A brief report.
Journal of Health Communication, 17(Suppl 1), 54-61. doi:
10.1080/10810730.2011.649102

Miller, L. M. S., Sutter, C. A., Wilson, M. D., Bergman, J. J., Beckett, L. A., & Gibson, T. N.
(2017). An evaluation of an eHealth tool designed to improve college students' label-
reading skills and feelings of empowerment to choose healthful foods. *Front Public
Health, 5*, 359. doi: 10.3389/fpubh.2017.00359

Ministry of Health, Singapore. (2017). Better health, better care, better life. The war on
diabetes. Retrieved 09/09/2017, from
http://www.moh.gov.sg/content/dam/moh_web/PressRoom/Highlights/2016/cos/facts
heets/COS_Factsheet - Diabetes.pdf

Moattari, M., Ebrahimi, M., Sharifi, N., & Rouzbeh, J. (2012). The effect of empowerment
on the self-efficacy, quality of life and clinical and laboratory indicators of patients
treated with hemodialysis: A randomized controlled trial. *Health and Quality of Life
Outcomes, 10*, 115. doi: 10.1186/1477-7525-10-115

Moustakis, V. S., Litos, C., Dalivigas, A., & Tsironis, L. (2004). *Website quality assessment
criteria*. Paper presented at the 9th International Conference on Information Quality
(IQ).

Muralidharan, S., Ranjani, H., Anjana, R. M., Allender, S., & Mohan, V. (2017). Mobile
health technology in the prevention and management of type 2 diabetes. *Indian
Journal of Endocrinology and Metabolism, 21*(2), 334. doi:
10.4103/ijem.IJEM_407_16

Murphy, K., Casey, D., Dinneen, S., Lawton, J., & Brown, F. (2011). Participants'
perceptions of the factors that influence diabetes self-management following a
structured education (DAFNE) programme. *Journal of Clinical Nursing, 20*(9-10),
1282-1292. doi: 10.1111/j.1365-2702.2010.03564.x

Murray, E., Lo, B., Pollack, L., Donelan, K., Catania, J., Lee, K., . . . Turner, R. (2003). The
impact of health information on the internet on health care and the physician-patient
relationship: National U.S. Survey among 1.050 U.S. Physicians. *Journal of Medical
Internet Research, 5*(3), e17. doi: 10.2196/jmir.5.3.e17

Nacinovich, M. (2011). Defining mHealth. *Journal of Communication In Healthcare, 4*(1), 1-
3. doi: 10.1179/175380611x12950033990296

Naeem, A. G. (2016). The role of culture and religion in the management of diabetes: A
study of Kashmiri men in Leeds. *The Journal of the Royal Society for the Promotion
of Health, 123*(2), 110-116. doi: 10.1177/146642400312300216

National Diabetes Information Clearinghouse, NDIC. (2011, 12/05/2011). The diabetes
dictionary: Diabetes. Retrieved 02/20/2015, from
http://diabetes.niddk.nih.gov/dm/pubs/dictionary/pages/a-d.aspx

Nelson, L. A., Mayberry, L. S., Wallston, K., Kripalani, S., Bergner, E. M., & Osborn, C. Y. (2016). Development and usability of reach: A tailored theory-based text messaging intervention for disadvantaged adults with type 2 diabetes. *JMIR Human Factors, 3*(2), e23. doi: 10.2196/humanfactors.6029

Norris, S. L., Engelgau, M. M., & Narayan, K. M. (2001). Effectiveness of self-management training in type 2 diabetes: A systematic review of randomized controlled trials. *Diabetes Care, 3*, 561-587.

Nørgaard, S. K., Nichum, V. L., Barfred, C., Juul, H. M., Secher, A. L., Ringholm, L., . . . Mathiesen, E. R. (2017). Use of the smartphone application "pregnant with diabetes". *Danish Medical Journal, 64*(11), pii: A5417.

Odoom, R., Anning-Dorson, T., & Acheampong, G. (2017). Antecedents of social media usage and performance benefits in small- and medium-sized enterprises. *Journal of Enterprise Information Management, 30*(3). doi: 10.1108/JEIM-04-2016-0088

Office of Disease Prevention and Health Promotion. (2014). Determinants of health. Retrieved 12/16/2017, from http://www.healthypeople.gov/2020/about/foundation-health-measures/Determinants-of-Health

Oftedal, B., Bru, E., & Karlsen, B. (2011). Motivation for diet and exercise management among adults with type 2 diabetes. *Scandinavian Journal of Caring Sciences, 25*(4), 735-744. doi: 10.1111/j.1471-6712.2011.00884.x

Oh, H. J., & Lee, B. (2012). The effect of computer-mediated social support in online communities on patient empowerment and doctor-patient communication. *Health Communication, 27*(1), 30-41. doi: 10.1080/10410236.2011.567449

Omboni, S., Caserini, M., & Coronetti, C. (2016). Telemedicine and m-health in hypertension management: Technologies, applications and clinical evidence. *High Blood Pressure & Cardiovascular Prevention, 23*(3), 187-196. doi: 10.1007/s40292-016-0143-6

Osmani, V., Forti, S., Mayora, O., & Conforti, D. (2017). *Enabling prescription-based health apps*. Cornell University Library.

Oxford Dictionaries. (2016). Definition of empower in English. Retrieved 05/07/2016, from http://www.oxforddictionaries.com/definition/english/empower

Ozbas, A. A., & Tel, H. (2016). The effect of a psychological empowerment program based on psychodrama on empowerment perception and burnout levels in oncology nurses: Psychological empowerment in oncology nurses. *Palliative & Supportive Care, 14*(4), 393-401. doi: 10.1017/S1478951515001121

Paglialonga, A., Lugo, A., & Santoro, E. (2018). An overview on the emerging area of identification, characterization, and assessment of health apps. *Journal of Biomedical Informatics*. doi: 10.1016/j.jbi.2018.05.017

Palazuelos, D., Diallo, A. B., Palazuelos, L., Carlile, N., Payne, J. D., & Franke, M. F. (2013). User perceptions of an mHealth medicine dosing tool for community health workers. *Journal of Medical Internet Research, 1*(1), e2. doi: 10.2196/mhealth.2459

Park, S., Burford, S., Hanlen, L., Dawda, P., Dugdale, P., Nolan, C., & Burns, J. (2016). An integrated mHealth model for type 2 diabetes patients using mobile tablet devices. *Journal of Mobile Technology in Medicine, 5*(2), 24-32. doi: 10.7309/jmtm.5.2.4

Park, S., Burford, S., Lee, J. Y., & Toy, L. (2016). *Mobile health: Empowering people with type 2 diabetes using digital tools*. Canberra: News & Media Research Centre, University of Canberra.

Parkin, C. G., & Davidson, J. A. (2009). Value of self-monitoring blood glucose pattern analysis in improving diabetes outcomes. *Journal of Diabetes Science and Technology, 3*(3), 500-508. doi: 10.1177/193229680900300314

Pereira-Azevedo, N., Osorio, L., Cavadas, V., Fraga, A., Carrasquinho, E., Cardoso de Oliveira, E., . . . Roobol, M. J. (2016). Expert involvement predicts mHealth app downloads: Multivariate regression analysis of urology apps. *JMIR mHealth uHealth,* *4*(3), e86. doi: 10.2196/mhealth.5738

Peyrot, M., Rubin, R. R., Lauritzen, T., Skovlund, S. E., Snoek, F. J., Matthews, D. R., & Landgraf, R. (2006). Patient and provider perceptions of care for diabetes: Results of the cross-national DAWN study. *Diabetologia, 49*(2), 279-288. doi: 10.1007/s00125-005-0048-8

Peyrot, M., Rubin, R. R., Lauritzen, T., Snoek, F. J., Matthews, D. R., & Skovlund, S. E. (2005). Psychosocial problems and barriers to improved diabetes management: Results of the cross-national diabetes attitudes, wishes and needs (DAWN) study. *Diabetic Medicine, 22*(10), 1379-1385. doi: 10.1111/j.1464-5491.2005.01644.x

Rai, A., Chen, L., Pye, J., & Baird, A. (2013). Understanding determinants of consumer mobile health usage intentions, assimilation, and channel preferences. *Journal of Medical Internet Research, 15*(8), e149. doi: 10.2196/jmir.2635

Ramirez, A. G., & Turner, B. J. (2010). The role of peer patients in chronic disease management. *Annals of Internal Medicine, 153*(8), 544-545. doi: 10.7326/0003-4819-153-8-201010190-00014

Ramirez, V., Johnson, E., Gonzalez, C., Ramirez, V., Rubino, B., & Rossetti, G. (2016). Assessing the use of mobile health technology by patients: An observational study in primary care clinics. *JMIR mHealth uHealth, 4*(2), e41. doi: 10.2196/mhealth.4928

Rappaport, J. (1987). Terms of empowerment/exemplars of prevention: Toward a theory for community psychology. *American Journal of Community Psychology, 15*(2), 121-148.

Research2guidance. (2014a). Currently, only 1,2% of diabetics that have a smartphone use a diabetes app. Until 2018 the share will rise to 7,8% globally. Retrieved 09/22/2017, from http://research2guidance.com/currently-only-12-of-diabetics-that-have-a-smartphone-use-a-diabetes-app-until-2018-the-share-will-rise-to-78-globally/

Research2guidance. (2014b). Diabetes app market report 2014. Retrieved 03/07/2015, from http://www.research2guidance.com/shop/index.php/diabetes-app-market-report-2014

Research2guidance. (2016). Diabetes app market report 2016-2021. Retrieved 05/28/2018, from http://research2guidance.com/wp-content/uploads/2016/10/r2g_2016_diabetes-_app_market_report-Preview.pdf

Riley, W. T., Rivera, D. E., Atienza, A. A., Nilsen, W., Allison, S. M., & Mermelstein, R. (2011). Health behavior models in the age of mobile interventions: Are our theories up to the task? *Translational Behavioral Medicine, 1*(1), 53-71. doi: 10.1007/s13142-011-0021-7

Robbins, R., Krebs, P., Jagannathan, R., Jean-Louis, G., & Duncan, D. T. (2017). Health app use among US mobile phone users: Analysis of trends by chronic disease status. *JMIR mHealth uHealth, 5*(12), e197. doi: 10.2196/mhealth.7832

Robinson, T. N., Patrick, K. , Eng, T. R., & Gustafson, D. (1998). An evidence-based approach to interactive health communication: A challenge to medicine in the information age. Science panel on interactive communication and health. *Journal of American Medical Association, JAMA, 280*(14), 1264-1269.

Rodger, W. (1991). Insulin-dependent (type I) diabetes mellitus. *Canadian Medical Association Journal, 145*(10), 1227-1237.

Rodgers, W. M., Markland, D., Selzler, A. M., Murray, T. C., & Wilson, P. M. (2014). Distinguishing perceived competence and self-efficacy: An example from exercise. *Research Quarterly for Exercise and Sport, 85*(4), 527-539. doi: 10.1080/02701367.2014.961050

Rodriguez, J. A., & Singh, K. (2018). The Spanish availability and readability of diabetes apps. *Journal of Diabetes Science and Technology, 12*(3), 719-724. doi: 10.1177/1932296817749610

Rodriguez, K. M. (2013). Intrinsic and extrinsic factors affecting patient engagement in diabetes self-management: Perspectives of a certified diabetes educator. *Clinical Therapeutics, 35*(2), 170-178. doi: 10.1016/j.clinthera.2013.01.002

Rogers, E. M. (2003). *Diffusion of innovations* (5th ed.). New York: Free Press.

Rose, K. J., König, M., & Wiesbauer, F. (2013). *Evaluating success for behavioral change in diabetes via mHealth and gamification: Mysugr's keys to retention and patient engagement.* INSEAD, Social Innovation Centre. Fontainebeau. Retrieved from https://assets.mysugr.com/website/mysugr.com-wordpress/uploads/2017/03/attd-2013-poster.pdf

Rosland, A. M., Kieffer, E., Israel, B., Cofield, M., Palmisano, G., Sinco, B., . . . Heisler, M. (2008). When is social support important? The association of family support and professional support with specific diabetes self-management behaviors. *Journal of General Internal Medicine, 23*(12), 1992-1999. doi: 10.1007/s11606-008-0814-7

Rossi, M. G., & Bigi, S. (2017). mHealth for diabetes support: A systematic review of apps available on the Italian market. *mHealth, 3*, 16-16. doi: 10.21037/mhealth.2017.04.06

Rossmann, C., & Karnowski, V. (2014). eHealth & mHealth: Gesundheitskommunikation online und mobil [health communication online and mobile]. In K. Hurrelmann & E. Baumann (Eds.), *Handbuch Gesundheitskommunikation [handbook health communication]* (pp. 271-285). Bern: Huber.

Rossmann, C., Riesmeyer, C., Brew-Sam, N., Karnowski, V., Joeckel, S., Chib, A., & Ling, R. (2019). Appropriation of mHealth for diabetes self-management: Lessons from two qualitative studies. *JMIR Diabetes, 4*(1), e10271. doi: 10.2196/10271

Roter, D. L., & Hall, J. A. (1989). Studies of doctor-patient interaction. *Annual Review of Public Health, 10*(1), 163-180.

Ryan, R. M., & Deci, E. L. (2000). Intrinsic and extrinsic motivations: Classic definitions and new directions. *Contemporary Educational Psychology, 25*(1), 54-67.

Sanjari, M., Peyrovi, H., & Mehrdad, N. (2015). Managing children with diabetes within the family: Entering into the diabetes orbit. *Journal of Diabetes and Metabolic Disorders, 15*, 7. doi: 10.1186/s40200-016-0228-8

San Martín, H., & Herrero, Á. (2012). Influence of the user's psychological factors on the online purchase intention in rural tourism: Integrating innovativeness to the UTAUT framework. *Tourism Management, 33*(2), 341-350. doi: 10.1016/j.tourman.2011.04.003

Sarstedt, M., & Mooi, E. (2014). Cluster analysis. In M. Sarstedt & E. Mooi (Eds.), *A concise guide to market research* (pp. 273-324). Berlin, Heidelberg: Springer.

Scambler, S., Newton, P., & Asimakopoulou, K. (2014). The context of empowerment and self-care within the field of diabetes. *Health (London), 18*(6), 545-560. doi: 10.1177/1363459314524801

Scheibe, M., Reichelt, J., Bellmann, M., & Kirch, W. (2015). Acceptance factors of mobile apps for diabetes by patients aged 50 or older: A qualitative study. *Medicine 2.0, 4*(1), e1. doi: 10.2196/med20.3912

Scheier, M. F., Carver, C. S., & Bridges, M. W. (1994). Distinguishing optimism from neuroticism (and trait anxiety, self-mastery, and self-esteem): A reevaluation of the life orientation test. *Journal of Personality and Social Psychology, 67*(6), 1063-1078. doi: 10.1037/0022-3514.67.6.1063

Schoeppe, S., Alley, S., Rebar, A. L., Hayman, M., Bray, N. A., Van Lippevelde, W., . . . Vandelanotte, C. (2017). Apps to improve diet, physical activity and sedentary behaviour in children and adolescents: A review of quality, features and behaviour change techniques. *International Journal of Behavioral Nutrition and Physical Activity, 14*(1). doi: 10.1186/s12966-017-0538-3

Schoville, R. R. (2015). *Exploring the implementation process of technology adoption in long-term care nursing facilities* (PhD thesis), University of Michigan, Michigan.

Schreier, G., Eckmann, H., Hayn, D., Kreiner, K., Kastner, P., & Lovell, N. (2012). Web versus app: Compliance of patients in a telehealth diabetes management programme using two different technologies. *Journal of Telemedicine and Telecare, 18*(8), 476-480. doi: 10.1258/jtt.2012.GTH112

Schulz, P. J., & Nakamoto, K. (2013). Health literacy and patient empowerment in health communication: The importance of separating conjoined twins. *Patient Education and Counseling, 90*(1), 4-11. doi: 10.1016/j.pec.2012.09.006

Schwarzer, R., & Jerusalem, M. (1999). *Skalen zur Erfassung von Lehrer- und Schülermerkmalen: Dokumentation der psychometrischen Verfahren im Rahmen der wissenschaftlichen Begleitung des Modellversuchs selbstwirksame Schulen [scales for assessing teacher and student characteristics: Documentation of the psychometric methods in the context of the scientific monitoring of the experiment "self-effective schools"]*. Berlin: R. Schwarzer.

Seeman, T. (2008). Support & social conflict: Section one – social support. Retrieved 04/18/2018, from http://www.macses.ucsf.edu/research/psychosocial/socsupp.php

Sen, A. (1999). *Development as freedom*. Oxford: Oxford University Press.

Shakespeare, T., & Watson, N. (2002). The social model of disability: An outdated ideology? *Research in Social Science and Disability, 2*, 9-28.

Shao, Y., Liang, L., Shi, L., Wan, C., & Yu, S. (2017). The effect of social support on glycemic control in patients with type 2 diabetes mellitus: The mediating roles of self-efficacy and adherence. *Journal of Diabetes Research, 2017*, 2804178. doi: 10.1155/2017/2804178

Shaw, S. J., Huebner, C., Armin, J., Orzech, K., & Vivian, J. (2008). The role of culture in health literacy and chronic disease screening and management. *Journal of Immigrant and Minority Health, 11*(6), 531-531. doi: 10.1007/s10903-008-9149-z

Shetty, A. S., Chamukuttan, S., Nanditha, A., Raj, R. K., & Ramachandran, A. (2011). Reinforcement of adherence to prescription recommendations in Asian Indian diabetes patients using short message service (SMS) – a pilot study. *Journal of the Association of Physicians of India, 59*, 711-714.

Signorelli, C., Wakefield, C. E., Johnston, K. A., Fardell, J. E., Brierley, M. E., Thornton-Benko, E., . . . Cohn, R. J. (2018). 'Re-engage' pilot study protocol: A nurse-led eHealth intervention to re-engage, educate and empower childhood cancer survivors. *BMJ Open, 8*(4), e022269. doi: 10.1136/bmjopen-2018-022269

Sigurdardottir, A. K., & Jonsdottir, H. (2008). Empowerment in diabetes care: Towards measuring empowerment. *Scandinavian Journal of Caring Sciences, 22*(2), 284-291. doi: 10.1111/j.1471-6712.2007.00506.x

Singapore Government. (2015). The straits times – Singapore 'has 2nd-highest proportion of diabetics'. Retrieved 12/16/2015, from http://www.gov.sg/news/content/the-straits-times-singapore-has-2nd-highest-proportion-of-diabetics

Singh, K., Bates, D., Drouin, K., Newmark, L. P., Rozenblum, R., Lee, J., . . . Klinger, E. V. . (2016). Developing a framework for evaluating the patient engagement, quality, and safety of mobile health applications. *The Commonwealth Fund, 1863*(5).

SingHealth, Singapore General Hopsital. (2017). Dose adjustment for normal eating (DAFNE). Retrieved 05/14/2017, from http://www.sgh.com.sg/clinical-departments-centers/endocrinology/pages/doseadjustmentfornormaleating.aspx

Sleigh, A., Chng, A., Mayberry, T., & Ryan, M. (2012). Surfing South East Asia's powerful digital wave. Retrieved 06/15/2015, from http://www.accenture.com/SiteCollectionDocuments/PDF/Accenture-Surfing-ASEAN-Digital-Wave-Survey.pdf

Smahel, D., Elavsky, S., & Machackova, H. (2017). Functions of mHealth applications: A user's perspective. *Health Informatics Journal*, 1460458217740725. doi: 10.1177/1460458217740725

Smith, B. K., Frost, J., Albayrak, M., & Sudhakar, R. (2007). Integrating glucometers and digital photography as experience capture tools to enhance patient understanding and communication of diabetes self-management practices. *Personal and Ubiquitous Computing, 11*(4), 273-286.

Snoek, F. J. (2007). Self management of type 2 diabetes. *BMJ, 335*(7618), 458-459. doi: 10.1136/bmj.39315.443160.BE

Solomon, M. R. (2008). Information technology to support self-management in chronic care. *Disease Management & Health Outcomes, 16*(6), 391-401. doi: 10.2165/0115677-200816060-00004

Spreitzer, G. M. (1995). Psychological empowerment in the workplace: Dimensions, measurement, and validation. *Academy of Management Journal, 38*(5), 1442-1465. doi: 10.2307/256865

Spreitzer, G. M. (1996). Social structural characteristics of psychological empowerment. *Academy of Management Journal, 35*, 483-504.

St. George, S. M., Delamater, A. M., Pulgaron, E. R., Daigre, A., & Sanchez, J. (2016). Access to and interest in using smartphone technology for the management of type 1 diabetes in ethnic minority adolescents and their parents. *Diabetes Technology and Therapeutics, 18*(2), 104-109. doi: 10.1089/dia.2015.0086

Statista. (2014). Prevalent features of the diabetes apps on the United Kingdom (UK) market in 2014, by factor. Retrieved 09/21/2017, from http://www.statista.com/statistics/450086/diabetes-management-by-health-app-united-kingdom-uk/

Statista. (2015). Number of free and paid mobile app store downloads worldwide from 2011 to 2017 (in billions). Retrieved 10/15/2015, from http://www.statista.com/statistics/271644/worldwide-free-and-paid-mobile-app-store-downloads/

Statista. (2017). Smartphone penetration rate as share of the population in Singapore from 2015 to 2022. Retrieved 08/19/2017, from http://www.statista.com/statistics/625441/smartphone-user-penetration-in-singapore/

Statista. (2018). Diabetes. Retrieved 06/15/2018, from http://www.statista.com/outlook/314/100/diabetes/worldwide

Statistics Solutions. (2018). Structural equation modeling. Retrieved 06/09/2018, from http://www.statisticssolutions.com/structural-equation-modeling/

Stoyanov, S. R., Hides, L., Kavanagh, D. J., Zelenko, O., Tjondronegoro, D., & Mani, M. (2015). Mobile app rating scale: A new tool for assessing the quality of health mobile apps. *JMIR mHealth uHealth, 3*(1), e27. doi: 10.2196/mhealth.3422

Strom, J. L., & Egede, L. E. (2012). The impact of social support on outcomes in adult patients with type 2 diabetes: A systematic review. *Current Diabetes Reports, 12*(6), 769-781. doi: 10.1007/s11892-012-0317-0

Sundar, S. S., Bellur, S., & Jia, H. (2012). Motivational technologies: A theoretical framework for designing preventive health applications. In D. Hutchison, T. Kanade, J. Kittler, J. M. Kleinberg, F. Mattern, J. C. Mitchell, M. Naor, O. Nierstrasz, C. Pandu Rangan, B. Steffen, M. Sudan, D. Terzopoulos, D. Tygar, M. Y. Vardi, G. Weikum, M. Bang & E. L. Ragnemalm (Eds.), *Lecture notes in computer science* (pp. 112-122). Berlin; Heidelberg: Springer Berlin Heidelberg.

Sunyaev, A., Dehling, T., Taylor, P. L., & Mandl, K. D. (2015). Availability and quality of mobile health app privacy policies. *Journal of the American Medical Informatics Association, 22*(e1), e28-33. doi: 10.1136/amiajnl-2013-002605

Talukder, M., & Quazi, A. (2011). The impact of social influence on individuals' adoption of innovation. *Journal of Organizational Computing and Electronic Commerce, 21*(2), 111-135. doi: 10.1080/10919392.2011.564483

Tan, S. S., & Goonawardene, N. (2017). Internet health information seeking and the patient-physician relationship: A systematic review. *Journal of Medical Internet Research, 19*(1), e9. doi: 10.2196/jmir.5729

Tattersall, R. (2002). The expert patient: A new approach to chronic disease management for the twenty-first century. *Clinical Medicine, 2*(3), 227-229. doi: 10.7861/clinmedicine.2-3-227

Te Boveldt, N., Vernooij-Dassen, M., Leppink, I., Samwel, H., Vissers, K., & Engels, Y. (2014). Patient empowerment in cancer pain management: An integrative literature review. *Psychooncology, 23*(11), 1203-1211. doi: 10.1002/pon.3573

Thabrew, H., Stasiak, K., Garcia-Hoyos, V., & Merry, S. N. (2016). Game for health: How eHealth approaches might address the psychological needs of children and young people with long-term physical conditions. *Journal of Paediatrics and Child Health*. doi: 10.1111/jpc.13271

The Lancet. (2012). Patient empowerment – who empowers whom? *The Lancet, 379*(9827), 1677. doi: 10.1016/S0140-6736(12)60699-0

Thomas, K. W., & Velthouse, B. A. (1990). Cognitive elements of empowerment: An "interpretive" model of intrinsic task motivation. *Academy of Management Review, 15*(4), 666-681.

Thornton, L., Quinn, C., Birrell, L., Guillaumier, A., Shaw, B., Forbes, E., . . . Kay-Lambkin, F. (2017). Free smoking cessation mobile apps available in Australia: A quality review and content analysis. *Australian and New Zealand Journal of Public Health, 41*(6), 625-630. doi: 10.1111/1753-6405.12688

Tol, A., Alhani, F., Shojaeazadeh, D., Sharifirad, G., & Moazam, N. (2015). An empowering approach to promote the quality of life and self-management among type 2 diabetic patients. *Journal of Education and Health Promotion, 4*, 13. doi: 10.4103/2277-9531.154022

Toobert, D. J., Hampson, S. E., & Glasgow, R. E. (2000). The summary of diabetes self-care activities measure. *Diabetes Care, 23*(7), 943-950.

Torbjornsen, A., Jenum, A. K., Smastuen, M. C., Arsand, E., Holmen, H., Wahl, A. K., & Ribu, L. (2014). A low-intensity mobile health intervention with and without health counseling for persons with type 2 diabetes, part 1: Baseline and short-term results from a randomized controlled trial in the Norwegian part of Renewing Health. *JMIR mHealth uHealth, 2*(4), e52. doi: 10.2196/mhealth.3535

Trentini, F., Malgaroli, M., Camerini, A.-L., Di Serio, C., & Schulz, P. J. (2015). Multivariate determinants of self-management in health care: Assessing health empowerment model by comparison between structural equation and graphical models approaches. *Epidemiology Biostatistics and Public Health, 12*(1), 1-13. doi: 10.2427/18334

United Nations, UN. (2005). Gender equality and empowerment of women through ICT. In UnitedNations (Ed.), *Women 2000 and beyond*: UnitedNations.

van Dam, H. A., van der Horst, F. G., Knoops, L., Ryckman, R. M., Crebolder, H. F., & van den Borne, B. H. (2005). Social support in diabetes: A systematic review of controlled intervention studies. *Patient Education and Counseling, 59*(1), 1-12. doi: 10.1016/j.pec.2004.11.001

van Uden-Kraan, C. F., Drossaert, C. H., Taal, E., Seydel, E. R., & van de Laar, M. A. (2009). Participation in online patient support groups endorses patients' empowerment. *Patient Education and Counseling, 74*(1), 61-69. doi: 10.1016/j.pec.2008.07.044

Vatankhah, M., & Tanbakooei, N. (2014). The role of social support on intrinsic and extrinsic motivation among Iranian EFL learners. *Procedia – Social and Behavioral Sciences, 98*, 1912-1918. doi: 10.1016/j.sbspro.2014.03.622

Veazie, S., Winchell, K., Gilbert, J., Paynter, R., Ivlev, I., Eden, K. B., . . . Helfand, M. (2018). Rapid evidence review of mobile applications for self-management of diabetes. *Journal of General Internal Medicine.* doi: 10.1007/s11606-018-4410-1

Venkatesh, V., & Davis, F. D. (1996). A model of the antecedents of perceived ease of use: Development and test. *Decision Sciences, 27*(3), 451-481. doi: 10.1111/j.1540-5915.1996.tb00860.x

Venkatesh, V., Morris, M. G., Davis, G. B., & Davis, F. D. (2003). User acceptance of information technology: Toward a unified view. *MIS Quarterly, 27*(3), 425-478.

Venkatesh, V., Thong, J., & Xu, X. (2012). Consumer acceptance and use of information technology: Extending the unified theory of acceptance and use of technology. *MIS Quarterly, 36*(1), 157-178.

Viennot, N., Garcia, E., & Nieh, J. (2014). *A measurement study of Google Play.* Paper presented at the ACM International Conference on Measurement and Modeling of Computer Systems.

Villanti, A. C., Cantrell, J., Pearson, J. L., Vallone, D. M., & Rath, J. M. (2014). Perceptions and perceived impact of graphic cigarette health warning labels on smoking behavior among U.S. young adults. *Nicotine and Tobacco Research, 16*(4), 469-477. doi: 10.1093/ntr/ntt176

Wallace, D. D., Gonzalez Rodriguez, H., Walker, E., Dethlefs, H., Dowd, R. A., Filipi, L., & Barrington, C. (2018). Types and sources of social support among adults living with type 2 diabetes in rural communities in the Dominican Republic. *Global Public Health*, 1-12. doi: 10.1080/17441692.2018.1444782

Wang, Y., Xue, H., Huang, Y., Huang, L., & Zhang, D. (2017). A systematic review of application and effectiveness of mHealth interventions for obesity and diabetes treatment and self-management. *Advances in Nutrition: An International Review Journal, 8*(3), 449-462. doi: 10.3945/an.116.014100

Wehmeyer, M. (2004). Self-determination and the empowerment of people with disabilities. *American Rehabilitation, 28*(1), 22-29.

Welch, G. W., Jacobson, A. M., & Polonsky, W. H. (1997). The problem areas in diabetes scale: An evaluation of its clinical utility. *Diabetes Care, 20*(5), 760-766. doi: 10.2337/diacare.20.5.760

Weymann, N., Harter, M., & Dirmaier, J. (2016). Information and decision support needs in patients with type 2 diabetes. *Health Informatics Journal, 22*(1), 46-59. doi: 10.1177/1460458214534090

White, M. (2001). Receiving social support online: Implications for health education. *Health Education Research, 16*(6), 693-707. doi: 10.1093/her/16.6.693

Whitehead, L., Jacob, E., Towell, A., Abu-Qamar, M., & Cole-Heath, A. (2018). The role of the family in supporting the self-management of chronic conditions: A qualitative systematic review. *Journal of Clinical Nursing, 27*(1-2), 22-30. doi: 10.1111/jocn.13775

Wiederhold, B. K. (2015). mHealth apps empower individuals. *Cyberpsychology, Behavior and Social Networking, 18*(8), 429-430. doi: 10.1089/cyber.2015.29006.bkw

Wilkinson, A., Whitehead, L., & Ritchie, L. (2014). Factors influencing the ability to self-manage diabetes for adults living with type 1 or 2 diabetes. *International Journal of Nursing Studies, 51*(1), 111-122. doi: 10.1016/j.ijnurstu.2013.01.006

Williams, G. C., Grow, V. M., Freedman, Z. R., Ryan, R. M., & Deci, E. L. (1996). Motivational predictors of weight loss and weight-loss maintenance. *Journal of Personality and Social Psychology, 70*(1), 115-126. doi: 10.1037/0022-3514.70.1.115

Williams, G. C., McGregor, H. A., Zeldman, A., Freedman, Z. R., & Deci, E. L. (2004). Testing a self-determination theory process model for promoting glycemic control through diabetes self-management. *Health Psychology, 23*(1), 58-66. doi: 10.1037/0278-6133.23.1.58

Wirth, W., von Pape, T., & Karnowski, V. (2008). An integrative model of mobile phone appropriation. *Journal of Computer-Mediated Communication, 13*(3), 593-617. doi: 10.1111/j.1083-6101.2008.00412.x

Wittenberg, E., Xu, J., Goldsmith, J., & Mendoza, Y. (2019). Caregiver communication about cancer: Development of a mHealth resource to support family caregiver communication burden. *Psychooncology, 28*(2), 365-371. doi: 10.1002/pon.4950

Woldeyohannes, H. O., & Ngwenyama, O. K. (2017). *Factors influencing acceptance and continued use of mHealth apps.* Paper presented at the HCI in Business, Government and Organizations. Interacting with Information Systems: 4th International Conference, Vancouver, BC, Canada.

World Health Organization, WHO. (2009). Patient empowerment and health care. In World Health Organization (Ed.), *Guidelines on hand hygiene in health care: First global patient safety challenge clean care is safer care.* Geneva: WHO, World Health Organization.

World Health Organization, WHO. (2011). mHealth – new horizons for health through mobile technologies. *Global Observatory for eHealth Series* (Vol. 3). Geneva: WHO.

World Health Organization, WHO. (2015). Diabetes programme. World diabetes day 2014. Retrieved 03/23/2015, from http://www.who.int/entity/diabetes/en/index.html

World Health Organization, WHO. (2016a). *Global report on diabetes.* Geneva, Switzerland: World Health Organization.

World Health Organization, WHO. (2016b). *International classification of health interventions (ICHI).* Geneva, Switzerland: World Health Organization.

Wright, K. B. (2006). Researching internet-based populations: Advantages and disadvantages of online survey research, online questionnaire authoring software packages, and web survey services. *Journal of Computer-Mediated Communication, 10*(3), 00-00. doi: 10.1111/j.1083-6101.2005.tb00259.x

Wright, K. B., Rains, S., & Banas, J. (2010). Weak-tie support network preference and perceived life stress among participants in health-related, computer-mediated support groups. *Journal of Computer-Mediated Communication, 15*(4), 606-624. doi: 10.1111/j.1083-6101.2009.01505.x

Wu, Y., Yao, X., Vespasiani, G., Nicolucci, A., Dong, Y., Kwong, J., . . . Li, S. (2017). Mobile app-based interventions to support diabetes self-management: A systematic review of randomized controlled trials to identify functions associated with glycemic efficacy. *JMIR mHealth uHealth, 5*(3), e35. doi: 10.2196/mhealth.6522

Wyatt, J. C., Thimbleby, H., Rastall, P., Hoogewerf, J., Wooldridge, D., & Williams, J. (2015). What makes a good clinical app? Introducing the RCP health informatics unit checklist. *Clinical Medicine, 15*(6), 519-521. doi: 10.7861/clinmedicine.15-6-519

Wysocki, T., Taylor, A., Hough, B. S., Linscheid, T. R., Yeates, K. O., & Naglieri, J. A. (1996). Deviation from developmentally appropriate self-care autonomy: Association with diabetes outcomes. *Diabetes Care, 19*(2), 119-125. doi: 10.2337/diacare.19.2.119

Yang, S., Hsue, C., & Lou, Q. (2015). Does patient empowerment predict self-care behavior and glycosylated hemoglobin in Chinese patients with type 2 diabetes? *Diabetes Technology and Therapeutics, 17*(5), 343-348. doi: 10.1089/dia.2014.0345

Ye, Q., Boren, S. A., Khan, U., Simoes, E. J., & Kim, M. S. (2018). Experience of diabetes self-management with mobile applications: A focus group study among older people with diabetes. *European Journal for Person Centered Healthcare, 6*(2), 262. doi: 10.5750/ejpch.v6i2.1451

Ye, Q., Khan, U., Boren, S. A., Simoes, E. J., & Kim, M. S. (2018). An analysis of diabetes mobile applications features compared to AADE7: Addressing self-management behaviors in people with diabetes. *Journal of Diabetes Science and Technology, 12*(4), 808-816. doi: 10.1177/1932296818754907

Zaires, S., Perrakis, G., Bekri, E., Katrakazas, P., Lambrou, G., & Koutsouris, D. (2017). Chronic disease management via mobile apps: The diabetes case. In H. Eskola, O. Väisänen, J. Viik & J. Hyttinen (Eds.), *EMBEC & NBC 2017, IFMBE proceedings* (Vol. 65, pp. 177-180). Singapore: Springer.

Zapata, B. C., Fernandez-Aleman, J. L., Idri, A., & Toval, A. (2015). Empirical studies on usability of mHealth apps: A systematic literature review. *Journal of Medical Systems, 39*(2), 1. doi: 10.1007/s10916-014-0182-2

Zhang, M. W. B., & Ho, R. C. M. (2017). M-health and smartphone technologies and their impact on patient care and empowerment. In L. Menvielle, A. F. Audrain-Pontevia & W. Menvielle (Eds.), *The digitization of healthcare* (pp. 277-291). London: Palgrave Macmillan.

Zhao, J., Freeman, B., & Li, M. (2016). Can mobile phone apps influence people's health behavior change? An evidence review. *Journal of Medical Internet Research, 18*(11), e287. doi: 10.2196/jmir.5692

Zhu, Z., Liu, Y., Che, X., & Chen, X. (2017). Moderating factors influencing adoption of a mobile chronic disease management system in China. *Informatics for Health and Social Care*, 1-20. doi: 10.1080/17538157.2016.1255631

Zoffmann, V., & Kirkevold, M. (2012). Realizing empowerment in difficult diabetes care: A guided self-determination intervention. *Qualitative Health Research, 22*(1), 103-118. doi: 10.1177/1049732311420735

Printed in the United States
By Bookmasters